AF768839

Veterinary Science

Veterinary Science

Edited by **Mel Roth**

SYRAWOOD
PUBLISHING HOUSE
New York

Published by Syrawood Publishing House,
750 Third Avenue, 9th Floor,
New York, NY 10017, USA
www.syrawoodpublishinghouse.com

Veterinary Science
Edited by Mel Roth

© 2016 Syrawood Publishing House

International Standard Book Number: 978-1-68286-364-0 (Hardback)

This book contains information obtained from authentic and highly regarded sources. Copyright for all individual chapters remain with the respective authors as indicated. All chapters are published with permission under the Creative Commons Attribution License or equivalent. A wide variety of references are listed. Permission and sources are indicated; for detailed attributions, please refer to the permissions page and list of contributors. Reasonable efforts have been made to publish reliable data and information, but the authors, editors and publisher cannot assume any responsibility for the validity of all materials or the consequences of their use.

The publisher's policy is to use permanent paper from mills that operate a sustainable forestry policy. Furthermore, the publisher ensures that the text paper and cover boards used have met acceptable environmental accreditation standards.

Trademark Notice: Registered trademark of products or corporate names are used only for explanation and identification without intent to infringe.

Printed in China.

Contents

Preface

Recent progress in the fields of biology and medicine has led to rapid advancements in veterinary science. It has emerged as a self-sustained discipline in past few decades. It includes the anatomical and physiological study of both domestic as well as wild animals. It serves as a monitoring aid to human health through control of zoonotic diseases. The book encompasses contemporary developments and trends in therapeutic treatment of animals and livestock. Some of the topics included in this book like veterinary anatomy, physiology, epidemiology, etc. are bound to provide incredible insights to the students and researchers engaged in this field.

The information contained in this book is the result of intensive hard work done by researchers in this field. All due efforts have been made to make this book serve as a complete guiding source for students and researchers. The topics in this book have been comprehensively explained to help readers understand the growing trends in the field.

I would like to thank the entire group of writers who made sincere efforts in this book and my family who supported me in my efforts of working on this book. I take this opportunity to thank all those who have been a guiding force throughout my life.

Editor

Filarial Nematode Infection in *Ixodes scapularis* Ticks Collected from Southern Connecticut

Pabbati Namrata, Jamie M. Miller, Madari Shilpa, Patlolla Raghavender Reddy, Cheryl Bandoski, Michael J. Rossi and Eva Sapi *

Department of Biology and Environmental Science, University of New Haven, West Haven, CT 06516, USA; E-Mails: namratapabbati@yahoo.com (P.N.); j_miller0109@hotmail.com (J.M.M.); shilpa.madari@gmail.com (M.S.); raaghavenderreddy@gmail.com (P.R.R.); cband1@unh.newhaven.edu (C.B.); Mrossi@newhaven.edu (M.J.R.)

* Author to whom correspondence should be addressed; E-Mail: esapi@newhaven.edu;

Abstract: It was recently demonstrated that the lone star tick *Amblyomma americanum* could harbor filarial nematodes within the genus *Acanthocheilonema*. In this study, *Ixodes scapularis* (deer) ticks collected from Southern Connecticut were evaluated for their potential to harbor filarial nematodes. Non-engorged nymphal and adult stage *Ixodes scapularis* ticks were collected in Southern Connecticut using the standard drag method. *In situ* hybridization with filarial nematode specific sequences demonstrated the presence of filarial nematodes in *Ixodes* ticks. Filarial nematode specific DNA sequences were amplified and confirmed by direct sequencing in *Ixodes* nymphal and adult ticks using either general filarial nematode or *Onchocercidae* family specific PCR primers. Phylogenetic analysis of the 12S rDNA gene sequence indicated that the filarial nematode infecting *Ixodes scapularis* ticks is most closely related to the species found in *Amblyoma americanum* ticks and belongs to the genus of *Acanthocheilonema.* Our data also demonstrated that infection rate of these filarial nematode in *Ixodes* ticks is relatively high (about 22% and 30% in nymphal and adult *Ixodes* ticks, respectively). In summary, the results from our studies demonstrated that filarial nematode infection was found in *Ixodes* ticks similar to what has been found in *Amblyomma americanum* ticks.

Keywords: *Ixodes scapularis*; hard ticks; *Onchocercidae* family; mtDNA marker

---

1. Introduction

The tick *Ixodes scapularis* is the host of variety pathogens with medical and veterinary importance such as bacterial pathogens belonging to genera *Borrelia, Anaplasma, Bartonella, Rickettsia, Francisella* and *Coxiella* [1–7]. *Ixodes* ticks can also harbor protozoan parasites; the best known being *Babesia* spp [8]. In 1984, W. Burgdorfer reported the presence of parasitic worms in *Ixodes* ticks collected from Shelter Island, NY. He discovered 30 microfilarial worms (species was not identified) in one adult *Ixodes dammini* tick [9]. The presence of microfilarial nematodes has been reported in ticks such as the soft tick *Ornithodoros*, the hard tick *Rhipicephalus*, and recently in *Amblyoma americanum* (lone star) ticks [10–12]. The species they identified in those studies were closely related to *Acanthocheilonema* (formerly *Dipetalonema*) filarial nematodes which are known animal parasites. Development and transmission of *Acanthocheilonema* species by both soft and hard ticks has also been demonstrated [10,11].

In this study, we further investigated the potential presence of filarial nematodes in the *Ixodes scapularis* (deer tick) collected from Southern Connecticut. The goal was to visualize filarial nematode infections in *Ixodes scapularis* using filarial nematode DNA specific *in situ* hybridization techniques. Polymerase chain reaction (PCR) combined with direct sequencing methods were used to characterize the potential genus and species as well as the rate of microfilarial infection in nymphal and adult ticks collected from Southern Connecticut.

2. Experimental Section

2.1. Tick Collection and DNA Preparation

Non-engorged nymphal- and adult-stage ticks were collected by the standard drag method from Southern Connecticut (Fairfield County, five different sites) in Spring/Summer 2009–2010 and transferred to 15 mL polypropylene Falcon tubes with or without 70% alcohol. Ticks were washed extensively with 70% alcohol to remove any external contaminants and crushed in liquid nitrogen. Genomic DNA was prepared using the DNeasy Blood and Tissue kit (Qiagen) following the manufacturer's instructions. DNA concentration was measured using the Nanodrop 3300 Fluorophore following the manufacturer's instructions.

2.2. PCR Protocols

The isolated genomic DNA was used as a template for the various PCR experiments. To confirm the tick species, each sample was first assessed using *Ixodes scapularis*-specific primers targeting the mitochondrial 16S rDNA gene (Ixo-F 5'-TAAACAATTAAAAG-3' and Ixo-R 5'-AATCGCTAAAAACG-3') as described previously [4]. The PCR amplifications were performed using standard PCR buffer (Promega buffer B), plus 2.5 μL of 25 mM $MgCl_2$, 1 μL dNTPs mix (10 mM each), 1 μL of each PCR primer (50 pmol/μL) and 0.25 μL of *Taq* DNA Polymerase (Promega) in a 25 μL reaction volume. PCR reaction included an initial denaturation at 94 °C for 5 min, 35 cycles of 94 °C for 45 sec, 50 °C for 45 sec, 72 °C for 1 min, and a final extension step at 72 °C for 2 min.

Initial filarial nematode-specific PCR reactions were carried out using previously described filarial nematode genus-specific primers FL1 and ITSR (18S and 5.8S rDNA containing an internal transcribed sequence region) [13], FL1: 5'-TTCCGTAGGTGAACCTGC-3' and ITSR: 5'-ACCCTCAACCAGACGTAC-3'). Cycling conditions consisted of an initial denaturation at 94 °C for 5 min and 35 subsequent cycles of 45 sec at 94 °C, 45 sec at 54 °C and 1 min at 72 °C.

For further PCR characterization, *Onchocerciadea* family-specific primers were designed for conserved mitochondrial 12S rDNA regions (5'-TGACTGACTTTAGATTTTTCTTTGG-3' and 5'-AATTACTTTCTTTTCCAATTTCACA-3'). Cycling conditions consisted of an initial denaturation at 94 °C for 5 min and 40 subsequent cycles of 45 sec at 94 °C, 45 sec at 56 °C and 1 min at 72 °C, followed by a final extension step at 72 °C for 2 min.

All primers were custom made using Eurofins MWG Operon oligonucleotide service. All PCR reactions included a negative control using water in the place of template DNA. PCR products were evaluated by standard 2% agarose gel electrophoresis.

2.3. Sequencing and Sequence Analyses

PCR products were extracted from the agarose gel using QIAquick Gel Extraction kit (Qiagen) according to the manufacturer's instructions. The eluates from each sample were sequenced in both directions using the primers that generated the products. Sequencing reactions were performed by Keck Sequencing Laboratory at Yale University (New Haven, CT, USA). Obtained sequences were compared by searching the GenBank database (National Center for Biotechnology Information) using the Basic Local Alignment Tool (BLAST). Sequence alignment (Clustel W) and neighbor-joining phylogenetic analyses were conducted using MEGA version 5 [14]. Tree support was evaluated by bootstrapping with 500 replications.

2.4. Nucleotide Sequence Accession Numbers

Nucleotide sequences for the 18S/5.8S internal transcribed spacer sequence (ITS) and for the 12S rDNA loci have been deposited in GenBank (http://www.ncbi.nlm.nih.gov) with the following accession numbers: JX117890 and JF701608 through JF701611 respectively.

2.5. In Situ Hybridization

In situ hybridization was used to confirm the presence of filarial nematodes in ticks. Adult ticks were dissected under a dissecting microscope. The live ticks were first fixed in wax on the slides and dissected starting from the thoracic region to downward to the anus region and then the slides were reversed to continue dissecting from anus region to thoracic region on the other side. The mouthpart region was dissected carefully to remove the dorsal side of the hard body. A drop of double distilled sterile water was put on the dissected tick and whole gut region along with the salivary glands were separated. The whole gut was transferred to another clean slide. They were separated and fixed with freshly made paraformaldehyde (4%, w/v) and in alcohol:formaline:aldehyde solution (1:2:1, v/v/v) for 24 hours at 4 °C.

A 27-base long oligonucleotide probe was designed to the 18S/5.8S rDNA internal transcribed sequence (5'-GAAACATTCAATTACCTCAAACTTGGG-3') based on the sequence obtained for the filarial-specific PCR reaction (see above). As a negative control, a 27-base long random oligonucleotide probe (5'-GCATAGACATGAGATATACTGTACTAG-3') was also designed. Both probes were synthesized and labeled with FITC at 5' end by Eurofins MWG Operon oligonuclotide services. For the *in situ* experiments, 100 ng of labeled probe was mixed first with 2.5 μg of salmon sperm DNA (Sigma) and precipitated at −20 °C for 30 min with 0.1 volume of 3 M sodium acetate and two volumes of ice-cold ethanol. The mixture was then centrifuged at 22,000 × g for 20 min. The resultant pellet was resuspended in 1XTE buffer pH 8.0. The probe was incubated at 95 °C for 10 min, immediately placed on ice for 5 min and then incubated at 37 °C for 15 min. The prefixed whole gut tissue sections first were treated with 1 mg/mL Proteinase K in Proteinase K Buffer at 56 °C for 5 min and then denatured in denaturating solution (70% v/v formamide, 2× SSC, 0.1 mM EDTA pH 7) at 95 °C before hybridization. The sections were hybridized with the probe mixture 56 °C overnight. They were then washed thrice in 2× SSC for 3 min each at room temperature followed by two 20 min washes in 0.1× SSC at 42 °C and a final wash in 0.1× SSC at room temperature. Sections were then washed with freshly made blocking solution (3% w/v BSA in 4× SSC, Triton X-100) for 3 min and wash solution (4× SSC, 0.05% v/v Triton X-100) for 3 min. To visualize the structures of the tick tissue, all tissue samples were counterstained with 300 ng/mL DAPI for 90 seconds in dark and washed with 1× PBS pH 7.4 (phosphate buffer saline) once and mounted with Permafluor mounting medium (Thermo Scientific). All steps were repeated with several controls such as: (1) 100 ng negative control, random oligonucleotide, (2) 200 ng of a competing oligonucleotide present during the hybridization step (5'-CCCAAGTTTGAGGTAATTGAATGTTTC-3'), (3) RNase treatment of the sections before the hybridization step (20 μg/mL for 30 min at 37 °C) and (4) no DNA probe control. Images were acquired using a Leica DM2500 biomedical microscope equipped with dark field, differential interference contrast (DIC) and epifluorescent illumination.

3. Results and Discussion

3.1. PCR

To demonstrate the presence of filarial nematodes in *Ixodes scapularis* ticks, genomic DNA from 20 nymphal ticks collected from Southern Connecticut was then tested for the presence of filarial nematode DNA using a universal filarial nematode-specific PCR technique. Previously published [13] filarial nematode primers FIL and ITSR were then used to amplify the 18S and 5.8S rDNA regions for all species in the phylum *Filaria.* The expected bands of 400 bp were successfully amplified in 3 tick samples (data not shown) and positive DNA fragments were isolated for direct sequencing. A representative sequence was deposited into NCBI Genbank (JX117890). The sequences were further analyzed by the BLAST sequence analysis program (NCBI). The resulting sequences revealed that the amplified products had the highest similarity with various genera of the *Onchocercidae* family in *Filarial* phylum showing greatest similarities to *Onchocerca, Dirofilarie*, *Brugia, Mansonella* and *Acanthocheilonema* genera. Total scores were used to identify the greatest similarity. *Onchocerca/Dirofilarie* genera had the maximum query coverage ranging from 60% to 86% and 60%

to 63% respectively. Sequences had maximum identity of 71%–81% for *Onchocerca species* and 78%–79% for *Dirofilarie species*. However, based on these similarity scores, assignment of the sequence found in *Ixodes* ticks to a specific genus was not possible.

3.2. In Situ Confirmation

To further provide evidence for the presence of filarial nematodes in *Ixodes* ticks, *in situ* hybridization was performed with an *Onchocercidae* family specific oligonucleotide derived from the sequences identified above. The probe was labeled with an FITC fluorescent dye and hybridized on tick gut sections of *Ixodes scapularis* (Figure 1). DIC microscopy and DAPI counterstain were used to visualize the structure and the nuclei of the tissue (Figure 1, Panel A and F respectively). The *in situ* staining revealed that filarial nematode-like structures could be observed in tick guts using *Onchocercidae* family DNA specific probes (Figure 1B). As controls; an FITC labeled random probe sequence, a competing oligonucleotide and RNAase treated samples were utilized in consecutive sections as described in the experimental section (Panel C–E respectively). No positive staining was seen on sections with an FITC labeled random sequence probe, or with the experiment with competing oligonucleotide (Figure 1, Panel C and D). Significant signals were observed even when the sections were RNAse treated demonstrating DNA staining on the section (Panel E). Also, in the "no DNA control" experiments, there were no detectable fluorescent signals on the slides (data not shown).

Figure 1. Representative image of an *in situ* hybridization experiment using *Onchocercidae* family filarial nematode specific probe (18S/5.8S internal transcribed spacer sequence) on whole mount tick consecutive sections. Panel A and Panel F show the structure and the nuclei of the tissue using differential interphase microscopy (DIC) and DAPI staining (blue staining) respectively. Panel B show the filarial specific probe staining (bright green staining) while Panels C–E show different control experiments: Panel C = random probe, Panel D = competing oligonucleotide and Panel D = RNase treated sections). 400× magnification.

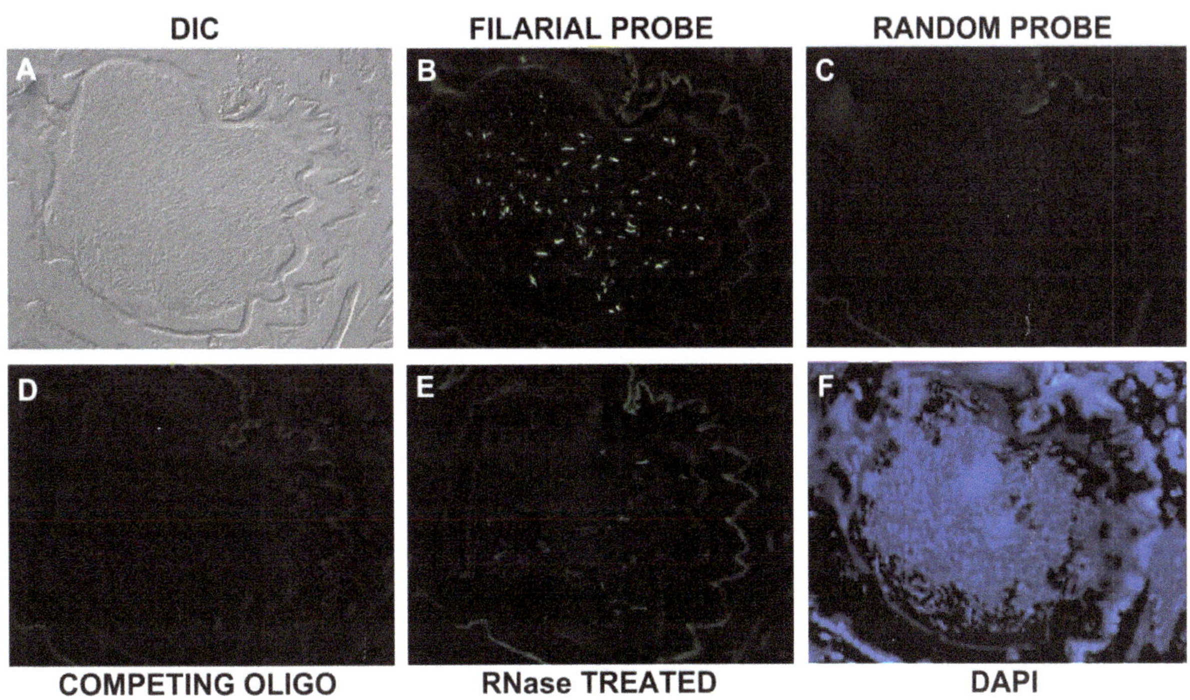

3.3. Additional PCR and Sequencing Analyses

In order to further narrow down the potential species for this microfilaria discovered in *Ixodes* tick samples, the *Onchocercidae* family was targeted using *Onchocercidae* family-specific mitochondrial 12S rDNA PCR primers in the 20 individual nymphal tick samples. PCR experiments with previously published 12S rDNA primer sets did not produce the predicted PCR target [13,15,16], therefore a novel 12S rDNA primer set was designed and used in *Ixodes* nymphal tick samples. Figure 2 shows a representative PCR experiment with five individual nymphal tick samples showing the successful amplification of a 218 bp fragment of an *Onchocercidae* family specific 12 rDNA (Figure 2, lanes 2–5). As positive controls, the same tick DNA samples were also analyzed for *Ixodes scapularis* specific 16S rDNA sequence and found to be positive (Figure 2, lanes 2–5). As a negative control no tick DNA added to lane 6 samples, which showed no amplifications for either the *Onchocercidae* family specific filarial or *Ixodes scapularis* specific PCR experiments. BLAST analyses identified three types of isolates with 99% identity (1 or 2 nucleotide differences in the 218 bp sequence). Representative sequences were submitted to the NCBI National Genome Database (Accession numbers: JF701608-11). Sequence alignment (ClustelW) and neighbor-joining phylogenetic analysis were conducted on a 200 bp alignment of the three types of 12S rDNA sequences obtained and compared to corresponding genomic segments of the 12S rDNA gene sequences from different genera of *Onchocercidae* family using MEGA 5 Evolutionary Genetics Analysis program [14]. Tree support was evaluated by bootstrapping with 500 replications. Figure 3 shows that the result of the phylogenetic analysis indicated that the filarial nematode infecting *Ixodes scapularis* ticks were most closely related to filarial nematodes in the genus *Acanthocheilonema.*

Figure 2. Polymerase chain reaction (PCR) performed using *Onchocercidae* family specific primers for mitochondrial 12S rDNA gene (upper panel) and for *Ixodes scapularis* specific 16S rDNA (lower panel). DNA isolated from five individual nymphal tick DNA samples (lanes 1–5). Lane 6 shows the negative control (no DNA) for both PCR reactions. Lane M is a 50 bp molecular weight ladder from Fisher Scientific.

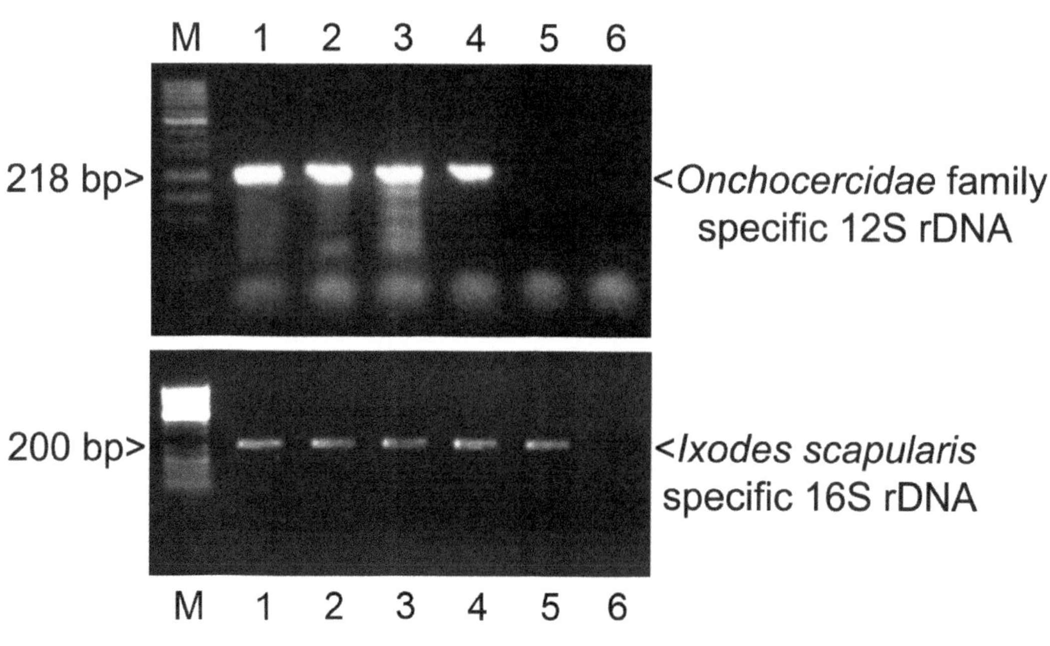

Figure 3. A neighbor-joining phylogenetic analysis of a 200 bp alignment of the mitochondrial 12S rDNA gene of the three microfilarial nematode isolates obtained from our study (JF70108-11) compared to other species in *Onchocercidae* family using MEGA 5 Evolutionary Genetics Analysis program. Alphanumeric codes represent GenBank (NCBI) ID numbers. Numbers at nodes indicate bootstrap support values (500 replicates).

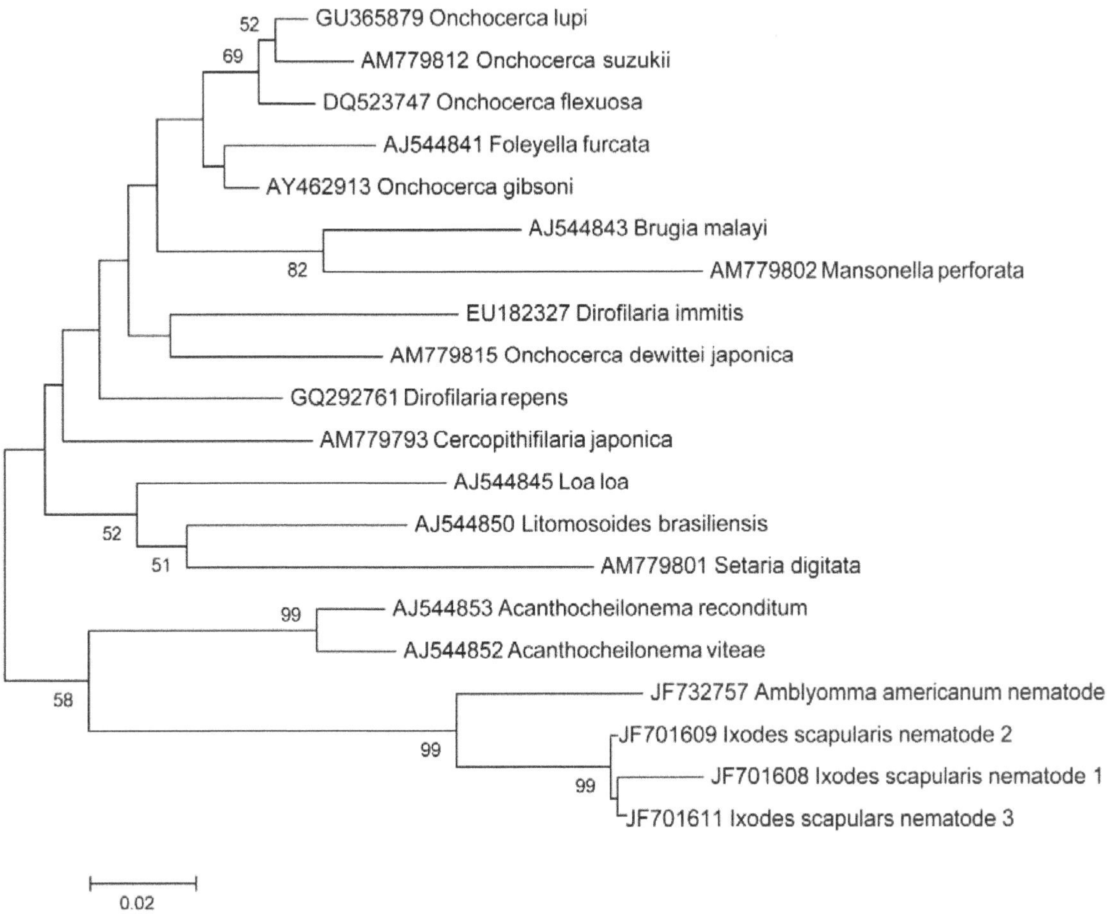

The closest potential filarial species to what was found in *Ixodes* ticks were the filarial species found in *Amblyoma* ticks (92% identity). Comparing filarial species to known *Acanthocheilonema species* such as *Acanthocheilonema vita*, and *Acanthocheilonema reconditum* we have found 85 and 84% identity in the 200 bp region of 12S rDNA gene respectively. We attempted to further identify the species found in *Ixodes* ticks using additional published primer sets targeting *Onchocerciadea* genus specific genes such as loci for mitochondrial nicotinamide adenine dehydrogenase (NADH) and cytochrome oxidase I (COI) major sperm protein 1 and 2 (OVMSP1 and OVMSP2) [15–18], with no successful amplification (data not shown).

3.4. Rate of Infection

To determine the rate of infection, a total of 100 nymphal and 100 adults tick samples were tested individually to evaluate the percentage of deer ticks (*Ixodes scapularis*) infected with filarial nematodes using the same *Onchocercidae* family specific primers for mitochondrial 12S rDNA gene. Our results found that 22% of the *Ixodes scapularis* nymphal ticks and 30% of the adults tick samples were positive for this filarial gene.

In this paper, we identified an *Acanthocheilonema spp* filarial infection in *Ixodes scapularis* ticks collected in Southern Connecticut. Our PCR results showed that filarial nematode DNA sequence could be amplified from *Ixodes* nymphal and adult ticks using either filarial nematode or *Onchocercidae* family specific PCR primers. Direct sequencing of the resulting sequences further confirmed *Onchocercidae* family specific sequences. *In situ* hybridization with an *Onchocercidae* specific DNA probe also demonstrated the presence of filarial nematodes in tick tissue sections. Phylogenetic analysis of the 12S mitochondrial rDNA gene sequence indicated that the filarial nematodes infecting *Ixodes scapularis* ticks were most closely related to the species found in *Amblyoma americanum* ticks and in the genus *Acanthocheilonema.* Comparing the 12S rDNA filarial sequences found in *Ixodes* ticks to well characterized species in the genus *Acanthocheilonema,* we have the most similarity to *Acanthocheilonema reconditum* (formerly *Dipetalonema reconditum*) and *Acanthocheilonema vitae* (formerly *Dipetalonema viteae*).

Acanthocheilonema reconditum is a known parasite found in dogs while *Acanthocheilonema viteae* is a rodent parasite [19,20]. The latter is used as a model system for human filarial infections because it shares antigenic homology with the human filarial worm *Onchocerca volvulus* [20]. Based on this information, one can speculate that the species found in *Ixodes* tick is most likely an animal parasite. Interestingly, an *Acanthocheilonema reconditum* infection was also found in human subjects [21,22], therefore further investigation is necessary to identify the potential host(s) of the filarial species found in *Ixodes* ticks.

In this study, we attempted to further identify the filarial nematode species found in *Ixodes* ticks using published PCR primer sets targeting *Onchocerciadea* specific genes other than those targeting ribosomal DNA genetic segments, with no success, suggesting that filarial nematodes found in *Ixodes* ticks have unique sequences for those targets. In future projects, we will use a second-generation whole genome sequencing approach to more specifically identify this potential species.

We have visualized the filarial nematodes with *in situ* hybridization. In the literature, the filarial nematodes are usually found to be in the hindgut portion of the arthropod's body after a blood meal [21,22]. They either remain in the hindgut and accessory glands or they migrate to the salivary glands for manifestation of the disease to the human host. Our *in situ* staining results with whole mount tick sections of nymphal *Ixodes scapularis* ticks showed the hindgut regions of the ticks were the primary location of these filarial nematodes. Stage specific development of *Acanthocheilonema* filarial nematodes was already found in nymphal brown dog ticks (Rhipicephalus sanguineus) [11]. Our sequencing data shows that filarial nematodes found in *Amblyomma and Ixodes* ticks are closely related. This data combined with our *in situ* data further suggest it is likely that hard ticks can support the stage specific development of these filarial nematodes.

Our 12S rDNA *Onchocercidae* specific PCR results further revealed that 22% nymphal and 30% adult ticks, collected from the Southern Connecticut area were infected with filarial nematodes. Comparing to the filarial infection rate found in *Amblyomma* ticks collected in Maryland (~3.5%), this rate is significantly higher, however it is comparable to a recent report where ~29% of another haematophagous arthropod, *Culicidae* mosquities, were found to be positive for *Setaria* and unidentified filarial nematodes in Germany [23].

4. Conclusions

Our study concludes that *Ixodes scapularis* tick can indeed be a potential vector for filarial nematodes. Based on our *in situ* and additional data from the literature, it is probable that *Ixodes* ticks can support the different developmental stages of this filarial nematode as well as its transmission to animals or even humans in the endemic area where ticks are prevalent. Our study warrants further investigation regarding the potential transmission of this type of infection to different hosts.

Acknowledgments

This work was supported by grants from University of New Haven and from Tick-Borne Disease Alliance (TBDA, formally Turn the Corner) to ES. The Schwartz Foundation, the Lyme Disease Association and the Lyme Research Alliance donated microscope, microscope attachments and computers for image analyses. The funders had no role in study design, data collection and analysis, decision to publish, or preparation of the manuscript. The authors thank to Roman Zajac (University of New Haven, West Haven, CT, USA) for his helpful discussion in the preparation of the phylogenetic tree.

Author Contributions

NP: As part of her Master's thesis she conducted a significant part of the tick collection field-work, executed PCR and *in situ* staining works, analyzed the data and contributed to the manuscript drafting. JMM contributed in the designs and execution of PCR experiments, sequence analysis and phylogenetic tree output. SM and PRR extracted DNAs and performed PCR experiments. CB was involved in sample collection, additional *in situ* staining works and in manuscript drafting and MJR gave significant input to the study design and involved in manuscript drafting.

ES contributed to the overall study design and analyses of the data, supervised the laboratory work and wrote the manuscript. All authors read and approved the final version of the manuscript.

Conflicts of Interest

The authors declare no conflict of interest.

References

1. Piesman, J.; Hicks, T.C.; Sinsky, R.J.; Obiri, G. Simultaneous transmission of *Borrelia burgdorferi* and *Babesia microti* by individual nymphal *Ixodes dammini* ticks. *J. Clin. Microbiol.* **1987**, *25*, 2012–2013.
2. Levin, M.L.; Fish, D. Acquisition of coinfection and simultaneous transmission of *Borrelia burgdorferi* and *Ehrlichia phagocytophila* by *Ixodes scapularis* ticks. *Infect. Immun.* **2000**, *68*, 2183–2186.
3. Courtney, J.W.; Dryden, R.L.; Montgomery, J.; Schneider, BS.; Smith, G.; Massung, R.F. Molecular characterization of *Anaplasma phagocytophilum* and *Borrelia burgdorferi* in *Ixodes scapularis* ticks from Pennsylvania. *J. Clin. Microbiol.* **2003**, *41*, 1569–1573.

4. Adelson, M.E.; Rao, R.V.; Tilton, R.C.; Cabets, K.; Eskow, E.; Fein, L.; Occi. J.L.; Mordechai, E. Prevalence of *Borrelia burgdorferi*, *Bartonella* spp., *Babesia microti*, and *Anaplasma phagocytophila* in *Ixodes scapularis* Ticks collected in northern New Jersey. *J. Clin. Microbiol.* **2004**, *42*, 2799–2801.
5. Holman, M.S.; Caporale, D.A.; Goldberg, J.; Lacombe, E.; Lubelczyk, C.; Rand, P.W.; Smith, R.P. *Anaplasma phagocytophilum, Babesia microti,* and *Borrelia burgdorferi* in *Ixodes scapularis,* southern coastal Maine. *Emerg. Infect. Dis.* **2004**, *10*, 744–746.
6. Swanson, S.J.; Neitzel, D.; Reed, K.D.; Belongia, E.A. Coinfections acquired from *Ixodes* ticks. *Clin. Microbiol.* **2006**, *19*, 708–727.
7. Tokarz, R.; Jain, K.; Bennett, A.; Briese, T.; Lipkin, W.I. Assessment of polymicrobial infections in ticks in New York State. *Vector Borne Zoonotic Dis.* **2010**, *10*, 217–221.
8. Kjemtrup, AM.; Conrad, P.A. Human babesiosis: An emerging tick-borne disease. *Int. J. Parasitol.* **2000**, *30*, 1323–1337.
9. Beaver, P.C.; Burgdorfer W. A microfilaria of exceptional size from the Ixodid tick, *Ixodes dammini* from Shelter Island New York. *J. Parasitol.* **1984**, *70*, 963–966.
10. Londono, M.I. Behaviour and characteristics of the filarial *Dipetalonema viteae* in the tick *Ornithodoros tartakowskyi*. *Antioquia Medica* **1973**, *23*, 515–516.
11. Olmeda-García, A.S.; Rodríguez-Rodríguez, J.A. Stage specific development of filarial nematodes in vector ticks. *J. Helminthol.* **1994**, *68*, 231–235.
12. Zhang, X.; Norris, D.E.; Rasgon, J.L. Distribution and molecular characterization of *Wolbachia* endosymbionts and filarial nematodes in Maryland populations of the lone star tick (*Amblyomma americanum*). *FEMS Microbiol. Ecol.* **2011**, *77*, 50–56.
13. Nuchprayoon, S.; Junpee, A.; Poovorawn, Y.; Scott, A. Detection and differentiation of filarial parasites by universal primer and polymerase chain reaction–restriction fragment length polymorphism analysis. *Am. J. Trop. Med. Hy.* **2005**, *73*, 895–900.
14. Tamura, K.; Peterson, D.; Nei, M. MEGA5: Molecular evolutionary genetics analysis using maximum likelihood, evolutionary distance and maximum parsimony methods. *Mol. Biol Evol.* **2011**, *28*, 2731–2739.
15. Casiraghi, M.; Anderson, T.J.C.; Bandi, C.; Bazzocchi, C.; Genchi C. A Phylogenetic analysis of filarial nematode: Comparison with the phylogeny of *Wolbachia* endosymbionts. *Parasitology* **2001**, *122*, 93–103.
16. Otranto, D.; Brianti, E.; Dantas-Torres, F.; Weigl, S.; Latrofa, M.S.; Gaglio, G.; Cauquil, L.; Giannetto, S.; Bain, O. Morphological and molecular data on the dermal microfilariae of a species of *Cercopithi* filaria from a dog in Sicily. *Vet. Parasitol.* **2011**, *182*, 221–229.
17. Li, B.W.; Rush, A.C.; Tan, J.; Weil, G.J. Quantitative analysis of gender-regulated transcripts in the filarial Nematode *Brugia malayi* by real-time RT-PCR. *Mol. Biochem. Parasitol.* **2004**, *137*, 329–337.
18. Hojas, R.M.; Post R.J. Regional genetic variation in the major sperm protein genes of *Onchocerca volvulus* and *Mansonella ozzardi* (Nematoda: *Filarioidea). Int. J. Parasitol.* **2000**, *30*, 1459–1465.
19. Brianti, B.; Gagglio, G.; Napoli, E.; Giannetto, S.; Dantas-Torres, P.; Bain, O.; Otranto, D. New insights into the ecology and biology of *Acanthocheilonema reconditum* causing canine subcutaneous filariosis. *Parasitology* **2012**, *139*, 530–536.

20. Eisenbeiss, W.F.; Apfel, H.; Meyer, T.F. Recovery, distribution, and development of *Acanthocheilonema viteae* third- and early fourth-stage larvae in adult jirds. *J. Parasitol.* **1991**, *77*, 580–586.
21. Beaver, P.C.; Meyer, E.A.; Jarroll, E.L. *Dipetalonema* from the eye of a man in Oregon, USA. A case report. *Am. J. Trop. Med. Hyg.* **1980**, *29*, 367–372.
22. Huynh, T.; Thean, J.; Maini R. *Dipetalonema reconditum* in the human eye. *Br. J. Ophtalmol.* **2001**, *85*, doi:10.1136/bjo.85.11.1384i.
23. Czajka, C.; Becker, N.; Poppert, S.; Jöst, H.; Schmidt-Chanasit, J.; Krüge A. Molecular detection of *Setaria tundra* (Nematoda: Filarioidea) and an unidentified filarial species in mosquitoes in Germany. *Parasit. Vectors* **2012**, *5*, doi:10.1186/1756-3305-5-14.

2

Long-Term Changes in Pain Sensitivity in an Animal Model of Social Anxiety

Alessandra Berry [†,*], Veronica Bellisario [†], Sara Capoccia, Nadia Francia, Enrico Alleva and Francesca Cirulli

Section of Behavioural Neurosciences, Department of Cell Biology and Neurosciences, Istituto Superiore di Sanità, Viale Regina Elena 299, Rome 00161, Italy;
E-Mails: veronica.bellisario@guest.iss.it (V.B.); sara.capoccia@guest.iss.it (S.C.); nadia.francia@iss.it (N.F.); enrico.alleva@iss.it (E.A.); francesca.cirulli@iss.it (F.C.)

† These authors contributed equally to this work.

* Author to whom correspondence should be addressed; E-Mail: alessandra.berry@iss.it;

Abstract: Animal models with an eco-ethological relevance can help in identifying novel and reliable stress-related markers. To this end, 3-month-old C57BL/6J male mice were exposed to social defeat (SD) stress for 10 days as this stressor shows good face and predictive validity for several models of human affective disorders including depression, social phobia and post-traumatic stress disorder. Social avoidance and pain threshold were assessed 24 h and 4 weeks after the end of SD stress, while corticosterone was assayed at the beginning and at the end of the stressful procedure (days 1 and 10). SD subjects were characterized by increased corticosterone levels (30 min following stress exposure), increased latency to approach the social target in the short-term as well as increased emotionality in the long-term. Moreover, an increase in nociceptive threshold (stress-induced analgesia) was found both in the short-term and 4 weeks after the end of stress. These data indicate that the SD paradigm is able to induce emotional changes associated with a stressful/traumatic event. In addition, they indicate that variations in the nociceptive threshold might represent a physiological marker of both short- and long-term effects of stress.

Keywords: mice; animal model; stress-induced analgesia; pain sensitivity; social defeat stress; emotionality

1. Introduction

Animal models represent a key heuristic approach to identifying reliable markers and pathophysiological aspects of stress-related diseases, such as generalized anxiety, major depression, post-traumatic stress disorder (PTSD) and schizophrenia [1–5]. In an attempt to model pathologies associated with stress, powerful stressors such as cold, electric foot-shock, forced swimming, restraint and chronic unpredictable stress are commonly used. However, as many authors have pointed out, most of these stressful challenges used in the laboratory setting are not so relevant to situations that humans encounter in their everyday life, likewise they hardly resemble those usually faced by rodents in a natural context [6–9]. By contrast, social stressors are effective in triggering powerful physiological and, more importantly, emotional responses both in humans and in social animals such as rats and mice [5,10–15] also leading to avoidance/withdrawal, a behavioral trait which is common in several human affective disorders including depression, social phobia and also PTSD [16]. In particular, it has been proposed that, compared to models based on physical stressors, social defeat (SD) stress, which (in mice and rats) is based on the experimental induction of social conflicts through repeated exposures to a larger, dominant, conspecific might represent a reliable paradigm to model stress-induced human psychopathological traits [17]. Indeed, SD stress does not result in habituation upon repeated presentations, providing an ethologically and ecologically relevant form of persistent emotional distress [18]. Chronic exposure to this kind of stress profoundly alters the motivation for social interactions in rodents [19–21] and also leads to short- and long-term behavioral and physiological changes, such as decreased locomotion and exploratory activity [22,23], in addition to increased emotionality [10,24]. Berton and colleagues, using a modified version of the SD stress in mice, observed long-term effects on neural and behavioral plasticity in response to aversive social experiences including social avoidance up to 4 weeks from the end of the stressful procedure [16]. Intriguingly, these authors also showed that chronic treatment with antidepressants is able to normalize social withdrawal in this mouse model. Thus, SD stress appears as a solid animal model with good face and predictive validity that may help in identifying novel and reliable markers of stress-related psychosocial alterations.

Psychiatric pathologies in which stressful/traumatic events play a main role in their etiology, such as PTSD acute stress and borderline personality disorders (BPD), are characterized by common stress-induced features, such as intrusive memories and dissociative states, involving numbing and changes in pain perception [25–27]. A well characterized physiological response to stress is an increase in nociceptive threshold that relies upon the activation of different endogenous opioid and/or non-opioid pain inhibitory systems [28–32]. This phenomenon is commonly known as stress-induced analgesia (SIA) [33] and represents a key component of the organism's defense system against aversive stimuli, preparing for the "fight or flight" response [34]. Former experiments on social conflict have provided a biologically relevant model of SIA with decreased nociception in defeated mice [21,35–38]. However, current knowledge of this aspect of nociception refers mostly to acute responses occurring within a few hours from the end of stress exposure. Jackson and co-workers, in 1979, were the first to show that 24 h after exposure to electric foot shock rats still show an analgesic reaction [39].

The aim of this study was to compare the short- (24 h) and the long-term (4 weeks) effects of exposure to a chronic psychosocial stress (SD) on social anxiety with a main focus on specific changes in pain sensitivity resulting from SD. We hypothesized that defeated mice would show greater social avoidance and higher pain threshold than controls. In order to test this hypothesis, we investigated specific behavioral changes as a result of the social defeat experience (by means of the social avoidance test—SAT) and the nociceptive response (by means of the hot plate test) 24 h and, for the first time, 4 weeks after the end of SD. Physiological parameters, such as changes in plasma levels of corticosterone (CORT) and body weight, were assessed before and at the end of the 10-day stressful procedure to control for SD effectiveness.

2. Experimental Section

Animals: experimental subjects were male mice either from a C57BL/6J (n = 26; SD or control subjects—CTRL) or CD-1 (n = 32; aggressive resident mice) strain purchased from a commercial breeder (Charles River, Calco, Italy). Upon arrival, C57BL/6J mice were pair-housed in cages (37 × 21 × 19 cm) provided by a perforated Plexiglas partition allowing sensory but not physical contact, meaning they were housed in two compartments (18.5 × 21 × 19 cm) within the same cage, separated by a perforated partition wall for 7 days (acclimatization); CD-1 mice were single-housed. Animals were all kept in the same room provided by air conditioning (temperature 21 ± 1 °C, relative humidity 60% ± 10%) under a reversed 12/12 h light/dark cycle with lights off from 06:30 a.m. to 06:30 p.m. Pellet food (standard diet Altromin-R, purchased from Rieper, Italy) and tap-water were continuously available.

Following 1 week of acclimatization, experimental subjects were randomly assigned to the chronic social defeat condition (SD, n = 14; 10 days of SD stress) or to a control group (CTRL, n = 12; daily handling). SD mice were blood sampled by tail nick at the beginning (day 1) and at the end of the stressful procedure (day 10) to assess neuroendocrine activation. At the end of the 10-day stress paradigm, all subjects were tested for social avoidance (SAT) and nociceptive threshold (hot plate (HP) test) either under short- (24 h) or long-term (4 weeks) conditions (final number of subjects for each group: CTRLs, n = 6 both for short- and long-term conditions; SD, n = 7 both for short- and long-term conditions); see Figure 1 for a schematic representation of the experimental timeline. Behavioral performances were video-recorded and the behavioral analysis was carried out from the videotape, using commercial software ("The Observer 3.0"). At the end of each session, apparatuses were cleaned by cotton pads soaked with a 50% solution of ethanol and water. Since it has been shown that the effects of repeated psychosocial stress are more pronounced if the test is performed during the active circadian phase of mice [40], all tests were conducted between 9:30 a.m. and 12:30 p.m. under dim light (1 lux), during the dark period of a reversed light cycle.

Figure 1. Schematic representation of the experimental timeline. The experiment lasted 38 days in total. SD subjects underwent 10 days of daily bouts of social defeat, followed by continuous protected sensory contact with their aggressor. Body weight was assessed on the day before stress took place (day 0), on day 5 and on day 10 of SD. Blood samples for corticosterone assessment were collected on days 1 and 10. SD and CTRL subjects were either tested on day 11 (24 h following the end of the SD procedure, short-term effects of stress), or on day 38 (4 weeks following the end of the SD procedure, long-term effects of stress). b.w.: body weight; CORT: corticosterone; SAT: Social Avoidance Test; HP: Hot Plate Test; SD: Social Defeat.

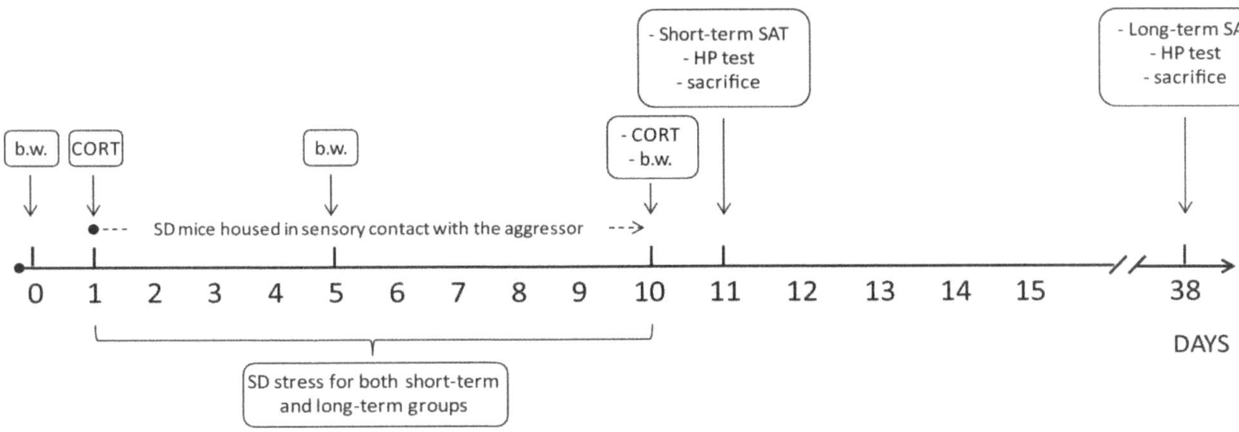

Animal handling and experimental procedures were performed in accordance with the Guidelines laid down by the European Communities Council Directive 2010/63/EU and with the Italian legislation on animal experimentation (Decreto L.vo 116/92).

Social Defeat Stress: C57BL/6J mice were randomly assigned to the chronic social defeat condition (SD, n = 14; 10 days of SD stress) or to a control group (CTRL, n = 12; daily handling). SD subjects underwent 10 days of daily bouts of social defeat, followed by continuous protected sensory contact with their aggressor [13,16]. More precisely, each SD mouse (C57BL/6J, n = 14) was introduced into the home cage of an unfamiliar resident (CD-1, n = 14) for 5 min and was physically defeated, soon after, residents and intruders were physically separated by a perforated transparent Plexiglas partition and maintained in sensory contact for 24 h until the next trial. Every day, each SD mouse was exposed to a different aggressor while CTRL subjects were housed in stable pairs with a same strain conspecific, under the same sensory conditions, and were daily handled by the time SD subjects underwent social stress. This housing was maintained throughout the study and was meant to avoid any bias related to changes in the housing conditions after the stressful procedure in the SD group. At the end of the 10 days of stress, SD mice were pair-housed with a same sex, same strain conspecific in a cage provided by a Plexiglas perforated partition for either 24 h or 4 weeks (28 days). Since C57BL/6J mice are usually smaller than same-age CD-1 conspecifics, in order to prevent excessive physical aggression possibly leading to a lethal outcome, intruders (C57BL/6J) were selected so to have a body size comparable to that of residents (CD-1). Resident mice were selected for their attack latencies reliably shorter than 30 s upon 3 consecutive screening tests [16]. CD-1 mice were housed alone at least 3 weeks prior to the SD stress procedure in order to increase aggressive behavior.

The intruder mouse was considered "defeated" when displaying submissive postures. Excessive aggressive behaviors (e.g., incessant biting that could lead to injuries) were interrupted by inserting the Plexiglas partition.

Body weight: to assess stress-related changes in body weight, SD mice were weighed the day before the stress started (day 0) and on days 5 and 10 of the SD procedure. The body weight of control subjects was also registered on the same days, *i.e.*, on handling days 0, 5 and 10.

Neuroendocrine activation: to assess the effect of the SD stress on hypothalamic-pituitary-adrenal (HPA) axis activation, plasma CORT levels were measured on the first (day 1) and on the last day (day 10) of the procedure at different time points, *i.e.*, soon before (0 min) and following (30 and 120 min) the defeat. Blood sampling was performed by means of the tail nick a standard minimally-invasive consolidated procedure in use in our laboratory and many others. Briefly: a mouse is taken from the cage and gently placed on the metal top of a clean cage; the experimenter holds the tip of the tail while the mouse that is not restrained is allowed to move. By means of a razor blade, a small nick is performed (approximately 2 mm wide × 0.5 mm deep) in the tail, perpendicular to the tail vein, approximately 2 cm from the tip of the tail. Blood droplets are directly collected into EDTA-coated capillary tubes. For further details on the procedure, see also [41,42]. To prevent bleeding before the test took place, the animals' tail was carefully dried and pinched for 10 s with a clean tissue.

Social Avoidance Test (SAT): social avoidance behavior is a widely used indicator of the effects of social stress, with defeated subjects decreasing the time spent investigating a novel conspecific [16]. Thus, to assess the short- (24 h) and long-term (4 weeks) effects of the exposure to a socially stressful event, experimental subjects (CTRL, $n = 6$ and SD, $n = 7$ for both short- and long-term assessment) underwent a SAT. More precisely, mice were introduced to a plastic open field arena (42 × 42 cm) for two consecutive 2.5 min sessions (a test duration chosen for its optimal sensitivity/throughput ratio [16]). During session I ("no target"), the open field contained an empty wire mesh cage (diameter = 10 cm, h = 10 cm) located in the middle of one side of the arena. During session II ("social target"), a social target (an unfamiliar CD-1 male mouse) was introduced into the wire mesh cage. Between the two sessions, the experimental subject was placed back into its home cage for 1 min. The time spent in the "interaction zone" (8 cm wide corridor surrounding the cage) *vs.* the "corners" (opposite to the location of the cage) was scored as a reliable measure of social avoidance. When data were analyzed, the arena was ideally divided into squares (7 × 7 cm) and latency and frequency of locomotion (crossings of squares) were scored, in addition to latency, frequency and duration of the risk assessment behavior (*stretched-attend posture—SAP*), *freezing* and exploration of the wire mesh cage (*touching object*).

Behaviors were defined as follows: *crossing*, crossing the square limits with all paws; *stretched-attend posture*, exploratory posture in which the body is stretched forward and then retracted to the original position without any forward locomotion; *freezing*, self-explanatory; *touching object*, self-explanatory.

Hot Plate Test (HP): two hours following the end of the SAT, subjects were placed on a hot metal plate set at 50 ± 1 °C enclosed by a 19 cm diameter Perspex cylinder (Model D837; Basile, Socrel Comerio, Italy), to prevent animals from jumping off the plate. Although many studies use higher temperatures, we have previously shown that already at 50 ± 1 °C it is possible to test differences in the sensitivity to a thermal noxious stimulus both in mice and rats by overall reducing suffering of experimental subjects [43,44]. Nociception was assessed by scoring latency, frequency and duration of *forepaw* and *hindpaw licking*, the latter behavioral item (*hindpaw licking*) being the most reliable measure of pain sensitivity [44]. A cut-off time of 60 s was used.

Radioimmunoassay for corticosterone determination (RIA): Blood samples (100 μL, approximate volume) were collected individually in potassium EDTA coated tubes (1.6 mg EDTA/mL blood; Sarstedt, Germany). All samples were kept on ice and later centrifuged at 3000 rpm for 15 min at +4 °C. Blood plasma was transferred to Eppendorf tubes for CORT determination and stored at −80 °C until further analysis. CORT was measured using commercially available radioimmunoassay (RIA) kit (MP Biomedicals, LLC, NY, USA) containing 125 iodine labelled CORT; 5 μL of plasma were sufficient to carry out CORT measurement. Sensitivity of the assay was 0.125 mg/dL, inter- and intra-assay variation was less than 10% and 5%, respectively. Vials were counted for 2 min in a gamma-scintillation counter (Packard Minaxi Gamma counter, Series 5000).

Statistical analysis: Data were analyzed using parametric analysis of variance (ANOVA) with group (stress (SD) *vs.* control (CTRL)) as between-subjects factor and days, minutes, sessions ("no target" *vs.* "social target") and zones ("center" *vs.* "corners" *vs.* "interaction zone") as within-subject repeated measures, when appropriate (body weight measurement, CORT assessment and SAT). Since subjects tested at 24 h and at 4 weeks belonged to two different groups of animals, we decided to run separate statistical analyses. Post hoc comparisons were performed using the Tukey's test. Data are expressed as mean +SEM. A significance level of 0.05 was chosen.

3. Results and Discussion

3.1. Body Weight

The SD paradigm affected body weight of the experimental subjects. In fact, on day 10 SD mice showed a significant decrease in body weight compared to CTRL subjects (interaction between days and stress condition: $F_{2,48} = 4.176$, $p = 0.0213$, see Figure 2).

Figure 2. Body weight. Social defeated (SD) subjects decreased their body weight following 10 days of chronic SD stress. Data are presented as mean + S.E.M. (CTRL, $n = 12$; SD, $n = 14$). ** $p < 0.01$.

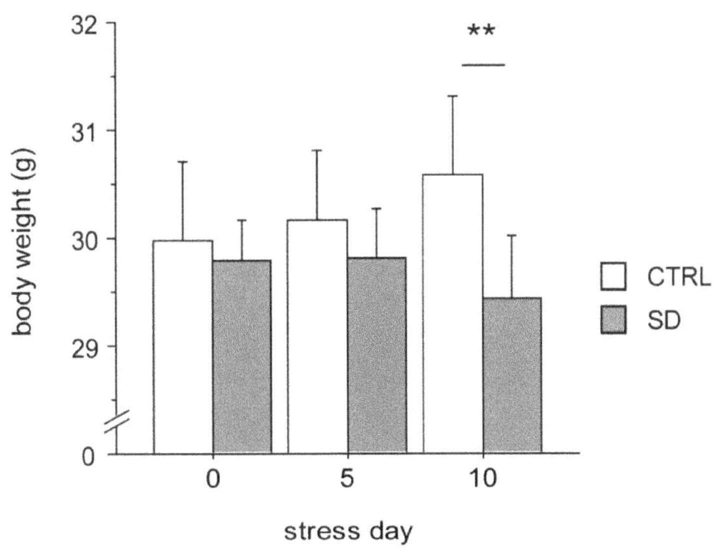

3.2. Neuroendocrine Activation

The social defeat paradigm was effective in challenging the HPA axis (main effect of repeated measures: $F_{2,26} = 78.342$, $p < 0.0001$). In particular, the SD procedure leads to an overall increase in CORT levels 30 min from the onset of stress (basal *vs.* 30, $p < 0.01$) and is followed by a smooth decrease 120 min later (30 *vs.* 120 min, $p < 0.05$). No difference was found between day 1 and day 10 that were overall characterized by a similar profile in the HPA axis activation during time (interaction between days and time course: $F_{2,26} = 0.921$, $p = 0.4106$, see Figure 3). CORT levels were not assessed in the CTRL group thus we cannot exclude that, although minimally-invasive, the blood sampling procedure might have contributed to the observed HPA axis activation.

Figure 3. Neuroendocrine activation following the first (day 1) and the last encounter (day 10). SD stress is able to challenge the HPA axis. Experimental subjects do not show a significant habituation to the stressful procedure following 10 days of SD, being characterized by a similar neuroendocrine profile on day 1 and on day 10. This lack of habituation is due to the fact that each day a different social stimulus was used, thus preventing a clear habituation profile. Data are presented as mean + S.E.M. (SD, $n = 14$). ** $p < 0.01$, time point 0 *vs.* both 30 and 120 min; * $p < 0.05$, 30 min *vs.* 120 min.

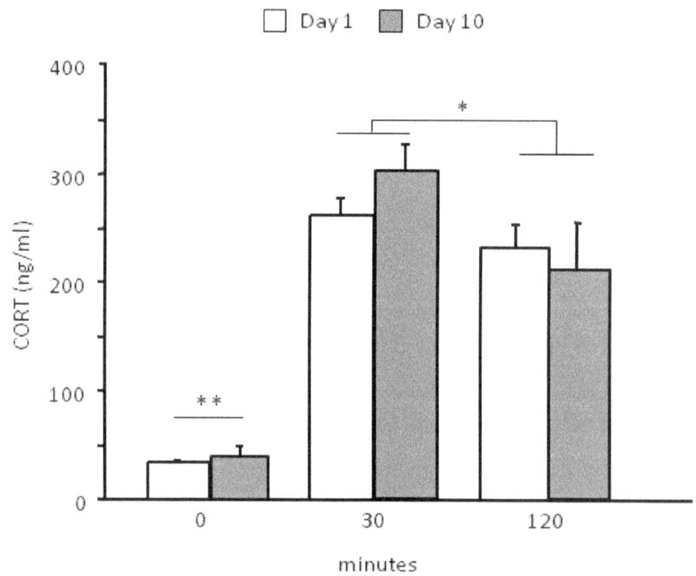

3.3. Social Avoidance Test—SAT

3.3.1. Short-Term Effects (24 h)

Analysis of sessions I and II of the SAT indicated that the behavior of SD mice was affected by previous exposure to a stressful experience since they showed a higher latency to touch the wire mesh cage when the social stimulus was present (interaction between stimulus and stress condition for *touching object* behavior: $F_{1,11} = 10.521$, $p = 0.0078$, see Figure 4A). By contrast, no difference was found in the time spent in the "interaction zone" between SD and CTRL mice (main effect of stress condition: $F_{1,11} = 0.658$, $p = 0.4343$, *i.e.*, average time spent either in the presence or in the absence of the social target, see Figure 4B).

Figure 4. Social Avoidance Test (SAT). The presence of a social stimulus increased the latency of SD mice to touch the wire mesh cage (*touching object*) 24 h (**A**) but not 4 weeks after the end of the stress procedure (**E**). Overall, independently from the presence of the social stimulus, in the long-term situation (4 weeks), SD subjects spent less *time in the interaction zone* than CTRLs (**F**), showed both a shorter latency to perform *SAP* (**G**) and to *freeze* (**H**). No difference was found between SD and CTRL mice in the short-term condition (**B**, **C** and **D**, respectively). Data are presented as mean + S.E.M. $n = 7$ (SD) and 6 (CTRL). Subjects were tested only once either at 24 h or 4 weeks from the end of SD. * $p < 0.05$. ** $p < 0.01$ (main effect of the social condition).

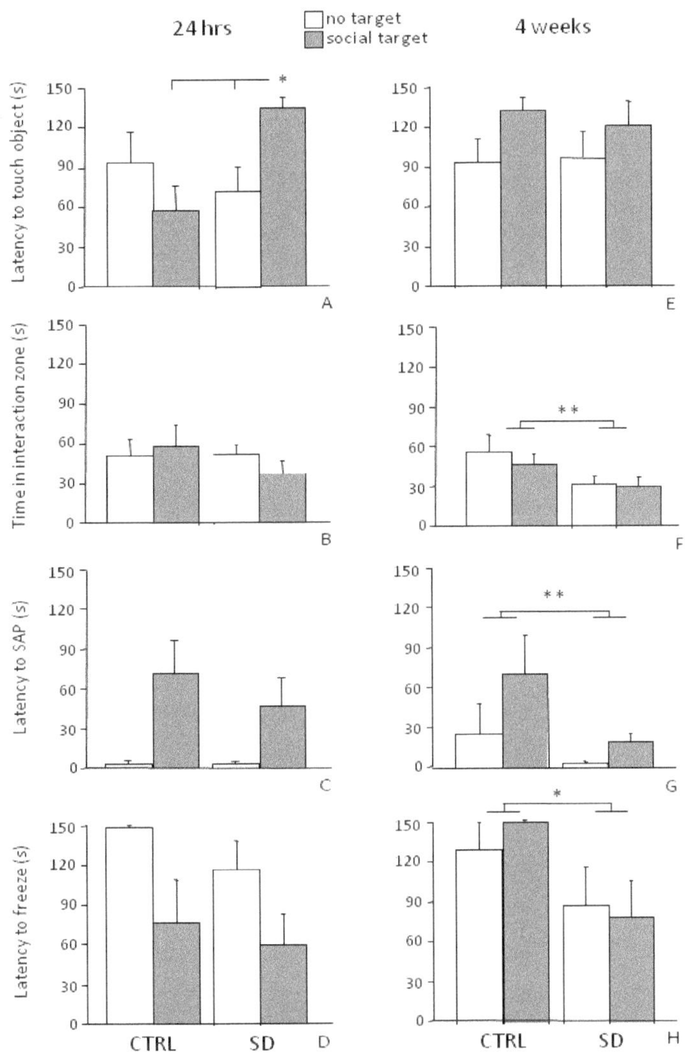

In general, all mice showed an increased locomotor activity in the interaction zone, *i.e.*, in the proximity of the wire mesh cage (main effect of the zone: $F_{2,22} = 20.863$, $p = 0.0001$, post hoc comparisons: "interaction zone" both *vs.* "center" and "corners", $p < 0.01$). All subjects, independently from CTRL or SD conditions, showed a decrease in locomotor activity (*crossing* frequency) when the social stimulus was present (main effect of stimulus: $F_{1,11} = 14.372$, $p = 0.0030$) and this effect was particularly apparent in the interaction zone (interaction between zone and stimulus: $F_{2,22} = 4.584$; $p = 0.0217$, post hoc comparisons: "interaction zone"-"no target" session *vs.* "interaction zone"-"social target" session, $p < 0.05$).

The stress procedure did not affect either the latency to the first episode of risk assessment (main effect of stress condition for *stretched-attend posture (SAP)* behavior: $F_{1,11} = 0.586$, $p = 0.4602$, see Figure 4C) or freezing ($F_{1,11} = 0.915$, $p = 0.3592$, see Figure 4D). By contrast, regardless of the stress procedure, the presence of an aggressive CD-1 male mouse reduced the latency to *freeze* in all subjects (main effect of stimulus: $F_{1,11} = 10.409$, $p = 0.0081$, data not shown in figure) and increased both frequency and duration of this behavior particularly in the corners (interaction between stimulus and zone: $F_{2,22} = 7.095$; 6.699, $p = 0.0042$; 0.0053, respectively for frequency and duration of *freezing*; post hoc comparisons: "corners"-"social target" session *vs.* "corners"-"no target" session, $p < 0.01$; "corners" both *vs.* "center" and "interaction zone", during the "social target" session $p < 0.01$).

3.3.2. Long-Term Effects (4 Weeks)

Four weeks from the end of the SD procedure, when mice were tested in the SAT, an increase in the latency to the first approach to the object and a reduction in the frequency of *touching object* in all experimental subjects (main effect of stimulus: $F_{1,11} = 7.250$; 5.241, $p = 0.0209$; 0.0428, respectively for latency and frequency) was found. In particular, no effect of the stress experience was found on the latency to approach the cage both in sessions I and II (interaction between stimulus and stress condition $F_{1,11} = 0.378$, $p = 0.5513$, see Figure 4E). However, in general, SD mice spent less time in the "interaction zone" compared to the CTRLs (main effect of the stress condition: $F_{1,11} = 7.147$, $p = 0.0217$, see Figure 4F).

As for locomotor activity, all mice showed an increased frequency of *crossings* in the interaction zone (main effect of zone: $F_{2,22} = 20.650$; $p < 0.0001$). However, this behavior decreased in this specific portion of the arena from session I to II, *i.e.*, when the CD-1 mouse was introduced in the wire mesh cage (interaction between session and zone for *crossings* frequency: $F_{2,22} = 3.505$, $p = 0.0477$, post hoc comparisons: "interaction zone"-"no target" session *vs.* "interaction zone"-"social target", $p < 0.05$).

Overall exposure to the SD procedure reduced the latency to first *SAP* episode (main effect of stress condition: $F_{1,11} = 6.612$, $p = 0.0260$, see Figure 4G) as well as the latency to *freeze* (main effect of stress condition: $F_{1,11} = 7.796$, $p = 0.0175$, see Figure 4H).

3.4. Hot Plate (HP) Test

Twenty-four hours after the end of the social stress (short-term condition), SD mice showed a higher pain threshold than controls, being characterized by lower latency, frequency and duration of *hindpaw licking*, suggesting overall a SIA profile (main effect of stress: $F_{1,11} = 5.302$; 4.838; 5.201; $p = 0.0418$; 0.0500; 0.0435; respectively for latency, frequency and duration, see Figure 5A–C). Interestingly, a similar profile was still evident in SD mice 4 weeks from the end of stress (long-term condition), as shown by a persistent lower frequency of *hindpaw licking* (main effect of stress: $F_{1,11} = 6.769$; $p = 0.0246$, see Figure 5E) while no difference was found as for latency and duration (main effect of stress: $F_{1,11} = 2.187$; 1.118, $p = 0.1673$; 0.3130, respectively for latency and duration, see Figure 5D,F). CTRL and SD mice did not differ in *forepaw licking* behavior either when tested 24 h or 4 weeks following the end of the stressful procedure (main effect of stress: 24 h, $F_{1,11} = 0.525$; 0.880; 0.243, $p = 0.4840$; 0.3683; 0.6318, respectively for latency, frequency and duration; 4 weeks, $F_{1,11} = 2.015$; 0.035; 0.128, $p = 0.1834$; 0.8544; 0.7275, respectively for latency, frequency and duration).

Figure 5. Hot Plate (HP) Test. Twenty-four h after the end of stress, SD mice were characterized by an increase in pain threshold (SIA) showing a higher latency (**A**) and a reduced frequency (**B**) and duration (**C**) to perform *hindpaw licking*. A SIA profile was still apparent 4 weeks after the end of the stress procedure, when SD mice performed *hindpaw licking* with a lower frequency than CTRLs (**E**). No effect was observed as for the latency (**D**) and duration (**F**). Data are presented as mean +S.E.M. $n = 7$ (SD) and 6 (CTRL). * $p < 0.05$. ** $p < 0.01$. Subjects were tested only once either at 24 h or after 4 weeks after the end of SD.

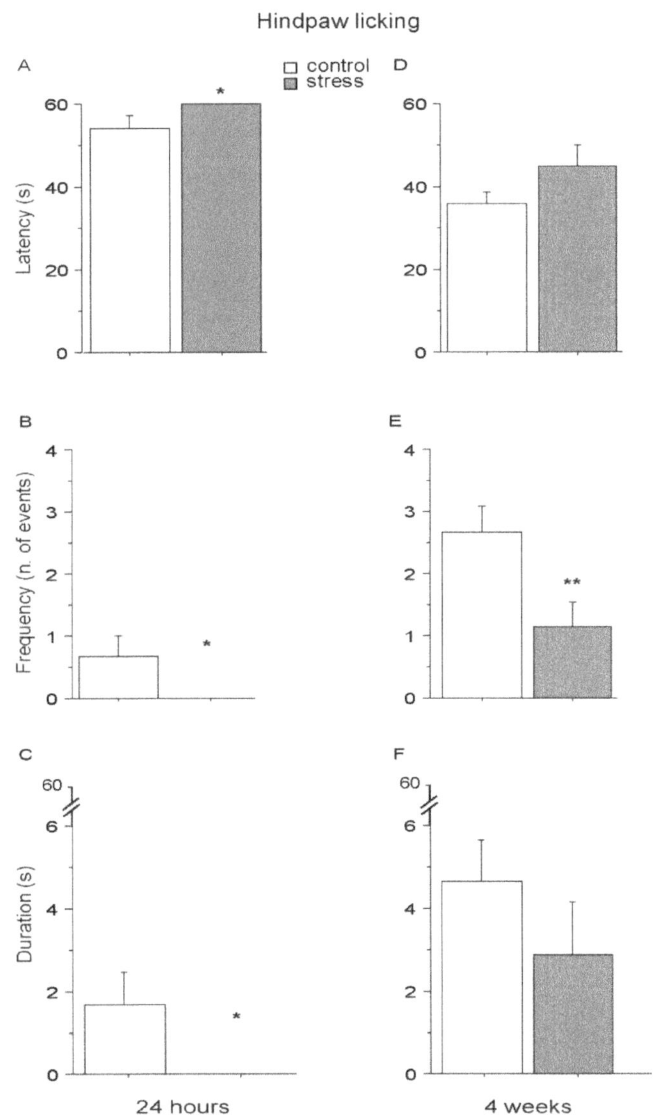

Results from this study show that a chronic social stress paradigm affects the emotional profile of C57BL/6J adult male mice as well as their nociceptive response to stressful stimuli. In addition, they provide evidence for SIA as a specific and adaptive biological mechanism with persistent long-term effects that might be elicited and/or reinforced by exposure to stressful stimuli with a similar salience as those previously experienced.

These data suggest that SIA might be useful to assess long-lasting physiological effects of stress-induced vulnerability, such as those characterizing human psychopathological conditions.

As shown by the increase in corticosterone levels 30 min following the onset of stress, experimental subjects do not show a significant habituation to the stressful procedure after 10 days of SD, being characterized by a similar neuroendocrine profile on day 1 and on day 10. This lack of habituation is due to the fact that each day a different social stimulus was used, thus preventing a clear habituation curve, SD representing a significant challenge for the neuroendocrine system. This piece of data was associated to a decrease in body weight (day 10). Adaptive metabolic responses to stress may vary according to the sensitivity to the procedure, duration and intensity of the stressful experience as well as to the mouse strain tested [45]. In our stress paradigm, C57BL/6J subjects, apart from the physical interaction with aggressors, were also in a continuous/chronic visual and olfactive contact with CD-1 subjects during the entire 10-day procedure. A decrease in body weight has been described to result from exposure to chronic social stress [46–48]. In line with these data, our results might indicate a catabolic effect of the daily exposure to the aggressive mouse. Alternatively, although we did not measure it, it is possible that mice undergoing SD were characterized by a decrease in food consumption during the stress administration.

In the SAT, SD subjects were characterized by a higher latency to approach the wire mesh cage in the presence of the CD-1 aggressor (*touching object*) soon after the end of stress (24 h). This is a clear indication that the SD procedure was effective in eliciting avoidance of a social target that had acquired salience as a threatening stimulus. Differently from previous studies [16], we did not find a difference in the "*time spent in the interaction zone*" at this time point neither in the SD nor in the CTRL group. As pointed out by Golden and co-workers, recent evidence suggests that C57BL/6J mice appear to be less susceptible to stress when compared with other strains [49,50]. In addition, these authors argue that in this test "a social interaction ratio equal to 1, in which equal time is spent in the presence *versus* absence of a social target, has been used as the threshold for dividing defeated mice into the susceptible and resilient categories [16,48]. Control C57BL/6J mice show a strong tendency to spend greater than or equal amounts of time in the interaction zone in each session. Mice below this criterion are grouped as susceptible, whereas mice above are grouped as resilient" [51]. Therefore, we cannot exclude that by using a larger number of experimental subjects we could have identified subgroups of mice "resilient" or "vulnerable" to the SD procedure. No change was observed overall in the general emotional behavior as we found no difference in the latency to *freeze* and to perform risk assessment behaviors (*SAP*).

The higher latency to approach the social target was not found at 4 weeks. However, at this time point, SD mice displayed a general avoidance for the interaction zone, regardless of the presence of the social target, and this was associated with an overall enhancement in their emotional profile as shown by the reduced latency to perform *SAP* and to *freeze* upon introduction in the arena. As for *freezing*, this behavior can be considered as a component of the classic anxiogenic pattern as assessed both in rats and mice as well as a measure of associative fear intensity [52,53]; therefore, we suggest that the behavioral profile observed 4 weeks from the end of SD likely reflects the long-term effects of the social defeat-related stressful experience. This result is further strengthened by the persistence of SIA only in mice that underwent chronic SD stress and up to 4 weeks (increased *hindpaw licking* frequency).

Indeed, a further main stress-induced change in the physiology of SD mice is the increase in pain threshold, as measured in the hot plate test. This alteration in nociception, also known as SIA, was observed not only under acute/short-term (24 h) conditions but also, and more intriguingly, up until 4 weeks from the end of the SD procedure. In the acute situation, the stress-induced analgesic profile was associated with behaviors indicative of social anxiety/avoidance (increased latency to *touching object*) while, in the long-term, with an overall increase in emotionality (decreased latency to *freeze* and to perform *SAP*). It is interesting to note that the assessment of nociceptive threshold was performed following the SAT *i.e.*, after the exposure of the experimental subjects to a social stimulus (unfamiliar CD-1 mouse) which had been associated with a stressful/traumatic experience (chronic defeat). Although on the one hand the SAT required the animal to come into contact with the aggressive CD-1 mouse in a different context from the SD procedure—and thus we cannot refer to contextual memory [54] in this case—on the other hand, as pointed out by Berton and co-workers, in defeated mice an associative process is required for a social target to progressively acquire salience as a threatening stimulus [16]. Therefore, re-exposure (without physical contact) to an aggressive mouse was able to induce analgesia, as revealed in the hot plate test. Worth noticing, very few studies have investigated the long-term effects of changes in thermal pain sensitivity as a result of stress exposure. As an example, Zhang and co-workers recently found a decrease in the nociceptive threshold (both thermal and mechanical) of Sprague-Dawley rats up to 21 days following the end of heterotypic stress consisting of the exposure of experimental subjects to restraint stress, forced swimming, diethyl ether and prolonged social isolation [55]. However, to our knowledge, this is the first time that such a long-term effect of SIA is reported in mice following the exposure to a repeated homotipic stressor such as SD.

It has been suggested that SD stress might be used as a reliable procedure to model PTSD for its relevance in reproducing some of the symptoms characterizing this pathology or some co-morbid disorders often associated to it [16,52]. Psychiatric pathologies in which stressful/traumatic events play a main role in their etiology, such as PTSD and BPD, are characterized by common stress-induced features such as intrusive memories and dissociative states involving also numbing and SIA [27,56]. Although the presence of persistent chronic pain has been often reported in people affected by PTSD [57–59], SIA in these patients appears as a specific response to the re-exposure to a stimulus resembling the original trauma [25,26]. A well-established relationship links pain sensitivity endogenous opioids and the SIA [60,61] and a great body of evidence reports specific changes in this biological system as a result of chronic stress [62] and severe physical or psychological traumas [63–65]. In addition, increased pain tolerance has been reported in individuals who self-injure [66] (an aberrant behavior also observed in abused children [67–69]). Likewise, in PTSD patients the secretion of endogenous opioids, as a result of re-exposure to a stimulus resembling the traumatic stress (combat videotapes), was indirectly measured as naloxone reversible anesthesia [25,26]. In a very recent and interesting review, Naomi Eisenberger suggests that "the experiences of social pain—the painful feelings associated with social disconnection—rely on some of the same neurobiological substrates that underlie experiences of physical pain" sharing therefore common signaling pathways leading to the modulation of nociceptive threshold throughout life as fine adaptation to emotional life events [70]. Indeed, chronic pain has been also found to be co-morbid with anxiety and depression [71] in a cause–effect vicious circle and recent evidence reports pain relief in a mouse model of stress as a result of chronic treatment with the selective serotonin reuptake inhibitor fluoxetine (an antidepressant able to reverse anxiety/depressive-like state) [72]. Interestingly, Berton and co-workers found that chronic administration of either fluoxetine or imipramine improved social interaction in mice undergoing SD stress, suggesting a link between neuronal pathways involved in the circuitry of reward and sociality [16]; similarly it has been proposed that common pathways involving pain and reward systems might have evolved to support complex social experiences [70,73–76]. Thus, an intriguing hypothesis is that pain, reward and sociality might share common basic mechanisms playing a main role in the etiology, onset and progression of psychiatric disorders.

4. Conclusions

Taken together, our data show that the SD stress paradigm is able to induce ethologically and ecologically relevant forms of persistent emotional disruption associated with short- and long-term changes in the nociceptive threshold. In addition, they reinforce previous evidence for SIA as a specific and adaptive biological mechanism with persistent long-term effects that might be elicited and/or reinforced by the exposure to stressful stimuli with similar salience as those previously experienced.

Taking into account all the limitations of our study, also related to the small number of experimental subjects and physiological parameters evaluated, these data suggest that SIA might represent a good physiological response to assess the long-lasting effects of stress-induced vulnerability such as that characterizing human psychopathological conditions.

Indeed, strong epidemiological evidence relates changes in pain perception with disorder of mood and anxiety. In particular, PTSD is associated with significantly elevated prevalence of chronic pain [57,58]. Despite this feature, SIA in PTSD patients appears as a specific response to the re-exposure to a stressful stimulus resembling the original trauma [25,26,77]. By contrast, BPD has been associated with reduced pain sensitivity both under stress and non-stress conditions in humans [78–80].

Future studies should further characterize changes in pain sensitivity in animal models of stress in order to design relevant preclinical studies of specific human psychopathologies. Progress in understanding the pathophysiology of human psychopathologies would greatly benefit from preclinical studies incorporating SIA as a physiological marker of stress.

Acknowledgments

We kindly acknowledge Carla Raggi for technical support in the preparation of this manuscript. Funding for this study was provided by the Italian Ministry of Health (Italia–USA Project) Fasc.11US/14/1 to E.A.

Author Contributions

A. Berry and V. Bellisario wrote the manuscript; F. Cirulli, E. Alleva and A. Berry designed the experimental protocol; F. Cirulli and E. Alleva, revised the manuscript, V. Bellisario, S. Capoccia and N. Francia performed the experiments.

Conflicts of Interest

All authors declare that no conflict of interests, financial or otherwise, exists with regard to this research.

References

1. Anisman, H.; Merali, Z.; Stead, J.D. Experiential and genetic contributions to depressive- and anxiety-like disorders: Clinical and experimental studies. *Neurosci. Biobehav. Rev.* **2008**, *32*, 1185–1206.
2. Cirulli, F.; Alleva, E. The NGF saga: From animal models of psychosocial stress to stress-related psychopathology. *Front Neuroendocrinol.* **2009**, *30*, 379–395.
3. Cryan, J.F.; Holmes, A. The ascent of mouse: Advances in modelling human depression and anxiety. *Nat. Rev. Drug Discov.* **2005**, *4*, 775–790.
4. Koolhaas, J.M.; de Boer, S.F.; Buwalda, B.; van Reenen, K. Individual variation in coping with stress: A multidimensional approach of ultimate and proximate mechanisms. *Brain Behav. Evol.* **2007**, *70*, 218–226.
5. Miczek, K.A.; de Wit, H. Challenges for translational psychopharmacology research—Some basic principles. *Psychopharmacology (Berl.)* **2008**, *199*, 291–301.
6. Koolhaas, J.M.; de Boer, S.F.; de Rutter, A.J.; Meerlo, P.; Sgoifo, A. Social stress in rats and mice. *Acta Physiol. Scand Suppl.* **1997**, *640*, 69–72.
7. Tamashiro, K.L.; Nguyen, M.M.; Sakai, R.R. Social stress: From rodents to primates. *Front Neuroendocrinol.* **2005**, *26*, 27–40.
8. Willner, P. The validity of animal models of depression. *Psychopharmacology (Berl.)* **1984**, *83*, 1–16.
9. Berry, A.; Bellisario, V.; Capoccia, S.; Tirassa, P.; Calza, A.; Alleva, E.; Cirulli, F. Social deprivation stress is a triggering factor for the emergence of anxiety- and depression-like behaviours and leads to reduced brain BDNF levels in C57BL/6J mice. *Psychoneuroendocrinology* **2012**, *37*, 762–772.
10. Kudryavtseva, N.N.; Bakshtanovskaya, I.V.; Koryakina, L.A. Social model of depression in mice of C57BL/6J strain. *Pharmacol. Biochem. Behav.* **1991**, *38*, 315–320.
11. Sheridan, J.F.; Stark, J.L.; Avitsur, R.; Padgett, D.A. Social disruption, immunity, and susceptibility to viral infection. Role of glucocorticoid insensitivity and NGF. *Ann. N. Y. Acad. Sci.* **2000**, *917*, 894–905.
12. Vialou, V.; Robison, A.J.; Laplant, Q.C.; Covington, H.E., 3rd.; Dietz, D.M.; Ohnishi, Y.N.; Mouzon, E.; Rush, A.J., 3rd; Watts, E.L.; Wallace, D.L.; *et al.* DeltaFosB in brain reward circuits mediates resilience to stress and antidepressant responses. *Nat. Neurosci.* **2010**, *13*, 745–752.
13. Bartolomucci, A.; Palanza, P.; Sacerdote, P.; Panerai, A.E.; Sgoifo, A.; Dantzer, R.; Parmigiani, S. Social factors and individual vulnerability to chronic stress exposure. *Neurosci. Biobehav. Rev.* **2005**, *29*, 67–81.
14. Beitia, G.; Garmendia, L.; Azpiroz, A.; Vegas, O.; Brain, P.F.; Arregi, A. Time-dependent behavioral, neurochemical, and immune consequences of repeated experiences of social defeat stress in male mice and the ameliorative effects of fluoxetine. *Brain Behav. Immun.* **2005**, *19*, 530–539.
15. Fuchs, E. Social stress in tree shrews as an animal model of depression: An example of a behavioral model of a CNS disorder. *CNS Spectr.* **2005**, *10*, 182–190.

16. Berton, O.; McClung, C.A.; Dileone, R.J.; Krishnan, V.; Renthal, W.; Russo, S.J.; Graham, D.; Tsankova, N.M.; Bolanos, C.A.; Rios, M.; *et al.* Essential role of BDNF in the mesolimbic dopamine pathway in social defeat stress. *Science* **2006**, *311*, 864–868.
17. Brown, G.W. Social roles, context and evolution in the origins of depression. *J. Health Soc. Behav.* **2002**, *43*, 255–276.
18. Tidey, J.W.; Miczek, K.A. Acquisition of cocaine self-administration after social stress: Role of accumbens dopamine. *Psychopharmacology (Berl.)* **1997**, *130*, 203–212.
19. Avgustinovich, D.F.; Kovalenko, I.L.; Kudryavtseva, N.N. A model of anxious depression: Persistence of behavioral pathology. *Neurosci. Behav. Physiol.* **2005**, *35*, 917–924.
20. Huhman, K.L.; Solomon, M.B.; Janicki, M.; Harmon, A.C.; Lin, S.M.; Israel, J.E.; Jasnow, A.M. Conditioned defeat in male and female Syrian hamsters. *Horm. Behav.* **2003**, *44*, 293–299.
21. Siegfried, B.; Frischknecht, H.R.; Waser, P.G. Defeat, learned submissiveness, and analgesia in mice: Effect of genotype. *Behav. Neural. Biol.* **1984**, *42*, 91–97.
22. Koolhaas, J.M.; Meerlo, P.; de Boer, S.F.; Strubbe, J.H.; Bohus, B. The temporal dynamics of the stress response. *Neurosci. Biobehav. Rev.* **1997**, *21*, 775–782.
23. Meerlo, P.; de Boer, S.F.; Koolhaas, J.M.; Daan, S.; van den Hoofdakker, R.H. Changes in daily rhythms of body temperature and activity after a single social defeat in rats. *Physiol. Behav.* **1996**, *59*, 735–739.
24. Ruis, M.A.; te Brake, J.H.; Buwalda, B.; de Boer, S.F.; Meerlo, P.; Korte, S.M.; Blokhuis, H.J.; Koolhaas, J.M. Housing familiar male wildtype rats together reduces the long-term adverse behavioural and physiological effects of social defeat. *Psychoneuroendocrinology* **1999**, *24*, 285–300.
25. Van der Kolk, B.A.; Greenberg, M.S.; Orr, S.P.; Pitman, R.K. Endogenous opioids, stress induced analgesia, and posttraumatic stress disorder. *Psychopharmacol. Bull.* **1989**, *25*, 417–421.
26. Pitman, R.K.; van der Kolk, B.A.; Orr, S.P.; Greenberg, M.S. Naloxone-reversible analgesic response to combat-related stimuli in posttraumatic stress disorder. A pilot study. *Arch. Gen. Psychiatry* **1990**, *47*, 541–544.
27. Ludascher, P.; Valerius, G.; Stiglmayr, C.; Mauchnik, J.; Lanius, R.A.; Bohus, M.; Schmahl, C. Pain sensitivity and neural processing during dissociative states in patients with borderline personality disorder with and without comorbid posttraumatic stress disorder: A pilot study. *J. Psychiatry Neurosci.* **2010**, *35*, 177–184.
28. Amir, S.; Brown, Z.W.; Amit, Z. The role of endorphins in stress: Evidence and speculations. *Neurosci. Biobehav. Rev.* **1980**, *4*, 77–86.
29. Bodnar, R.J.; Kelly, D.D.; Brutus, M.; Glusman, M. Stress-induced analgesia: Neural and hormonal determinants. *Neurosci. Biobehav. Rev.* **1980**, *4*, 87–100.
30. Chance, W.T. Autoanalgesia: Opiate and non-opiate mechanisms. *Neurosci. Biobehav. Rev.* **1980**, *4*, 55–67.
31. Lewis, J.W.; Cannon, J.T.; Liebeskind, J.C. Opioid and nonopioid mechanisms of stress analgesia. *Science* **1980**, *208*, 623–625.
32. Watkins, L.R.; Mayer, D.J. Organization of endogenous opiate and nonopiate pain control systems. *Science* **1982**, *216*, 1185–1192.
33. Butler, R.K.; Finn, D.P. Stress-induced analgesia. *Prog. Neurobiol.* **2009**, *88*, 184–202.

34. Bolles, R.C.; Fanselow, M.S. A perceptual-defensive-recuperative model of fear and pain. *Behav. Brain Sci.* **1980**, *3*, 291–301.
35. Miczek, K.A.; Thompson, M.L.; Shuster, L. Opioid-like analgesia in defeated mice. *Science* **1982**, *215*, 1520–1522.
36. Rodgers, R.J.; Hendrie, C.A. Social conflict activates status-dependent endogenous analgesic or hyperalgesic mechanisms in male mice: Effects of naloxone on nociception and behaviour. *Physiol. Behav.* **1983**, *30*, 775–780.
37. Rodgers, R.J.; Hendrie, C.A.; Waters, A.J. Naloxone partially antagonizes post-encounter analgesia and enhances defensive responding in male rats exposed to attack from lactating conspecifics. *Physiol. Behav.* **1983**, *30*, 781–786.
38. Teskey, G.C.; Kavaliers, M.; Hirst, M. Social conflict activates opioid analgesic and ingestive behaviors in male mice. *Life Sci.* **1984**, *35*, 303–315.
39. Jackson, R.L.; Maier, S.F.; Coon, D.J. Long-term analgesic effects of inescapable shock and learned helplessness. *Science* **1979**, *206*, 91–93.
40. Bartlang, M.S.; Neumann, I.D.; Slattery, D.A.; Uschold-Schmidt, N.; Kraus, D.; Helfrich-Forster, C.; Reber, S.O. Time matters: Pathological effects of repeated psychosocial stress during the active, but not inactive, phase of male mice. *J. Endocrinol.* **2012**, *215*, 425–437.
41. Fluttert, M.; Dalm, S.; Oitzl, M.S. A refined method for sequential blood sampling by tail incision in rats. *Lab. Anim.* **2000**, *34*, 372–378.
42. Sadler, A.M.; Bailey, S.J. Validation of a refined technique for taking repeated blood samples from juvenile and adult mice. *Lab. Anim.* **2013**, *47*, 316–319.
43. Berry, A.; Capone, F.; Giorgio, M.; Pelicci, P.G.; de Kloet, E.R.; Alleva, E.; Minghetti, L.; Cirulli, F. Deletion of the life span determinant p66Shc prevents age-dependent increases in emotionality and pain sensitivity in mice. *Exp. Gerontol.* **2007**, *42*, 37–45.
44. Cirulli, F.; Berry, A.; Alleva, E. Intracerebroventricular administration of brain-derived neurotrophic factor in adult rats affects analgesia and spontaneous behaviour but not memory retention in a Morris Water Maze task. *Neurosci. Lett.* **2000**, *287*, 207–210.
45. Savignac, H.M.; Finger, B.C.; Pizzo, R.C.; O'Leary, O.F.; Dinan, T.G.; Cryan, J.F. Increased sensitivity to the effects of chronic social defeat stress in an innately anxious mouse strain. *Neuroscience* **2011**, *192*, 524–536.
46. Reber, S.O.; Obermeier, F.; Straub, R.H.; Falk, W.; Neumann, I.D. Chronic intermittent psychosocial stress (social defeat/overcrowding) in mice increases the severity of an acute DSS-induced colitis and impairs regeneration. *Endocrinology* **2006**, *147*, 4968–4976.
47. Savignac, H.M.; Hyland, N.P.; Dinan, T.G.; Cryan, J.F. The effects of repeated social interaction stress on behavioural and physiological parameters in a stress-sensitive mouse strain. *Behav. Brain Res.* **2011**, *216*, 576–584.
48. Krishnan, V.; Han, M.H.; Graham, D.L.; Berton, O.; Renthal, W.; Russo, S.J.; Laplant, Q.; Graham, A.; Lutter, M.; Lagace, D.C.; *et al.* Molecular adaptations underlying susceptibility and resistance to social defeat in brain reward regions. *Cell* **2007**, *131*, 391–404.
49. Razzoli, M.; Carboni, L.; Andreoli, M.; Ballottari, A.; Arban, R. Different susceptibility to social defeat stress of BalbC and C57BL6/J mice. *Behav. Brain Res.* **2010**, *216*, 100–108.

50. Razzoli, M.; Carboni, L.; Andreoli, M.; Michielin, F.; Ballottari, A.; Arban, R. Strain-specific outcomes of repeated social defeat and chronic fluoxetine treatment in the mouse. *Pharmacol. Biochem. Behav.* **2010**, *97*, 566–576.
51. Golden, S.A.; Covington, H.E., 3rd.; Berton, O.; Russo, S.J. A standardized protocol for repeated social defeat stress in mice. *Nat. Protoc.* **2011**, *6*, 1183–1191.
52. Hammamieh, R.; Chakraborty, N.; De Lima, T.C.; Meyerhoff, J.; Gautam, A.; Muhie, S.; D'Arpa, P.; Lumley, L.; Carroll, E.; Jett, M. Murine model of repeated exposures to conspecific trained aggressors simulates features of post-traumatic stress disorder. *Behav. Brain Res.* **2012**, *235*, 55–66.
53. Litvin, Y.; Murakami, G.; Pfaff, D.W. Effects of chronic social defeat on behavioral and neural correlates of sociality: Vasopressin, oxytocin and the vasopressinergic V1b receptor. *Physiol. Behav.* **2011**, *103*, 393–403.
54. Girardi, C.E.; Tiba, P.A.; Llobet, G.B.; Levin, R.; Abilio, V.C.; Suchecki, D. Contextual exploration previous to an aversive event predicts long-term emotional consequences of severe stress. *Front. Behav. Neurosci.* **2013**, *7*, doi:10.3389/fnbeh.2013.00134.
55. Zhang, Y.; Gandhi, P.R.; Standifer, K.M. Increased nociceptive sensitivity and nociceptin/orphanin FQ levels in a rat model of PTSD. *Mol. Pain* **2012**, *8*, doi:10.1186/1744-8069-8-76.
56. Ludascher, P.; Bohus, M.; Lieb, K.; Philipsen, A.; Jochims, A.; Schmahl, C. Elevated pain thresholds correlate with dissociation and aversive arousal in patients with borderline personality disorder. *Psychiatry Res.* **2007**, *149*, 291–296.
57. Beckham, J.C.; Crawford, A.L.; Feldman, M.E.; Kirby, A.C.; Hertzberg, M.A.; Davidson, J.R.; Moore, S.D. Chronic posttraumatic stress disorder and chronic pain in Vietnam combat veterans. *J. Psychosom. Res.* **1997**, *43*, 379–389.
58. Shipherd, J.C.; Keyes, M.; Jovanovic, T.; Ready, D.J.; Baltzell, D.; Worley, V.; Gordon-Brown, V.; Hayslett, C.; Duncan, E. Veterans seeking treatment for posttraumatic stress disorder: What about comorbid chronic pain? *J. Rehabil. Res. Dev.* **2007**, *44*, 153–166.
59. Asmundson, G.J.; Katz, J. Understanding the co-occurrence of anxiety disorders and chronic pain: State-of-the-art. *Depress Anxiety* **2009**, *26*, 888–901.
60. Rubinstein, M.; Mogil, J.S.; Japon, M.; Chan, E.C.; Allen, R.G.; Low, M.J. Absence of opioid stress-induced analgesia in mice lacking beta-endorphin by site-directed mutagenesis. *Proc. Natl. Acad. Sci. USA* **1996**, *93*, 3995–4000.
61. Yamada, K.; Nabeshima, T. Stress-induced behavioral responses and multiple opioid systems in the brain. *Behav. Brain Res.* **1995**, *67*, 133–145.
62. Pike, J.L.; Smith, T.L.; Hauger, R.L.; Nicassio, P.M.; Patterson, T.L.; McClintick, J.; Costlow, C.; Irwin, M.R. Chronic life stress alters sympathetic, neuroendocrine, and immune responsivity to an acute psychological stressor in humans. *Psychosom. Med.* **1997**, *59*, 447–457.
63. Birrell, A.M.; Heffernan, S.J.; Ansselin, A.D.; McLennan, S.; Church, D.K.; Gillin, A.G.; Yue, D.K. Functional and structural abnormalities in the nerves of type I diabetic baboons: Aminoguanidine treatment does not improve nerve function. *Diabetologia* **2000**, *43*, 110–116.
64. Van Goozen, S.H.; van den Ban, E.; Matthys, W.; Cohen-Kettenis, P.T.; Thijssen, J.H.; van Engeland, H. Increased adrenal androgen functioning in children with oppositional defiant disorder: A comparison with psychiatric and normal controls. *J. Am. Acad. Child Adolesc. Psychiatry* **2000**, *39*, 1446–1451.

65. Bremner, J.D. Long-term effects of childhood abuse on brain and neurobiology. *Child Adolesc. Psychiatr. Clin. North Am.* **2003**, *12*, 271–292.
66. Claes, L.; Vandereycken, W.; Vertommen, H. Pain experience related to self-injury in eating disorder patients. *Eat. Behav.* **2006**, *7*, 204–213.
67. Zanarini, M.C.; Yong, L.; Frankenburg, F.R.; Hennen, J.; Reich, D.B.; Marino, M.F.; Vujanovic, A.A. Severity of reported childhood sexual abuse and its relationship to severity of borderline psychopathology and psychosocial impairment among borderline inpatients. *J. Nerv. Ment. Dis.* **2002**, *190*, 381–387.
68. Gratz, K.L.; Hepworth, C.; Tull, M.T.; Paulson, A.; Clarke, S.; Remington, B.; Lejuez, C.W. An experimental investigation of emotional willingness and physical pain tolerance in deliberate self-harm: The moderating role of interpersonal distress. *Compr. Psychiatry* **2011**, *52*, 63–74.
69. Joyce, P.R.; McKenzie, J.M.; Mulder, R.T.; Luty, S.E.; Sullivan, P.F.; Miller, A.L.; Kennedy, M.A. Genetic, developmental and personality correlates of self-mutilation in depressed patients. *Aust. N. Z. J. Psychiatry* **2006**, *40*, 225–229.
70. Eisenberger, N.I. The pain of social disconnection: examining the shared neural underpinnings of physical and social pain. *Nat. Rev. Neurosci.* **2012**, *13*, 421–434.
71. Moeller-Bertram, T.; Keltner, J.; Strigo, I.A. Pain and post traumatic stress disorder—Review of clinical and experimental evidence. *Neuropharmacology* **2012**, *62*, 586–597.
72. Hache, G.; Guiard, B.P.; le Dantec, Y.; Orvoen, S.; David, D.J.; Gardier, A.M.; Coudore, F. Antinociceptive effects of fluoxetine in a mouse model of anxiety/depression. *Neuroreport* **2012**, *23*, 525–529.
73. Moll, J.; Krueger, F.; Zahn, R.; Pardini, M.; de Oliveira-Souza, R.; Grafman, J. Human fronto-mesolimbic networks guide decisions about charitable donation. *Proc. Natl. Acad. Sci. USA* **2006**, *103*, 15623–15628.
74. Keysers, C.; Kaas, J.H.; Gazzola, V. Somatosensation in social perception. *Nat. Rev. Neurosci.* **2010**, *11*, 417–428.
75. Lamm, C.; Decety, J.; Singer, T. Meta-analytic evidence for common and distinct neural networks associated with directly experienced pain and empathy for pain. *Neuroimage* **2011**, *54*, 2492–2502.
76. Inagaki, T.K.; Eisenberger, N.I. Neural correlates of giving support to a loved one. *Psychosom. Med.* **2012**, *74*, 3–7.
77. Mickleborough, M.J.; Daniels, J.K.; Coupland, N.J.; Kao, R.; Williamson, P.C.; Lanius, U.F.; Hegadoren, K.; Schore, A.; Densmore, M.; Stevens, T.; Lanius, R.A. Effects of trauma-related cues on pain processing in posttraumatic stress disorder: An fMRI investigation. *J. Psychiatry Neurosci.* **2011**, *36*, 6–14.
78. Schmahl, C.; Bohus, M.; Esposito, F.; Treede, R.D.; Di Salle, F.; Greffrath, W.; Ludaescher, P.; Jochims, A.; Lieb, K.; Scheffler, K.; *et al*. Neural correlates of antinociception in borderline personality disorder. *Arch. Gen. Psychiatry* **2006**, *63*, 659–667.
79. Russ, M.J.; Roth, S.D.; Lerman, A.; Kakuma, T.; Harrison, K.; Shindledecker, R.D.; Hull, J.; Mattis, S. Pain perception in self-injurious patients with borderline personality disorder. *Biol. Psychiatry* **1992**, *32*, 501–511.

80. Bohus, M.; Limberger, M.; Ebner, U.; Glocker, F.X.; Schwarz, B.; Wernz, M.; Lieb, K. Pain perception during self-reported distress and calmness in patients with borderline personality disorder and self-mutilating behavior. *Psychiatry Res.* **2000**, *95*, 251–260.

3

Sublingual Immunotherapy in Human and Canine Atopic Dermatitis: A Mini Review

Ibrahim Ozmen [1] and Rosanna Marsella [2,*]

[1] Department of Dermatology, Corlu Military Hospital, 59850 Corlu, Tekirdag 59850, Turkey; E-Mail: ibrahimozmen@hotmail.com

[2] Department of Small Animal Clinical Sciences, College of Veterinary Medicine, University of Florida, Gainesville, FL 32610, USA

* Author to whom correspondence should be addressed; E-Mail: marsella@ufl.edu;

Abstract: Atopic Dermatitis (AD) is a prevalent disease that affects both humans and animals. Dogs share similar environments with the owners and spontaneously develop a disease that is clinically and immunologically identical to AD in humans. In past decades AD has become more and more common in both dogs and humans, possibly due to the increased exposure to indoor allergens and decreased exposure to parasites and beneficial bacteria. The allergic component plays an important role in both species. Allergen specific immunotherapy (ASIT) has been used with great success in veterinary medicine for decades for the treatment of AD and traditionally has been accomplished with subcutaneous injections. In human medicine, ASIT has been traditionally used for respiratory manifestations of atopic disease and only recently considered for the therapy of AD. Interestingly, dogs primarily express cutaneous manifestations of atopic disease and only rarely progress from cutaneous into respiratory disease, a process referred in human medicine as "atopic march". Recently, sublingual immunotherapy has been replacing subcutaneous immunotherapy both in human and veterinary medicine due to its ease and safety, leading to increased compliance. The purpose of this mini review is to focus on the use of sublingual immunotherapy for AD highlighting similarities and differences between humans and dogs.

Keywords: immunotherapy; sublingual; atopic dermatitis; dog; human

---

1. Introduction

Allergies are becoming increasingly common in westernized countries both in humans and dogs, possibly due to changes in life style conditions and decreased exposure to beneficial bacteria and parasites that help modulate the immune system. Allergies are chronic and progressive and can significantly impact the quality of life of affected individuals. It is very common for both humans and animals to build an allergic response to an increasing number of allergens over a lifetime requiring strategies to control symptoms in the long-term. In most individuals allergic disease is linked to some type of environmental exposure such as pollens, dust mites, molds, or food. While some allergens can be avoided (e.g., foods), others are difficult to avoid completely (e.g., dust or pollens). Due to the chronic nature, long-term sustainable alternatives are needed.

Many drugs that are effective in decreasing the symptoms also have undesirable long-term adverse effects (e.g., glucocorticoids). The concept of administering increasing doses of allergens with the intent of "re-educating" the immune system to shift from an "over-reactive" (or allergic response) to a more tolerant response is old and it is the base for allergen specific immunotherapy. Over the years many attempts have been done to refine this concept and to identify the most effective dosing regimen and the safest, least invasive, yet effective route of administration. Researchers have also tried to answer the question of threshold of allergens both in terms of number and amounts in order to obtain a clinical response thus trying to find a compromise between science and application of immunotherapy. Despite the multitude of studies and protocols, immunotherapy is still considered an art rather than an exact science and many controversies still exist.

Immunotherapy has been used in both veterinary medicine and human medicine for decades. The original route of administration has been the subcutaneous route with the idea of injecting progressively increasing doses of allergens. With this route of administration adverse effects are described and could be life-threatening such as anaphylactic reactions. The frequency of adverse systemic reactions varies between studies [1] and can range from 3.4% of patients [2] to one per 1600 visits or one per 47 patients [3]. One of the most recently published reports described a rate of 0.1% systemic reactions [4]. The need for increased safety while not jeopardizing efficacy, has led to the exploration of alternative routes of allergen administration. The sublingual route has gained interest in recent years thus the focus of this mini review is to selectively focus on sublingual immunotherapy in a comparative fashion highlighting similarities and differences between the experience in human medicine and the one in veterinary medicine.

2. The Experience in Human Medicine

Atopic dermatitis (AD) is a common, chronic, inflammatory, pruritic skin disease affecting flexural surfaces. The prevalence of AD ranges between 15% and 30% in children and 2%–10% in adults. Secondary Staphylococcal infections are common in atopic patients and further aggravate the severity of clinical signs. Dry skin due to genetically inherited epidermal barrier dysfunction is the main characteristic of the disease. Impaired epidermal barrier function can lead to penetration of allergens, susceptibility to infections and chronic inflammation [5]. Although AD is not considered as a typical allergic disorder, aeroallergens, food allergens, and house dust mites are known facilitating or aggravating factors of eczematous skin lesions in most of the patients [6]. It is also known that some of the patients with AD may manifest other signs of atopic disease besides skin and may experience an "atopic march" during their life. They may start with cutaneous disease (eczema) at young age and later develop allergic asthma and allergic rhinoconjunctivitis [7]. In about 80% of adult patients with AD, the disease may be associated with positive skin prick test, atopy patch test results, and increased serum IgE levels against specific allergens and concomitant allergic asthma and rhinitis [8]. These patients are described as having an allergic component to their eczema and are more amenable to treatments focused on control of allergen exposure as an allergic trigger is identifiable. Besides allergen avoidance, these patients are also ideal candidates for immunotherapy as their disease results from a combination of skin barrier defect and allergic sensitization.

Allergy treatment includes avoidance measures, pharmacotherapy and allergen-specific immunotherapy (ASIT). ASIT was first described by Noon in 1911 and remains the only treatment directed at the cause of IgE-mediated allergic diseases [9]. The main goal of ASIT is to induce allergen specific tolerance and stimulate T regulatory response. Peripheral T-cell tolerance is crucial for this [10]. ASIT induces important immunomodulatory effects, including induction of Treg with increased production of IL-10 and Transforming Growth Factor beta (TGF-β), Th1 and IgG. A decrease of IgE, Th2, and increase of blocking allergen specific IgG1 and IgG4 antibodies has been observed with ASIT although a decrease of IgE does not necessarily correlate with improvement of clinical signs. Decreased mediator release by mast cells and basophils and impaired IgE-facilitated antigen presentation by dendritic cells have been described after ASIT [11].

Unmodified or modified allergen extracts (allergoids) can be used in ASIT. Allergoids are produced by treating allergens with formaldehyde or glutaraldehyde, and these modified proteins are thought to have a reduced IgE-binding capacity. In most commercial allergens, aluminum serves as an adsorbent for delaying the release of extract. Some of the products contain adjuvants to increase the immunogenicity.

Allergen-specific immunotherapy induces not only symptomatic relief during the treatment, but also provides long-term clinical remission after discontinuation [12]. In addition to the clinical and cost-benefits during and after treatment, ASIT has been shown to prevent the development of asthma and new allergen sensitivities [13] thus it is the only treatment currently available that has the ability to halt the progression of the disease and have a protective effect from future worsening particularly when started at young age [14,15]. Currently ASIT is indicated for the treatment of allergic rhinitis, allergic asthma, and hymenoptera-induced anaphylaxis. Based on these clinical considerations ASIT was initiated to be used in the treatment of AD with limited data [5]. The traditional administration of allergens has been parenteral, and initial attempts to deliver allergens through other routes (e.g., orally) have provided unsatisfactory results [16,17]. As subcutaneous immunotherapy (SCIT) can induce severe adverse effects resulting in anaphylaxis and death, the interest in developing alternative, safer, and yet effective routes of allergen deliveries has grown over the past two decades. The investigation of the sublingual route (SLIT) was started due to the ease of administration. Some allergens, such as grass pollen and house dust mite (HDM) can be delivered through either route, whereas some, such as venoms, are only delivered subcutaneously [10]. Mucosal epithelium has no vasculature and yet contains dendritic cells, so the dendritic cells could be pulsed with less risk for systemic adverse reactions [13]. Thus, SLIT has a better safety profile than SCIT, which makes SLIT also useful for home administration [10]. The immunologic changes associated with SLIT are complex but reported to be similar to those of SCIT, ranging from modulation of cellular immunity, humoral response, and cytokine profile to promote tolerance.

SLIT has been commercially available and used in Europe with a satisfactory safety profile [8]. In 2014 a few SLIT formulations have been approved by the Federal Drug Administration (FDA) in the United States. Even before the official FDA approval of SLIT formulations, SLIT prescribers had already significantly increased from 5.9% in 2007 to 11.3% in 2011 [18]. The three approved formulations are Oralair® (a mix of five different grasses) produced by Greer, and Grastek® (timothy grass) and Ragwitek® (ragweed) both produced by Merck.

Based on the literature, SLIT is used in allergic rhinitis and asthma, which is associated with rhinitis in both adults and children [19]. Atopic dermatitis is being considered as a promising field of use of SLIT [19]. SLIT is currently accepted as an alternative to injections because of its satisfactory safety profile. Adverse effects are typically limited to itching in the oral cavity and, rarely, gastrointestinal effects. Systemic life-threatening adverse effects have been rarely reported with SLIT although they are still possible. SLIT's efficacy and safety in rhinitis and asthma in children has been confirmed in clinical trials [20]. Most of the clinical trials have focused on the efficacy and safety of SLIT for grass allergies, and fewer studies have been done to investigate other allergens. Based on the data available, the highest level of evidence for effectiveness of SLIT is given with grass pollen extract [12].

A meta-analysis was performed by Bae *et al.* [9], to assess the long-term efficacy of ASIT in patients with AD. They analyzed eight randomized controlled studies, six of which were performed with SCIT and two with SLIT. They demonstrated that ASIT has a significant positive effect on AD, also in long-term treatment for patients with severe AD when administered subcutaneously. Subgroup analyses of ASIT for children and of SLIT did not demonstrate significant effects. They explained these controversial results with the small number of studies and subjects [9].

Mastrandrea *et al.* [21], reported the results of a retrospective study with the treatment of SLIT in 35 patients with AD. Sixteen patients suffered from AD without respiratory allergic symptoms and 19 had AD associated with mild asthma and/or rhinitis. Allergy to respiratory allergens was diagnosed with a skin prick test. Allergens were prepared in a glycerol-saline solution and administered three times a week for 3 years. Only the complete disappearance of skin lesions was considered to indicate effectiveness. In the group without respiratory symptoms, complete remission of skin disease was demonstrated in 12.6% after 6 months, 31.2% after 12 months, and 68.8% of patients after 24 months. One patient developed asthma in this group 3 years after immunotherapy ended. In the group with AD associated to asthma or rhinitis complete remission of skin disease was seen in 0% after 6 months, 36.8% after 12 months and 73.7% of patients, respectively, after 24 months. The authors commented that SLIT was a safe treatment modality in AD and might favorably prevent the progression of atopic march [21]. Pajno *et al.* [6], designed a double-blind, placebo controlled (DBPC) study to assess the effect of SLIT in HDM sensitized children with AD. Patients were treated with SLIT or placebo for 18 months in addition to standard atopic dermatitis therapy. SLIT proved effective in reducing symptoms as presented by significant reduction of SCORAD (Scoring Atopic Dermatitis) index and use of standard medications [6]. However, SLIT did not demonstrate significant clinical benefits in patients with severe AD. The authors concluded that SLIT with a standardized mite extract could be considered safe and effective in children with mild to moderate AD.

In another open non-controlled trial pilot study, 86 patients with AD and IgE-proved HDM sensitization treated with SLIT (*Dermatophagoides pteronyssinus* and *Dermatophagoides farinae* extracts) for one year. At the end of 12 months a significant improvement, defined as a SCORAD reduction of >30%, was observed in 51 out of 86 patients (59%). In five patients (5.8%) SCORAD values did not change at the end of the observation period. Total and specific IgE levels were significantly decreased after SLIT [8]. The authors also reported that SLIT had allowed a gradual or complete withdrawal of concomitant therapies.

Zheng reported a study with 96 children suffering from AD. The patients were randomized into two treatment groups receiving HDM-SLIT drops or conventional therapy including antihistamines and topical medications. Clinical improvement and complete remission rates were significantly higher in the immunotherapy group than the medication group [22]. Limitations of this study included the lack of a control group and the lack of an objective definition of what was considered clinical improvement. Vanbervliet *et al.* [23], have tested the efficacy of SLIT against HDM in a mouse model of AD, as a proof of concept of using ASIT in type IV skin allergy. Mice were sensitized on the ear by application of HDM and they developed a specific ear inflammation and also distant challenge. After sensitization they were treated either with SLIT or placebo. Mice treated with SLIT did not develop HDM-induced skin inflammation in contrast to placebo [23].

A recently published study specifically addressed the efficacy and safety of SLIT with *Dermatophagoides farinae* drops in patients with AD and investigated related factors influencing the patients' compliance [24]. This was a randomized controlled study in which both groups were allowed pharmacotherapy, and the control group was allowed to receive medication and no vaccine. As there was no vehicle vaccine group the patients were aware of allocation to groups. Authors recorded the daily drug scores of the two groups, compliance and visual analogue scale (VAS) scores, and IgG4 level at various time points. Therapeutic efficacy was estimated by the change in SCORAD index. The reduction ratio of the SCORAD index was calculated by the score decrease from the first month divided by the first month. Patients with a reduction ratio of the SCORAD index ≥90% were considered cured, between 60% and 89% were deemed to gain a marked effect, between 20% and 59% were seen to improve, and ≤19% were believed to be ineffective. The authors defined the total effective rate of treatment as the ratio of cured cases plus cases with marked effect to total cases in each group. The total effective rate in the treatment group (77.78%) was significantly higher than the control group (53.85%) ($p < 0.05$). The treatment group was significantly reduced in daily drug scores and VAS scores compared with the control group at a 12-month follow-up. It is important to note that statistical significance may not always equate to clinically appreciable difference. For example in this study the control group had a VAS at the end of the study of 7.2 while the active ingredient group had a VAS of 6.1, a difference that is most likely not clinically appreciable. More importantly the amount of medications needed to control symptoms was different between the two groups. The authors reported that starting after the first month a significant different in drug scores was recorded between with two groups with the patients on SLIT needing fewer medications to control their clinical signs. Also, the SLIT group had a higher level of serum-specific IgG4 than the control group at 6 and 12 month of treatment ($p < 0.05$). In this report the authors concluded that *Dermatophagoides farinae* drops were a safe and effective SLIT for patients with AD, which was proven to reduce the need for rescue medications. The fact that significant improvement was noted after just the first month of therapy is considered a particularly encouraging result.

SLIT is also an effective treatment modality in food allergies. There have been three DBPC studies with hazelnut, peach, and peanut that suggest that SLIT represents a significant tolerance in allergic response of these foods [13].The potential use for food allergies is of great importance as currently there are no valid alternatives for patients with food allergies other than avoidance. Most recently both oral IT and SLIT have been evaluated for peanut allergy [25]. Peanut allergy is becoming increasingly common in children in westernized countries. Contrary to other food allergies, peanut allergy is rarely outgrown and can have fatal consequences. Thus it is crucial to identify safe and effective therapies for this allergy. In a recently published meta-analysis there was no difference in efficacy between the oral IT or SLIT group. Studies showed a statistically significant benefit of peanut IT in patients with peanut allergy. The main limitation is that these findings are based on an analysis of a small number of randomized controlled studies. It is important to emphasize that failure to demonstrate differences between different therapies is not necessarily the same as proving that there is no difference particularly when the power of the studies is low. In these types of situations all that can be stated is that the results are not conclusive either way. Thus controversy exists on whether there is already sufficient evidence to recommend this form of therapy in the clinics and on the risks for this type of recommendation. In order to make final recommendations, additional larger, well-designed and double-blinded randomized controlled studies are needed.

The preventive effects of SLIT on atopic march are also being studied [26] and it is currently hypothesized that early implementation of SLIT can halt the progression of allergic disease [27]. The preventative effect of SLIT was investigated [28] and showed that during the follow-up period, only 1% of non-asthma patients reported an onset of respiratory symptoms, and only 9.6% of patients undergoing new skin tests showed new sensitizations. It was also found that the clinical benefits were strongly linked to the length of treatment. The authors reported that patients with long-lasting benefits were treated for a mean length of over 2 years while patients that regressed to clinical signs similar to pre-SLIT condition had been treated for approximately 1 year. Thus it was concluded that it was beneficial to prolong SLIT and that the longer SLIT was done, the more likely it was that it could halt the progression of the disease and the development of new sensitizations. Although these findings were limited to the investigation of respiratory disease, they represent very encouraging results to help individuals that would be otherwise genetically predisposed to severe and progressive allergies.

Another longitudinal study evaluated the long lasting effect of SLIT over a 15-year period [29]. The authors reported that in the patients receiving SLIT for 3 years, clinical benefits persisted for 7 years. Patients receiving SLIT for 4 or 5 years showed clinical benefits for 8 years. Thus the authors concluded that a 4-year duration for SLIT was the optimal length of therapy. In terms of new sensitizations, they were reported in all the control subjects over a 15-year period and in less than a quarter of the patients receiving SLIT, thus confirming a positive effect to decrease the development of new allergies.

Effective SLIT doses for many allergens have not been established yet. The effective cumulative SLIT dose with grass pollen is 20 to 30 times higher than the SCIT dose. Most commonly SLIT is used in patients with a single allergen, and multi-allergen SLIT has not been well studied yet [10]. The safety of SLIT is reported to be superior to SCIT although systemic adverse effects can still occur. There are some rare reports of anaphylaxis with SLIT, and the most frequently reported side effects are oral itching, mild local edema, and throat irritation which generally occur within the few days of treatment and resolve spontaneously [17]. Only the first intake needs doctoral supervision. Patients in

SLIT treatment must have an intact oral mucosa and the treatment should not be carried out immediately after teeth brushing [12].

SLIT represents a significant advance because of its efficacy, safety, and convenience [30]. Very few small, randomized trials directly compared efficacy of SLIT with SCIT and could not demonstrate a significant difference in efficacy between the two routes [31]. Many clinical trials on SLIT and AD are ongoing to determine the most appropriate dosing regimen and provide high quality evidence of efficacy for AD [32]. It is important to remember that AD is a multifactorial disease, which includes complex genetic modifications, responsible for skin barrier impairment, and combinations of environmental and endogenous factors that can direct the disease course. For these reasons, we need more controlled and long-term studies to be able to assess the efficacy of SLIT in the treatment of human AD and disease-modifying potential on atopic march.

A recently published review [33] reviewed 266 articles to retrieve data on SLIT for a variety of allergies. One of the challenges in comparing the results of the various studies is that great variation in doses and protocol exists across studies making a direct comparison impossible. SLIT was reported to be effective at a wide range of doses, much larger than the doses used for SCIT. These doses range from the 5–300-fold of those for SCIT. SLIT was found to be very efficacious and the efficacy is sustained for a long time even after discontinuation. Clinical efficacy was maintained for at least one year after discontinuation and immunologic changes were detectable for up to 3 years after [34,35].

3. The Experience in Veterinary Medicine

Dogs are affected with a natural homologue of human AD that has striking clinical, immunologic, and skin barrier impairment similarities with the human counterpart [36,37]. Dogs also share the same environmental conditions, and concomitant occurrence of allergies has been shown in humans and their pets [38]. Interestingly, despite the fact that environmental sensitizations are extremely common in dogs with AD, this species does not experience the "atopic march" in the sense that no development of asthma occurs, even in the individuals with the most severe dermatitis [39]. It is common, however, for the disease to have a chronic progressive course with deterioration of dermatitis and complication by secondary skin infections. Disease starts in young adults and has a familial predilection. A subset of atopic dogs also has food allergies as triggering factor that aggravates the AD flare-ups. Dogs also have a skin barrier impairment, which leads to increased risk for allergic sensitization which progresses with age and pollen exposure. Areas typically affected are the flexural surfaces, and abnormal skin barrier function exists in those areas in young dogs even in absence of clinically appreciable disease. It is currently unknown whether the skin barrier defect is primary or secondary or both. Most dogs with AD have the extrinsic form of the disease with detectable allergen specific IgE to environmental allergens.

Allergen-specific immunotherapy has been successfully used for decades in veterinary medicine and has been recommended whenever feasible for the long-term management of canine AD [40–43]. Traditionally, ASIT in dogs was done by subcutaneous route and it is overall well tolerated [39]. Many protocols and regimen schedules are currently used for SCIT by different dermatologists and no robust studies have been done to compare different protocols. One study evaluated the efficacy between a low dose protocol and a standard protocol and found no significant differences in efficacy [44]. Some clinicians may consider rush protocols for special cases. Although this regimen has been proven to be reasonably safe and effective [45,46], it is not commonly adopted by most veterinary dermatologists in practice, as it is more labor intensive. Controversy also exists on the maximum number of allergens to be included in SCIT although a general assumption is that using too many allergens may not be ideal as it could possibly dilute the amount of each allergen used and therefore interfere with efficacy. Similarly it is typically not recommended to use mixes and it is preferred to use individual allergens. This recommendation is derived by studies done in human medicine [47,48]. Controlled studies should be done in veterinary medicine to specifically investigate this variable in veterinary medicine. No real standardization has been done in veterinary medicine regarding the extracts, and most of them are crude preparations whose strength is reported in weight/volume and protein content. In terms of mechanisms of action of ASIT in veterinary medicine, one of the investigated mechanisms in dogs is the shift from Th2 to a Th1 response [49] and stimulation of T regulatory response.

Despite the overall good efficacy and safety of subcutaneous ASIT, some owners are reluctant to give injections to their pets emphasizing the need in veterinary medicine for alternative routes of allergen delivery. SLIT is fairly new to veterinary medicine but is so far showing good promise. Great debate exists on how to best utilize SLIT, whether it should be given once daily or twice daily, the best concentration and how its efficacy may compare to SCIT. Due to these uncertainties SLIT is still considered by many dermatologists not the standard of care but a second line of therapy.

In one uncontrolled multi-centric study, 217 privately owned dogs with naturally occurring AD were enrolled to evaluate the efficacy of SLIT while allowing other treatments such as glucocorticoids and cyclosporine [50]. SLIT was administered twice daily in a non-aqueous vehicle using an escalating dosing regimen. Selection of allergens was based on allergy testing and was tailored to each individual patient. The response was recorded after a minimum of 6 months of therapy. Investigators reported a 55% good-to-excellent response to SLIT, meaning that some medication was still required to control symptoms but that the dose or frequency of rescue medications was decreased. Interestingly some dogs that had failed traditional SCIT were able to tolerate and have a favorable response to SLIT. Thus SLIT was effective in decreasing the need for rescue medications and was worth trying in patients that had not responded to SCIT. The reasons for why a patient may respond to SLIT and not SCIT are unknown at this time and need to be investigated. Compliance could be one of them as some owners are reluctant to give injections and are more likely to skip doses than with SLIT. Another interesting observation of this study was that the response to SLIT seemed to be faster than with traditional SCIT with some patients showing a positive response within a few months of therapy. Traditionally with SCIT minimal improvement is expected for the first 6–9 months of therapy. This study was uncontrolled, and it is likely that some placebo effect may have occurred. Placebo effect is well documented in medicine [51] and can be seen in owners' perception of improvement as well as investigator's assessment. Additionally in this open study no evaluation of the effect of immunologic parameters was done.

A vehicle controlled study using a validated experimental model for canine AD also showed a beneficial effect of SLIT [52]. For this study, which lasted one year, eighteen atopic beagles were experimentally sensitized to HDM, timothy grass, and ragweed. Although this study used a small number of patients, it had the strength of being vehicle-controlled, blinded, and controlled for confounding factors such as diet and type of allergy and allergen exposure. Six dogs were allocated to vehicle (glycerin) and twelve to active ingredient (allergens). Response was evaluated both clinically using a validated scoring system and immunologically, measuring allergen-specific IgE, IL-10, and

TGF-beta production by peripheral blood mononuclear cells at various time points. Allergens were administered once daily on an increasing dose over several months' period. Although both groups showed some clinical improvement at the end of the study, the improvement was twice as high in the active ingredient group as in the control group. The authors speculated that the improvement seen in the control group was possibly due to the fact that no allergen exposure was done for many months during the course of the study. Thus the lack of allergen exposure for a year may have led in itself to some improvement of clinical disease. The lack of statistical significance was possibly due to the small number of cases used for this study and the variability among subjects. From the clinical stand point the improvement in some dogs of the active group was considered clinically striking by the investigators as these dogs had been in the colony for a long time and had had a chronic history of severe disease. Larger controlled studies are needed to further investigate whether the lack of significance between vehicle and active ingredient group is real or simply due to small size. SLIT was found to be well tolerated, and no adverse effects were reported during the course of the study. Significant increases in the IL-10 and TGF-beta were found for several allergens in the active group when compared to vehicle supporting the hypothesis of increased T regulatory function. No significant changes in allergen-specific IgE response were noted in that study. A 2-month follow-up after the discontinuation of SLIT demonstrated that some of the immunologic changes induced during SLIT were partially reversed once SLIT was stopped suggesting the need for prolonged treatment.

Interestingly a previous study using oral IT using the same experimental model did not show any benefit [53]. Possible reasons for this reported lack of efficacy may include the short duration of the study (7 months rather than a full year) and the fact that swallowing the allergen immediately rather than placing it sublingually leads to decreased stimulation of the immune system in the oral cavity.

4. Conclusions and Directions for the Future

In conclusion, SLIT represents a safe and effective strategy to help with management of allergic diseases in both people and animals. Much work still needs to be done to standardize protocols and optimize success. The ease of administration and the safety and are all very favorable aspects. Although the ideal dose and protocol have not been established, overall the cumulative dose of allergen used is higher than what is used with SCIT. This could lead to increased cost for the patient.

In veterinary medicine SLIT is particularly new and has still a lot of unknowns. There is no study that has investigated the efficacy of SLIT for food allergies or respiratory disease representing an area where much work still needs to be done. No study has been done either to directly compare the efficacy of SCIT and SLIT, and uncertainty exists on the most effective protocol for SLIT. Practitioners and veterinary dermatologists are currently prescribing SLIT as alternative to SCIT for cases in which owners are reluctant to give injections and/or in case where adverse effects are noted with the SCIT. SLIT typically will require larger amounts of allergens and may not be the appropriate choice for owners with busy schedules due to the fact that it requires daily administration. Some practitioners prescribe SLIT twice daily while others prescribe it once daily. No direct comparison between these two protocols has been done thus the most effective treatment regimen to recommend is unknown. Finally no study has been done in veterinary medicine regarding rush protocols using SLIT. Thus there are a lot of unknowns in veterinary medicine about the best protocol in terms of doses, number of allergens, and frequency of administration of SLIT. Although SLIT is frequently recommended on the veterinary side, it is important to highlight that there are very few studies and a lot of variables that have not been investigated and that will need to be addressed in order to obtain strong evidence for or against the efficacy of this therapy. A list of some of the unmet needs for canine AD and SLIT is provided in Table 1. Thus, although SLIT has been shown to be effective in human medicine, it may be wise, in veterinary medicine, to recommend SLIT in specific cases rather than for all cases as a first line of treatment. Suitable cases may be cases in which the animal does not tolerate SCIT, did not respond to SCIT or when owners will not do ASIT altogether due to needle phobia.

Table 1. Unmet needs in canine atopic dermatitis (AD).

Evaluation of clinical efficacy of sublingual immunotherapy (SLIT) compared to subcutaneous immunotherapy (SCIT) in large controlled double blinded studies using dogs with naturally occurring disease and evaluation of differences in speed of action between the two routes
Evaluation of clinical efficacy of twice daily *versus* once daily protocol for SLIT
Evaluation of clinical efficacy of SLIT for mites *versus* grasses and single ingredient *versus* mixes
Evaluation of clinical efficacy of high doses *versus* low doses of SLIT
Evaluation of SLIT to decrease new sensitization over time compared to conventional pharmaceutical therapy

As we increase our knowledge in comparative medicine it is becoming more and more evident that the separation between veterinary and human medicine is not as marked as previously accepted and that we can benefit from knowledge that is developed on one species as it may have potential applications to another one. Although clearly more studies are needed in veterinary medicine to establish the most appropriate protocol and strength of allergens to use for SLIT, so far, this route of administration of allergens has been proven to be well tolerated and able to provide relief to canine patients as it does to humans. Of all therapies available for allergies, ASIT is the only one that can halt the progression of the disease, and even if this has not been demonstrated in dogs yet, it could be beneficial to encourage starting IT at young age in dogs to possibly minimize progression of severity.

Acknowledgements

The authors would like to acknowledge Ahrens for helping with the editing of the manuscript

Author Contributions

Ibrahim Ozmen, a human dermatologist, wrote the part of the manuscript on the human experience with SLIT. Rosanna Marsella, a veterinary dermatologist, wrote the veterinary aspect of the paper and took care of all the revisions and final editing.

Conflicts of Interest

The authors declare no conflict of interest.

References

1. Windom, H.H.; Lockey, R.F. An update on the safety of specific immunotherapy. *Curr. Opin. Allergy Clin. Immunol.* **2008**, *8*, 571–576.
2. Serrano, P.; Justicia, J.L.; Sánchez, C.; Cimarra, M.; Fernández-Távora, L.; Orovitg, A.; Moreno, C.; Guerra, F.; Alvà, V. Systemic tolerability of specific subcutaneous immunotherapy with index-of-reactivity-standardized allergen extracts administered using clustered regimens: A retrospective, observational, multicenter study. *Ann. Allergy Asthma Immunol.* **2009**, *102*, 247–252.
3. Tinkelman, D.G.; Cole, W.Q., 3rd; Tunno, J. Immunotherapy: A one-year prospective study to evaluate risk factors of systemic reactions. *J. Allergy Clin. Immunol.* **1995**, *95*, 8–14.
4. Epstein, T.G.; Liss, G.M.; Murphy-Berendts, K.; Bernstein, D.I. AAAAI/ACAAI surveillance study of subcutaneous immunotherapy, years 2008–2012: An update on fatal and nonfatal systemic allergic reactions. *J. Allergy Clin. Immunol. Pract.* **2014**, *2*, 161–167.
5. Compalati, E.; Rogkakou, A.; Passalacqua, G.; Canonica, G.W. Evidences of efficacy of allergen immunotherapy in atopic dermatitis: An updated review. *Curr. Opin. Allergy Clin. Immunol.* **2012**, *12*, 427–433.
6. Pajno, G.B.; Caminiti, L.; Vita, D.; Barberio, G.; Salzano, G.; Lombardo, F.; Canonica, G.W.; Passalacqua, G. Sublingual immunotherapy in mite-sensitized children with atopic dermatitis: A randomized, double-blind, placebo-controlled study. *J. Allergy Clin. Immunol.* **2007**, *120*, 164–170.
7. Bussmann, C.; Böckenhoff, A.; Henke, H.; Werfel, T.; Novak, N. Does allergen-specific immunotherapy represent a therapeutic option for patients with atopic dermatitis? *J. Allergy Clin. Immunol.* **2006**, *118*, 1292–1298.
8. Cadario, G.; Galluccio, A.G.; Pezza, M.; Appino, A.; Milani, M.; Pecora, S.; Mastrandrea, F. Sublingual immunotherapy efficacy in patients with atopic dermatitis and house dust mites sensitivity: A prospective pilot study. *Curr. Med. Res. Opin.* **2007**, *23*, 2503–2506.
9. Bae, J.M.; Choi, Y.Y.; Park, C.O.; Chung, K.Y.; Lee, K.H. Efficacy of allergen-specific immunotherapy for atopic dermatitis: A systematic review and meta-analysis of randomized controlled trials. *J. Allergy Clin. Immunol.* **2013**, *132*, 110–117.
10. Burks, A.W.; Calderon, M.A.; Casale, T.; Cox, L.; Demoly, P.; Jutel, M.; Nelson, H.; Akdis, C.A. Update on allergy immunotherapy: American Academy of Allergy, Asthma & Immunology/European Academy of Allergy and Clinical Immunology/PRACTALL consensus report. *J. Allergy Clin. Immunol.* **2013**, *131*, 1288–1296.
11. Akdis, M.; Akdis, C.A. Mechanisms of allergen-specific immunotherapy: Multiple suppressor factors at work in immune tolerance to allergens. *J. Allergy Clin. Immunol.* **2014**, *133*, 621–631.
12. Klimek, L.; Pfaar, O. A comparison of immunotherapy delivery methods for allergen immunotherapy. *Expert Rev. Clin. Immunol.* **2013**, *9*, 465–475.
13. Cox, L.; Compalati, E.; Kundig, T.; Larche, M. New directions in immunotherapy. *Curr. Allergy Asthma Rep.* **2013**, *13*, 178–195.
14. Tsilochristou, O.A.; Douladiris, N.; Makris, M.; Papadopoulos, N.G. Pediatric allergic rhinitis and asthma: Can the march be halted? *Paediatr. Drugs* **2013**, *15*, 431–440.
15. Fiocchi, A.; Fox, A.T. Preventing progression of allergic rhinitis: The role of specific immunotherapy. *Arch. Dis. Child Educ. Pract. Ed.* **2011**, *96*, 91–100.

16. Taudorf, E.; Laursen, L.; Lanner, A.; Björkstén, B.; Dreborg, S.; Weeke, B. Specific IgE, IgG and IgA antibody response to oral immunotherapy in birch pollinosis. *J. Allergy Clin. Immunol.* **1989**, *83*, 589–594.
17. Rebien, W.; Puttonen, E.; Maasch, H.J.; Stix, E.; Wahn, U. Clinical and immunological response to oral and subcutaneous immunotherapy with grass pollen extracts. A prospective study. *Eur. J. Pediatr.* **1982**, *138*, 341–344.
18. Sikora, J.M.; Tankersley, M.S. Perception and practice of sublingual immunotherapy among practicing allergists in the United States: A follow-up survey. *Ann. Allergy Asthma Immunol.* **2013**, *110*, 194–197.
19. Passalacqua, G.; Compalati, E.; Canonica, G.W. Sublingual immunotherapy: Clinical indications in the WAO-SLIT position paper. *World Allergy Organ J.* **2010**, *3*, 216–219.
20. Penagos, M.; Compalati, E.; Tarantini, F.; Baena-Cagnani, R.; Huerta, J.; Passalacqua, G.; Canonica, G.W. Efficacy of sublingual immunotherapy in the treatment of allergic rhinitis in pediatric patients 3 to 18 years of age: A meta-analysis of randomized, placebo-controlled, double-blind trials. *Ann. Allergy Asthma Immunol.* **2006**, *97*, 141–148.
21. Mastrandrea, F.; Serio, G.; Minelli, M.; Minardi, A.; Scarcia, G.; Coradduzza, G.; Parmiani, S. Specific sublingual immunotherapy in atopic dermatitis. Results of a 6-year follow-up of 35 consecutive patients. *Allergol. Immunopathol. (Madr)* **2000**, *28*, 54–62.
22. Zheng, J. Clinical study on sublingual immunotherapy for allergens of children with atopic dermatitis. *Hebei Med.* **2011**, *17*, 149–150.
23. Vanbervliet, B.; Tourdot, S.; Mascarell, L.; Rouzaire, P.; Vocanson, M.; Rozières, A.; Benetière, J.; Moingeon, P.; Nicolas, J.F.; Hennino, A. Sublingual immunotherapy prevents the development of eczema in percutaneous allergen-sensitized mice. *J. Invest. Dermatol.* **2012**, *132*, 244–246.
24. Qin, Y.E.; Mao, J.R.; Sang, Y.C.; Li, W.X. Clinical efficacy and compliance of sublingual immunotherapy with *Dermatophagoides farinae* drops in patients with atopic dermatitis. *Int. J. Dermatol.* **2014**, *53*, 650–655.
25. Sun, J.; Hui, X.; Ying, W.; Liu, D.; Wang, X. Efficacy of allergen-specific immunotherapy for peanut allergy: A meta-analysis of randomized controlled trials. *Allergy Asthma Proc.* **2014**, *35*, 171–177.
26. Esch, R.E. Sublingual immunotherapy. *Curr. Opin. Otolaryngol. Head Neck Surg.* **2008**, *16*, 260–264.
27. Scheinmann, P.; Pham, T.N.; Karila, C.; de Blic, J. Allergic march in children, from rhinitis to asthma: Management, indication of immunotherapy. *Arch. Pediatr.* **2012**, *19*, 330–334.
28. Madonini, E.; Agostinis, F.; Barra, R.; Berra, A.; Donadio, D.; Pappacoda, A.; Stefani, E.; Tierno, E. Long-term and preventive effects of sublingual allergen-specific immunotherapy: A retrospective, multicentric study. *Int. J. Immunopathol. Pharmacol.* **2003**, *16*, 73–79.
29. Marogna, M.; Spadolini, I.; Massolo, A.; Canonica, G.W.; Passalacqua, G. Long-lasting effects of sublingual immunotherapy according to its duration: A 15 year prospective study. *J. Allergy Clin. Immunol.* **2010**, *126*, 969–975.
30. Compalati, E.; Braido, F.; Canonica, G.W. Sublingual immunotherapy: Recent advances. *Allergol. Int.* **2013**, *62*, 415–423.

31. Dretzke, J.; Meadows, A.; Novielli, N.; Huissoon, A.; Fry-Smith, A.; Meads, C. Subcutaneous and sublingual immunotherapy for seasonal allergic rhinitis: A systematic review and indirect comparison. *J. Allergy Clin. Immunol.* **2013**, *131*, 1361–1366.
32. ClinicalTrials.gov. Sublingual immunotherapy in patients with atopic dermatitis. Available online: http://clinicaltrials.gov/show/NCT01471119 (accessed on 23 August 2014).
33. Dávila, I.; Navarro, A.; Domínguez-Ortega, J.; Alonso, A.; Antolín-Amérigo, D.; Diéguez, M.C.; González-Mancebo, E.; Martíns, C.; Martínez, C.; Núñez, B.; *et al.* SLIT: Indications, follow-up, and management. *J. Investig. Allergol. Clin. Immunol.* **2014**, *24*, S1–S35.
34. Durham, S.R.; Emminger, W.; Kapp, A.; Colombo, G.; de Monchy, J.G.; Rak, S.; Scadding, G.K.; Andersen, J.S.; Riis, B.; Dahl, R. Long-term clinical efficacy in grass pollen-induced rhinoconjunctivitis after treatment with SQ-standardized grass allergy immunotherapy tablet. *J. Allergy Clin. Immunol.* **2010**, *125*, 131–138.
35. Frølund, L.; Durham, S.R.; Calderon, M.; Emminger, W.; Andersen, J.S.; Rask, P.; Dahl, R. Sustained effect of SQ-standardized grass allergy immunotherapy tablet on rhinoconjunctivitis quality of life. *Allergy* **2010**, *65*, 753–757.
36. Marsella, R.; Girolomoni, G. Canine models of atopic dermatitis: A useful tool with untapped potential. *J. Invest Dermatol.* **2009**, *129*, 2351–2357.
37. Marsella, R.; Olivry, T.; Carlotti, D.N.; International Task Force on Canine Atopic Dermatitis. Current evidence of skin barrier dysfunction in human and canine atopic dermatitis. *Vet. Dermatol.* **2011**, *22*, 239–248.
38. Schäfer, T.; Merkl, J.; Klemm, E.; Wichmann, H.E.; Ring, J. We and our pets: Allergic together? *Acta Vet. Hung.* **2008**, *56*, 153–161.
39. Hill, P.B.; deBoer, D.J. The ACVD task force on canine atopic dermatitis (IV): Environmental allergens. *Vet. Immunol. Immunopathol.* **2001**, *81*, 169–186.
40. Olivry, T.; DeBoer, D.J.; Favrot, C.; Jackson, H.A.; Mueller, R.S.; Nuttall, T.; Prélaud, P.; International Task Force on Canine Atopic Dermatitis. Treatment of canine atopic dermatitis: 2010 clinical practice guidelines from the international task force on canine atopic dermatitis. *Vet. Dermatol.* **2010**, *21*, 233–248.
41. Olivry, T.; Foster, A.P.; Mueller, R.S.; McEwan, N.A.; Chesney, C.; Williams, H.C. Interventions for atopic dermatitis in dogs: A systematic review of randomized controlled trials. *Vet. Dermatol.* **2010**, *21*, 4–22.
42. Schnabl, B.; Bettenay, S.V.; Dow, K.; Mueller, R.S. Results of allergen-specific immunotherapy in 117 dogs with atopic dermatitis. *Vet. Rec.* **2006**, *158*, 81–85.
43. Griffin, C.E.; Hillier, A. The ACVD task force on canine atopic dermatitis (XXIV): Allergen-specific immunotherapy. *Vet. Immunol. Immunopathol.* **2001**, *81*, 363–383.
44. Colombo, S.; Hill, P.B.; Shaw, D.J.; Thoday, K.L. Effectiveness of low dose immunotherapy in the treatment of canine atopic dermatitis: A prospective, double-blinded, clinical study. *Vet. Dermatol.* **2005**, *16*, 162–170.
45. Mueller, R.S.; Bettenay, S.V. Evaluation of the safety of an abbreviated course of injections of allergen extracts (rush immunotherapy) for the treatment of dogs with atopic dermatitis. *Am. J. Vet. Res.* **2001**, *62*, 307–310.

46. Hobi, S.; Mueller, R.S. Efficacy and safety of rush immunotherapy with alum-precipitated allergens in canine atopic dermatitis. *Tierarztl. Prax. Ausg. K Kleintiere Heimtiere* **2014**, *42*, 167–173.
47. Nelson, H.S. Specific immunotherapy with allergen mixes: What is the evidence? *Curr. Opin. Allergy Clin. Immunol.* **2009**, *9*, 549–553.
48. Nelson, H.S.; Iklé, D.; Buchmeier, A. Studies of allergen extract stability: The effects of dilution and mixing. *J. Allergy Clin. Immunol.* **1996**, *98*, 382–388.
49. Shida, M.; Kadoya, M.; Park, S.J.; Nishifuji, K.; Momoi, Y.; Iwasaki, T. Allergen-specific immunotherapy induces Th1 shift in dogs with atopic dermatitis. *Vet. Immunol. Immunopathol.* **2004**, *102*, 19–31.
50. Deboer, D.J.; Morris, M. Multicenter open trial demonstrates efficacy of sublingual immunotherapy (SLIT) in canine atopic dermatitis. *Vet. Dermatol.* **2012**, *23*, S65.
51. Benedetti, F. Placebo and the new physiology of the doctor-patient relationship. *Physiol. Rev.* **2013**, *93*, 1207–1246.
52. Marsella, R.; Ahrens, K. Investigations on the effects of sublingual immunotherapy on clinical signs and immunological parameters using a canine model of atopic dermatitis: A double blinded, randomized, controlled study. *Vet. Dermatol.* **2012**, *23*, S66.
53. Marsella, R. Tolerability and clinical efficacy of oral immunotherapy with house dust mites in a model of canine atopic dermatitis: A pilot study. *Vet. Dermatol.* **2010**, *21*, 566–571.

4

Non-Human Primate Models of Orthopoxvirus Infections

Anne Schmitt, Kerstin Mätz-Rensing and Franz-Josef Kaup *

Pathology Unit, German Primate Center, Leibniz Institute for Primate Research, Kellnerweg 4, 37077 Göttingen, Germany; E-Mails: aschmitt@dpz.eu (A.S.); kmaetz@dpz.eu (K.M.-R.)

* Author to whom correspondence should be addressed; E-Mail: fkaup@gwdg.de;

Abstract: Smallpox, one of the most destructive diseases, has been successfully eradicated through a worldwide vaccination campaign. Since immunization programs have been stopped, the number of people with vaccinia virus induced immunity is declining. This leads to an increase in orthopoxvirus (OPXV) infections in humans, as well as in animals. Additionally, potential abuse of *Variola* virus (VARV), the causative agent of smallpox, or monkeypox virus, as agents of bioterrorism, has renewed interest in development of antiviral therapeutics and of safer vaccines. Due to its high risk potential, research with VARV is restricted to two laboratories worldwide. Therefore, numerous animal models of other OPXV infections have been developed in the last decades. Non-human primates are especially suitable due to their close relationship to humans. This article provides a review about on non-human primate models of orthopoxvirus infections.

Keywords: non-human primate; smallpox; monkeypox; cowpox; animal models

---

1. Introduction

The genus *Orthopoxvirus* (OPXV), as part of the *Poxviridae*, includes, among others, the species *variola* virus (VARV), monkeypox virus (MPXV), cowpox virus (CPXV), vaccinia virus (VACV), and mousepox virus. The causative agent of smallpox, VARV, was one of the most dangerous viruses known to mankind, being responsible for the death of 300 to 500 million people. Fortunately, smallpox has been successfully eradicated by a worldwide vaccination campaign under the leadership of the World Health Organization (WHO) [1]. Because of the inferior safety profile of the smallpox vaccine in immune compromised persons, pregnant women, or persons with atopic dermatitis, routine smallpox vaccinations were stopped in the 1980s following a recommendation from WHO. Only military personnel, selected healthcare, and laboratory workers still get the vaccine. Consequently, the number of people with lacking immunity, not only against smallpox, but also against other zoonotic OPXV infections is increasing [2], in humans, as well as in animals [3–7]. In the Democratic Republic of Congo there is a massive (20-fold) increase in human monkeypox incidence [8]. Additionally, it is feared that smallpox could be used as a biological weapon [9–11]. There is, thus far, no pharmaceutic treatment available and vaccines are partly unsafe, therefore, more research concerning orthopoxvirus infections is very important. Because of its high risk potential, research with VARV is limited to two BSL4 containments worldwide (Atlanta and Novosibirsk) and is, therefore, highly restricted. Suitable animal models are needed in which an orthopoxvirus causes a disease course, morbidity, and mortality, similar to human disease. Furthermore, the route of infection and transmission should be mimicked, and the infectious dose should be similar to that of humans. Unfortunately, no animal model fulfills all these criteria [12,13]. Nevertheless, these models can help to get an insight into the pathogenesis, and are a good tool to test the efficacy of antiviral compounds and of new vaccines. Furthermore, these animal models are important to fulfill the requirements of the animal efficacy rule. This rule was promulgated by the Food and Drug Administration (FDA) and demands a testing of medical countermeasures in at least two different animal models when clinical trials in humans are unethical or impossible [14].

In the last decades, considerable progress has been made in development of new animal models for OPXV infections [12,15–19]. CPXV, MPXV, VACV, VARV, ectromelia virus, rabbitpox virus, and camelpox virus have been used in animal models. Small animal models, other than non-human primates (NHP) models, have the advantage that large numbers of animals are available. Furthermore, maintenance costs are lower compared to monkeys. However, small animal models have limitations: Disease pathology, a shortened time course of disease, pharmacokinetic behavior of compounds, and tissue distribution can vary from human conditions [20]. Therefore, animals, which are closely related to humans, and whose physiological and pathological reactions are, therefore, more comparable to humans, are more suitable. NHP are the next relatives to humans, recapitulate human condition as closely as possible, and are, therefore, very appropriate to evaluate new vaccines, treatments, or pathogenesis [21]. Thus, NHP are the gold-standard for OPXV models, as their resemblance to humans allows the best predicative value for effects or side effects of new therapeutics or vaccines in humans [13].

In the following, we will review OPXV models in NHP, arranged by virus species and inoculation route (see Table 1).

2. Monkeypox

MPXV is an *Orthopoxvirus* which causes a zoonotic disease characterized by symptoms similar to smallpox but with a lethality rate of 1%–8% [2,22]. In all probability, some monkeypox infections were misinterpreted as smallpox because of the lack of laboratory testing [23]. One clinical symptom, which allows a differentiation from smallpox, is lymphadenopathy, which could lead to the conclusion that there is a more effective immune response [24,25]. MPXV was first detected in 1957 in captive primates in Denmark [26]. Not only are several species of NHP (rhesus macaques (see Figures 1 and 2), cynomolgus macaques, and chimpanzees), but also a broad spectrum of mammals, are susceptible to the disease [15,16]. In 1960, a naturally occurring MPXV outbreak was reported in cynomolgus and rhesus macaques [27]. Human monkeypox emerged in the 1970s in Western and Central Africa and today still leads to outbreaks in the rural villages near the rainforests [8]. The natural host is still unknown, but, with the utmost probability, African squirrels and/or other rodents play an important role [15]. Only once, the virus could be found in a carcass of a *Funiscirus* squirrel in Democratic Republic of the Congo [28]. Probably, the virus is transmitted via eating infected bushmeat, via saliva/respiratory excretions, or direct contact with crust material. However, the exact transmission route for MPXV is unclear. [12,15,22,24]. In 2003, the disease was accidentally introduced into the U.S. due to infected wild rodents imported from Africa, which transmitted the virus to prairie dogs (*Cynomys ludovicianus*) and then, via the prairie dogs, to approximately 40 humans [29–31]. Remarkably, the prairie dogs were the only infection source for the humans [15]. Discontinuation of vaccination after eradication of smallpox, inadequate health infrastructure and bushmeat consumption has given rise to increasing susceptibility to MPXV infection in the African population [23,32].

Studies with NHP are useful for understanding monkeypox disease. Additionally, NHP models of MPXV are a good alternative to VARV models, because they are less dangerous for laboratory workers and researchers. Compared to other MPXV susceptible species, such as prairie dogs, NHP are more suitable due to the close relationship to humans. Furthermore, they get better accustomed to the research conditions than other susceptible species, such as prairie dogs [15].

NHP can be infected with MPXV experimentally via different techniques, which are described below.

Figure 1. Monkeypox virus infected *Macaca mulatta* (*M. mulatta*) with multifocal severe papular dermatitis.

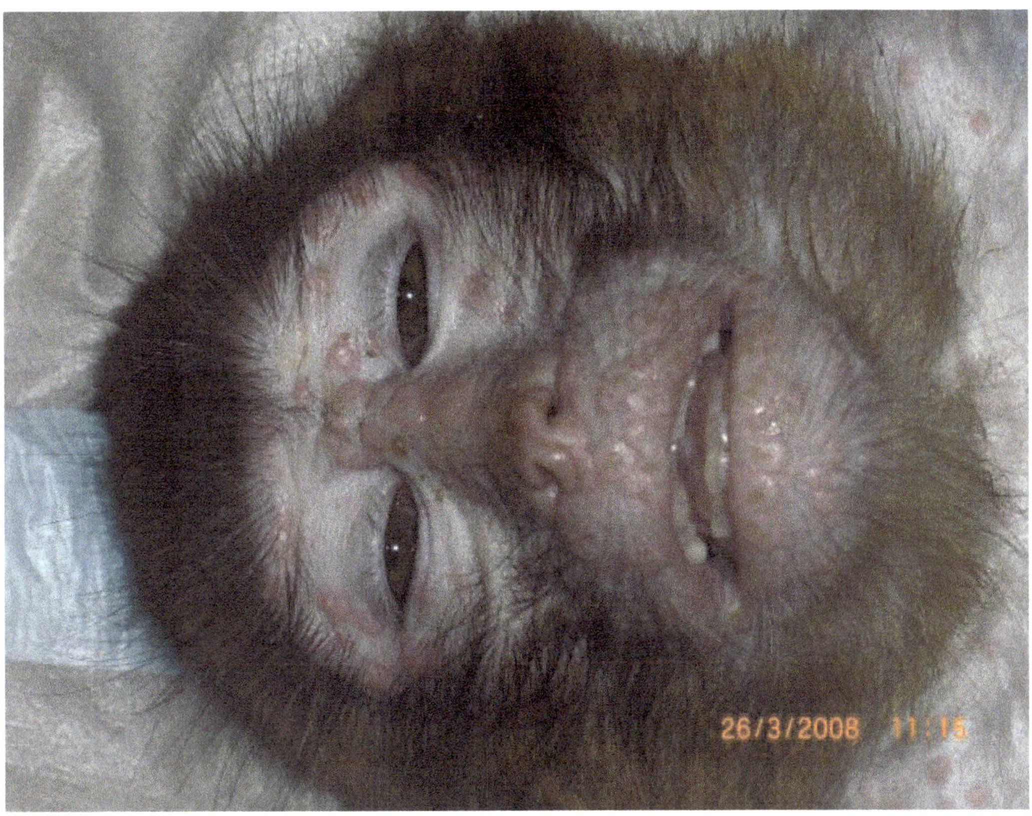

Figure 2. Skin of Monkeypox virus infected *M. mulatta* with multiple vesicular and erosive to ulcerative skin lesions.

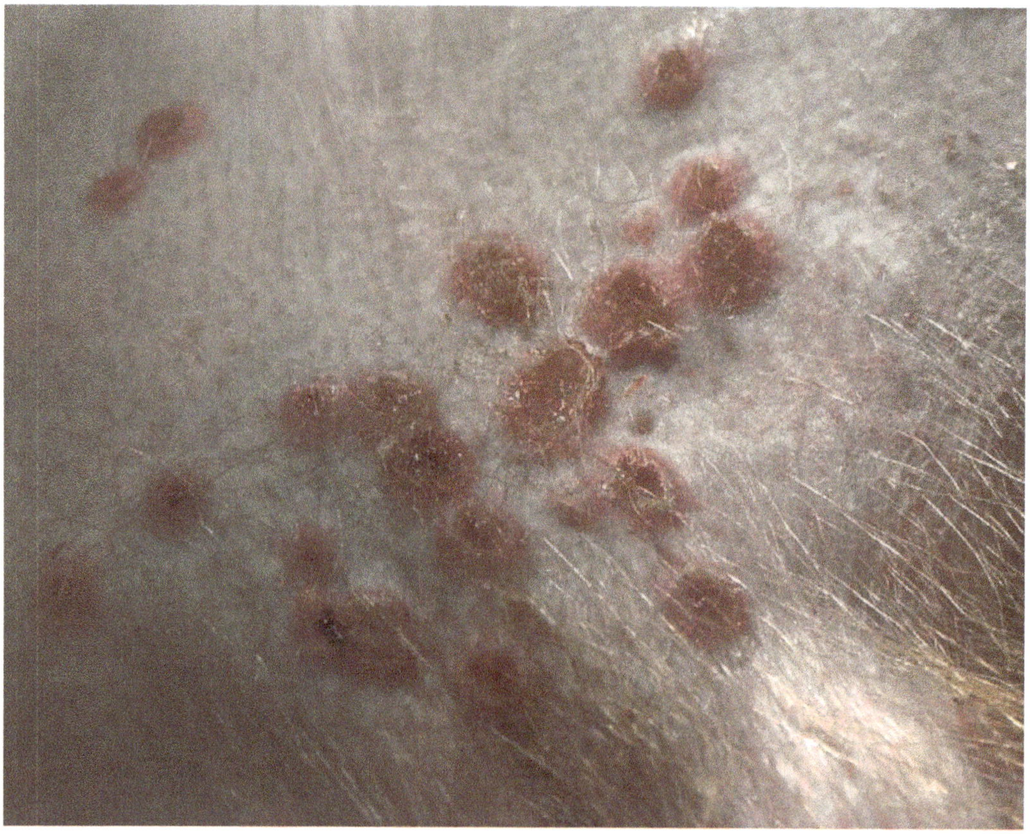

2.1. Intramuscular

In the late 1960s, Wenner and colleagues developed a model in which they inoculated 10^5 plaque-forming unit (PFU) of MPXV intramuscularly in cynomolgus and rhesus macaques [33]. Animals developed a vesicular to pustular rash and became diseased with a systemic viral infection. Disadvantages of this model are skin and muscle necrosis at the inoculation site [16].

In a study conducted in 1971, six baboons (*Papio cynocephalus*) were challenged intramuscularly with MPXV and all became infected. Typical lesions like vesicular pustules on the extremities, face, lips, and buccal mucosa, happened after around eight days post infection. One single animal succumbed to the disease. Challenging surviving animals with MPXV after first experiment proved the acquired immunity and the possibility to protect monkey colonies in captivity by immunizing [34].

2.2. Skin Scarification

In a following study, Heberling and Kalter challenged baboons with MPXV via skin scarification and showed an increased resistance to MPXV with ageing [35]. Baboons aged approximately one year developed typical pox lesions, fever, and lymphadenopathy, but did not die. The younger animals (approximately three-months old) showed a similar disease course, but five of ten animals succumbed to the disease.

2.3. Intravenous

Though the intravenous infection of MPXV causes a fulminant disease with severe lesions, which are very similar to smallpox, this model has several disadvantages: Key events like infection of the upper respiratory tract, primary viremia phase, and prodromal phases are skipped. Additionally, the route of transmission does not resemble the natural route of transmission of smallpox, which happens through close contact or inhaled aerosols. Furthermore, the infectious dose is much higher than the natural infection dose [36]. However, intravenous application of MPXV produces a course of disease that is appropriate to evaluate the efficacy and benefits of anti-OPXV therapeutics and vaccines.

Huggins and colleagues infected eight male cynomolgus macaques with a Zaire strain of MPXV via intravenous inoculation and proved the efficacy of the antiviral drug Tecovirimat (previously known as ST-246) dosed with 300 mg/kg/day. Tecovirimat was able to protect animals from disease and death. The infection with MPXV in the control group triggered a vesiculopustular rash accompanied by fever, elevated white blood cell count, lymphadenopathy, splenomegaly, and pulmonary edema [20]. Because of the fact that high drug doses at early times post infection were given, a follow-up study was conducted in which lower doses at later times were compared. The researchers conclude that 400 mg, once daily for 14 days after clinical diagnosis, can be an effective treatment for smallpox and monkeypox in humans [37].

To visualize viral infection, researchers inserted a gene encoding green fluorescent protein (GFP) into MPXV Zaire-79 and infected cynomolgus macaques intravenously. This way, initial lesions could be detected under fluorescent light one to two days earlier. Fluorescence was most intense in lesions of the oral cavity and weakest in skin of the palms and soles, which is protected by a thick layer of keratin [38].

Hooper and colleagues challenged rhesus macaques intravenously with MPXV after immunizing with a DNA vaccine consisting of four vaccinia virus genes. Unvaccinated control animals died on days seven, ten, and fourteen, showing hemorrhages in multiple organs, lymphadenopathy, and vesiculopustular rashes on the face and the hands. With a subunit vaccine, immunized animals did not develop severe disease and survived. This is a promising study, because a subunit vaccine does not have the feared side effects of the present smallpox vaccine [39]. In a following study, they tried to boost immune response to the gene-based vaccine using adjuvants like granulocyte macrophage-colony stimulating factor (GM-CSF) and *Escherichia coli* heat-labile enterotoxin. Unvaccinated control animals became severely ill, four of the five had to be euthanized, whereas all five animals vaccinated with gene-based vaccine with adjuvants survived without shedding virus, but one developed severe disease. Control animals which were vaccinated with modified Virus Ankara (MVA) shed virus, three of five became heavily ill [40].

To get more information about innate immunity in MPXV infection, Song and colleagues challenged rhesus macaques intravenously with MPXV and analyzed the changes in natural killer (NK) cell numbers, NK cell proliferation, chemokine receptor expression and cellular functions. They found that NK cell frequency and the absolute number in the blood and in the lymphoid tissues increase following MPXV infection. Interestingly, MPXV infection induces a reduced migrating capacity of NK cells and a reduced degranulation capacity. Thus, cytotoxic effects of cytokines were not reached [41].

Dyall and colleagues challenged cynomolgus macaques of both sexes intravenously, as well as intrabronchially, with 5×10^6 or 5×10^5 PFU of MPXV and observed progression and regression of the disease course with molecular imaging like positron emission tomography (PET) and computed tomography (CT). Animals that were infected intravenously did not show any signs of lung consolidation or inflammation in molecular imaging contrary to those infected intrabronchially. In these animals, PET/CT imaging revealed areas of necrosis, mixed inflammation, oedema, and some fibrosis in the lung. For both routes, clear manifestation of lymphadenopathy and manifestation in the axillary lymph nodes could be shown [42].

Earl and colleagues challenged cynomolgus macaques intravenously with MPXV at four, six, ten, and thirty days after immunization with MVA and Dryvax. The animals were protected against disease outbreak if they were challenged at least six days after immunization. The researchers found that a single dose of MVA induces a rapid immune response suggesting that it might be a countermeasure against a potential smallpox virus outbreak. A further result was that MVA produces a more rapid immune response compared to the licensed Dryvax vaccine [43].

To examine the question whether human immunodeficiency virus type 1 (HIV-1) infected creatures are protected by smallpox vaccination, researchers infected fourteen rhesus macaques with simian immunodeficiency virus (SIV) and immunized them with different combinations of MVA, NYVAC, and Dryvax. One and six months after immunization, the animals which had $CD4^+$ cell counts <300 mm^3 were challenged intravenously with 5×10^7 PFU of MPXV. All challenged monkeys showed a severe disease course with typical pox lesions on skin and the lining of the oropharynx. This lack of protection could be the consequence of the inability of the SIV-infected macaques to switch vaccinia-specific immunoglobulin (Ig) from IgM to IgG [44]. A further vaccination study with Dryvax conducted by Edghill-Smith and colleagues found that vaccinia-specific B-cell responses are indispensable for protection from lethal monkeypox disease, whereas $CD4^+$ and $CD8^+$ T cells do not play an important role. They immunized rhesus macaques with Dryvax and challenged them intravenously with a dose of 5×10^7 PFU of MPV [45].

Another study examined the use of subunit recombinant vaccine against MPXV in a rhesus macaque model. They immunized the monkeys with plasmid DNA alone, in combination with the equivalent recombinant proteins, or only with the proteins. Thirty-five weeks after the beginning of immunization, the animals were challenged intravenously with 5×10^7 PFU of MPXV. Immunization only with DNA did not lead to protection against MPXV challenge; the animals had to be euthanized due to severe disease. Animals which were immunized with proteins, developed mild to severe disease but survived. Animals that were immunized with a combination of DNA and proteins had only few lesions, which healed within days and showed only mild disease symptoms [46].

The integration of human cytokine IL15 into the genome of Wyeth strain of VACV confers long-term protection to cynomolgus macaques [47]. The researchers immunized the monkeys and challenged them three years later intravenously with 10^7 PFU of MPXV. By day 27 post challenge, all skin lesions of Wyeth-IL15 immunized animals were healed, whereas all unvaccinated control animals succumbed to the disease.

2.4. Intratracheal/Aerosolization

The transmission via aerosol is supposed to play an important role even if primary monkeypox infection is transmitted by direct cutaneous or mucosal contact [22,48]. Stittelaar and colleagues challenged cynomolgus macaques intratracheally with MPXV after vaccination with MVA and Elstree. One single animal developed a light course of disease but did not die. Unvaccinated control animals developed severe disease showing fibrinonecrotic bronchopneumonia, necrotizing dermatitis, glossitis, and splenitis with lymphoid depletion [49]. In a following study, the researchers again inoculated cynomolgus macaques intratracheally with a lethal dose of MPXV to evaluate the efficacy of post-exposure antiviral treatments and vaccination. In contrast to post-exposure vaccination with Elstree, antiviral treatment with cidofovir or with a nucleoside phosphonate analogue resulted in a reduced number of skin lesions and a reduced mortality rate. Untreated challenged control animals showed severe skin lesions, dyspnea and low blood oxygen saturation and died within 15 days after being challenged with MPXV [50].

One disadvantage of intratracheal models of MPXV infection is the huge amount of virus needed which does not resemble the natural infection. Intratracheal infection models do not take into consideration the physiological inhalation procedure, which is skipped by depositing virus directly into airways.

To infect monkeys more efficiently, researchers developed new aerosolization methods: Zaucha and colleagues established an aerosolized MPXV infection in cynomolgus monkeys using a head-only esposure chamber with a collision nebulizer. They exposed monkeys to four different doses of aerosolized MPXV, trying to imitate the natural route of transmission for human VARV infection. Fever, lymphadenopathy and depression were present around day six, post exposure. The animals died nine to seventeen days post exposure suffering from fibrinonecrotic bronchopneumonia. The pathogenesis of this route of infection is comparable to smallpox infection, which also starts in the respiratory mucosa, spreads to local lymph nodes, and is also followed by viremia [51].

To further characterize the pathogenesis of MPXV, Nalca and colleagues exposed cynomolgus macaques in the same way like described by Zaucha. Blood analysis revealed that complete blood count (CBC) and clinical chemistry of MPXV infected animals deviate from normal values—comparable to human monkeypox cases. Main pathological findings and cause of death were primary fibrinonecrotic bronchopneumonia, comparable to the results of Zaucha. Furthermore, they interestingly found that heavy males were more resistant [21].

Barnewall and colleagues performed a MPXV infection study with six cynomolgus macaques, also using the above described head-only aerosol exposure system. The most prominent pathological lesion was bronchopneumonia. They also found that weight and/or sex may be important for disease course. Furthermore they compared two sampling methods of MPXV aerosols and concluded that gelatin filters and impingers delivered comparable results [52]. One disadvantage of above described head-only chamber is the fact that each monkey inhales different doses of virus, which aggravates comparability [15].

To compare the protective effects of Imvamune and Acam2000 vaccines, Hatch and colleagues challenged cynomolgus macaques with a target dose of 10^5 PFU of MPXV. They used a flexible system, in which the challenge aerosol is delivered by a nebulizer over a modified veterinary anesthesia mask. Acam2000 protected the animals completely even if applicated only once, whereas Imvamune showed protection from severe disease and death only if applicated twice (prime and boost immunization) [53].

2.5. Microsprayer-Technique and Intrabronchial

A new challenge technique tries to refine the virus delivery. Goff and colleagues inserted a microsprayer attached to a bronchoscope into the trachea of cynomolgus macques and challenged the animals via a high-pressure syringe, which facilitates precise dosage. They could lower the dose of virus compared to the intravenous challenge dose and the infection resulted in a fatal disease course. The animals showed marked lobar fibrinonecrotic pneumonia and more cutaneous lesion compared to other aerosol models. This means a better comparability to smallpox. One disadvantage of this technique is the possible mechanical damage of the respiratory tissue causing an inflammation at the inoculation site [36].

Compared to the aerosol models, intrabronchial models have the advantage that inoculation via bronchoscope allows a measurable and exact deposit of virus. Furthermore, the technique is easy to conduct and does not require special expensive equipment.

Estep and colleagues proposed that monkeypox inhibitor of complement enzymes (MOPICE) is an important virulence factor in Central African strains of MPXV. To verify that, they inoculated rhesus monkeys intrabronchially with 2×10^5 PFU of MPXV-Zaire ($n = 4$) and with a recombinant MPXV-Zaire ($n = 4$), which does not express MOPICE. Both animals groups developed similar disease symptoms: typical pox skin lesions, fever, and respiratory symptoms. Interestingly, the animals which were infected with the knockout clade, showed more severe disease courses: One animal died at day 17 post infection due to MPXV-related disease complications, two animals had very low oxygen saturation levels at 14 and 28 days post infection, respectively, and two animals showed a delayed wound healing process. The knockout group had higher peak viral loads than the wild type infected group. The results suggest that MOPICE is not an important virulence factor, but that it is important to generate a successful adaptive immune response [54].

To find out if intrabronchial exposure to MPXV produces a disease course, which is comparable to human MPXV infection, researchers infected cynomolgus macaques with MPXV by the intravenous and the intrabronchial inoculation route. Although both routes produced typical pox-like disease, they concluded that the intrabronchial model is more adequate than the intravenous model: The whole disease course is delayed and, therefore, allows a deeper insight into pathogenesis [55].

To study host-pathogen interaction in bronchoalveolar lavage fluids (BALF), Brown and colleagues infected rhesus macaques intrabronchially with 2×10^5 PFU of MPXV and flushed lungs of infected animals with PBS. They found an increase in inflammatory and interestingly a decrease in structural and metabolic proteins after infection and conclude that inflammation is not the only contributor to disease course. Structural and metabolic proteins also seem to play in important role in pathogenesis of MPXV [56].

2.6. Intranasal

Saijo and colleagues showed that vaccination with Lister, as well as with LC16m8, protected cynomolgus macaques against a lethal MPXV infection. They infected the animals intranasally with MPXV strain Liberia or Zaire. Unvaccinated control animals featured loss of appetite, diarrhea, and papulovesicular skin lesions, but none of the animals died [57]. In a further study, they inoculated Congo Basin and West African strains of MPXV subcutaneously, respectively intranasally into cynomolgus monkeys. They found that the virulence of Congo Basin strain is much higher than of West African one, which could be explained by the difference in organ tropism and, thus, in the sites of virus replication. Congo Basin caused more organ dysfunction than West African and replicated more efficiently [58].

2.7. Subcutaneous

Subcutaneous infection seems to play in important role in MPXV infections [15] and is therefore a good model to test antiviral therapeutics. Early studies revealed that subcutaneous injection of MPXV in rhesus and cynomolgus macaques only caused locally restricted skin lesions or mild generalized disease without death [15,27,59]. Recent studies have obtained different results: In a vaccination study with Lister and LC16m8, cynomolgus macaques were challenged intranasally and subcutaneously. In non-immunized control animals, subcutaneous injection of MPXV has led to generalized, severe disease that required euthanasia. Histopathological investigations revealed alterations in the lymphoid system, respiratory, digestive and urinary tract and the skin [57]. A subsequent study compared Congo Basin and West African strains of MPXV. Three of four monkeys, which were subcutaneously infected with Congo Basin strain, showed a sharp decrease of body weight and succumbed to the disease. In the group that was subcutaneously infected with West African strain, one of three animals died [58].

Summary Monkeypox

Although MPXV has only been detected in African non-human primates, Asian macaques like rhesus and cynomolgus macques, which are not natural hosts, are the most often used species for MPXV models. This may be due to the fact that these species are widely spread in animal experiments, easy available and have been well investigated [15]. Both species are susceptible to MPXV, but rhesus macaques seem to be less susceptible than cynomolgus macaques, as observed in an US outbreak in 1960 [15,60]. Concerning the appropriate inoculation route, none mimics sufficiently natural infection with VARV or MPXV. The exact transmission route for MPXV is still not clear, which makes it more difficult to evaluate transmission routes. Additionally, the inoculum dose in natural infections may be lower than those inoculated experimentally. Intravenous models of MPXV infection skip infection of respiratory tissue and incubation phase and, therefore, do not mimic the natural route of transmission. Nevertheless, they cause systemic disease with mortality rates up to 100%. This makes the intravenous model interesting for vaccine and therapeutical studies concerning smallpox [15].

Respiratory NHP challenge models of MPXV have a slowed course of disease compared to intravenous models. They often cause fibrinonecrotic bronchopneumonia, which resembles human MPXV disease course. In addition, mortality rates of 100% rates are not reached in respiratory challenge models [15,36,51,55,57], which also resembles human MPXV. Thus, respiratory models are appropriate to get further insight into pathogenesis of human MPXV. Different techniques can be used to inoculate virus into the respiratory tract. Application via bronchoscope is easy, inexpensive and allows an exact deposition of the virus. However, there is the potential risk to damage tissue and to cause non-virus related inflammation [15]. This problem does not occur if virus is aerosolized. However, there is the disadvantage that quite high doses of virus are needed and it is not guaranteed that each monkey gets exact the same amount of virus.

Subcutaneous models closely mimic natural transmission of MPXV and are, therefore, a good tool to examine pathogenesis of human MPXV infections. Contrary to this, they do not mimic the transmission route for VARV, which happens via respiratory tract, and are therefore less suitable for VARV research.

3. Smallpox

Development of animal models for smallpox is very difficult, because natural VARV is restricted to humans. Additionally, it is unclear to what extent resultant pathology of animals compares with that of naturally happening smallpox disease in humans [61]. Due to their close relationship to humans, WHO and the U.S. National Academy of Sciences recommended the use of NHP models for smallpox research [62]. The VARV NHP models are reserved for *in vivo* experiments with antiviral drugs or vaccines that have already fulfilled the criteria required by FDA. Additionally, the research community hopes to get a deeper insight into the, thus far, unexplored pathogenesis of smallpox.

In 1906, Brinckerhoff and Tyzzer unsuccessfully tried to infect cynomolgus and pig-tailed macaques with VARV [61,63]. In the 1950s and 1960s, researchers still failed to develop efficient NHP models of smallpox. They challenged wild-caught monkeys with VARV via inhalation of a cloud of dried particles, but, beyond pulmonary lesions, they could detect no pathological changes in other tissues. The resulting mild disease did not resemble fulminant disease course of smallpox in humans [64]. Westwood challenged rhesus macaques via aerosol to VARV and succeeded in provoking a more pronounced clinical disease [65,66]. Ultimately, VARV studies with NHP were discontinued due to unsatisfying results. Sociopolitical changes and the fear of bioterrorism in the early 21st century reintensified VARV studies with NHP. First experiments again failed to produce lethal disease course: Cynomolgus macaques were challenged via aerosol with high doses of VARV strains. They only showed mild clinical signs without dying [67]. But a later experiment with two VARV strains (Harper and India 7124) resulted in a fulminant lethal disease course of cynomolgus macaques which were infected intravenously or intravenously in combination with aerosol exposure [68]. Disease course appeared to be dose dependent, as high doses administered intravenously (10^9 PFU) caused hemorrhagic diathesis ending in acute deaths whereas lower doses resulted in ordinary smallpox. A disadvantage regarding testing antiviral drugs is the fact that intravenous inoculation of VARV skips the incubation period which happens in natural human smallpox. Nevertheless, this model is the first that could produce a lethal VARV infection in cynomolgus macaques. It can be used as a model for hemorrhagic smallpox.

To get further insight into the molecular features of smallpox infection, researchers infected cynomolgus macaques intravenously or intravenously in combination with aerosol exposure with VARV (strain Harper and India 7124) and analyzed in serial blood samples the host gene expression in PBMCs (peripheral blood mononuclear cells). The animals had a severe clinical disease course developing fever, typical pox skin lesions, visceral and mucosal hemorrhage, and showed an upregulation of inflammatory cytokines [62].

To get more knowledge about the progression of smallpox disease and the differences between the ordinary and the hemorrhagic disease course, Wahl-Jensen and colleagues challenged cynomolgus macaques intravenously with VARV doses which either caused hemorrhagic or ordinary disease. They performed temporal pathology analysis and took serial samples. In the ordinary smallpox model, lymphoid and myeloid hyperplasia was observed. Only a few VARV particles in tissue could be detected compared to the hemorrhagic model. In hemorrhagic smallpox model lymphocytolysis and hematopoietic necrosis, as well marked antigen accumulation occurred. Furthermore, hemorrhagic disease was always accompanied by secondary bacterial infections [69].

Huggins and colleagues infected eight cynomolgus monkeys intravenously with 10^8 PFU of VARV (strain Harper). Two control animals, which did not receive drugs, had to be euthanized on day twelve. Their disease course resembled human smallpox infection, especially disease endpoints like lesions and death. Three animals were treated with Tecovirimat (300 mg/kg/day) immediately after infection and three animals 24 h post infection. Both groups were protected from disease and death [20].

A study conducted by Mucker and colleagues also evaluated the efficacy of Tecovirimat. They infected 18 male cynomolgus macaques intravenously with 10^8 PFU of VARV and showed that treatment with Tecovirimat two, as well as four, days post infection protected the animals from death, effected a significant reduction in total skin lesions, reduced viremia and virus shedding in the oropharynx. All non-treated control animals succumbed to the disease. The researchers conclude that Tecovirimat is an effective drug against smallpox disease [70].

Summary Smallpox

Due to fear of bioterrorism, efforts to develop smallpox NHP models have been intensified since the beginning of the 21st century leading to NHP models in which pathogenesis and antiviral drugs, especially Tecovirimat, have been investigated. Though intravenous inoculation of the virus does not represent the natural infection route, it causes a clinical course, which resembles the latter stage of human disease, and is, therefore, suitable to prove the efficacy of therapeutics. Working with smallpox virus to test the efficacy of antiviral drugs and vaccines against smallpox has the advantage that the original causative agent of the disease is used, even though NHP are not natural hosts. Because of its high zoonotic potential, research with this extremely dangerous virus is restricted to two biosafety-level four laboratories worldwide (CDC, USA and State Research Center of Virology and Biotechnology, Russia) and is, therefore, available to only a very small research community.

4. Cowpox

CPXV, which belongs to the OPXV, is a noteworthy virus. It has the broadest host range of all OPXV, the largest genetic repertoire and produces an array of gene products, which manipulate the immune system [7,71]. Cowpox is an emerging hazard. During the last decades, reports about CPXV infections in humans, as well as in animal are increasing [72–76]. As smallpox immunization has been stopped, human population is now getting more vulnerable to CPXV infections. Human cowpox is a zoonotic infection, which usually causes self-limiting, painful skin lesions, particularly located on the hands, face, or trunk. In immunocompetent people, they are healing within several weeks, leaving scars. Further symptoms are fever, depression, and lymphadenopathy. Ocular cowpox infection can, rarely, happen [77–79]. However, severe complications can occur in immunocompromised persons or persons with atopic dermatitis [80–84]. Unlike smallpox, which is transmitted via the respiratory route, cowpox has to be transmitted through direct contact with skin or mucosal lesions.

The name cowpox originates from infected domestic cattle, which transmitted the disease to milkers. The name is misleading [85], as transmission by cows is not the main transmission route any more. Nowadays, CPXV exists in many host species in Western Eurasia [86]. Asymptomatic carriers are wild infected rodents. A survey conducted by Kinnunen and colleagues, in which they screened wild rodents from Germany, Finland, and Siberia's Baikal region for OPV antibodies and for the presence of OPXV DNA, revealed a seroprevalence up to 33% and the presence of poxvirus antigen in three rodents [87]. Cats are infected by feeding on rodents that are carrying the virus [88]. Zoo animals and exotic animals like Llamas are also infected [4,86,89,90]. CPXV outbreaks in NHP in European zoos and sanctuaries have occurred [91,92].

Common marmosets (*Callithrix jacchus*) showed a fulminant disease course [91,92]. In a private husbandry in Germany, 30 of 80 New World Monkeys died within a week after onset of symptoms. They showed fever, depression, severe erosive-ulcerative lesions of the oral membranes, and lymphadenopathy. In this case, owners and animal caretakers did not become ill. Researchers from the German Primate Center and the Robert Koch Institute isolated an OPXV with close homology to CPXV and named it calpox, according to its host *Callithrix jacchus*. Pathologic examination showed hemorrhagic skin lesions on the face, scrotal region, soles and palms, facial oedema, and focal erosions and ulcerations of the oral mucous membranes (see Figure 3). Histopathologically, the hemorrhagic-to-pustular skin lesions were accompanied by vesiculation, epidermal acanthosis, and acantholysis and necrosis (see Figure 4). Eosinophilic intracytoplasmic inclusions bodies could be detected in degenerated keratinocytes. Transmission Electron Microscopy revealed particles with characteristic pox-like features. Kramski and colleagues succeeded in developing a common marmoset model for calpoxvirus infection. They infected marmosets via the intravenous and the intranasal route and produced a lethal disease course, in which the animals died within three days after onset of symptoms. The animals showed characteristic pox-like lesions in the skin and mucous membranes, subcutaneous oedema, splenic lymphoid hyperplasia, and lymphadenomegaly of different lymph nodes [93]. Histological investigations revealed vesicular dermatitis with necrosis, acanthosis, acantholysis, and syncytia formation of the basal keratinocytes [94]. Advantages of this model are firstly the low infectious dose, as even a very low dose of 5×10^2 PFU was effective. Secondly, CPXV can be handled under a lower biohazard level than MPXV or VARV, which facilitates research with this virus. Furthermore, common marmosets have several advantages compared to commonly used NHP: Their small size allows an easy handling. They can be housed in family groups, are not endangered and are inexpensive to keep [95].

As CPXV is genetically and, antigenically, quite comparable to VACV and related to MPXV and VARV (they share 19 immunomodulatory genes), CPXV models are an alternative to above presented models for smallpox and monkeypox [82,96,97]. In addition, gaining more knowledge of CPXV pathogenesis itself is also very important due to its increasing zoonotic potential.

Smith and colleagues present a CPXV model, in which they infect cynomolgus macaques intrabronchially with different dilutions of CPXV (5×10^4 to 5×10^5). Lymphoid hyperplasia up to oedema and histiocytosis in the lymph nodes (depending on the inoculated dose) and multifocal neutrophilic infiltrates in the liver showed similarity to histopathological changes in other OPXV infections like MPXV and VARV. Lesions in lung (like alveolar oedema, necrotizing fibrinous pleuritis, congestion, atelectasis, pneumonia) are more pronounced in comparison to human smallpox disease. Measuring of cytokines and chemokines revealed a heavy pro-inflammatory response [98].

Figure 3. *Callithrix jacchus* (*C. jacchus*) with marked subcutaneous oedema and erythema on the neck region and single papular lesions on mucocutaneous junctions after experimental infection with calpox.

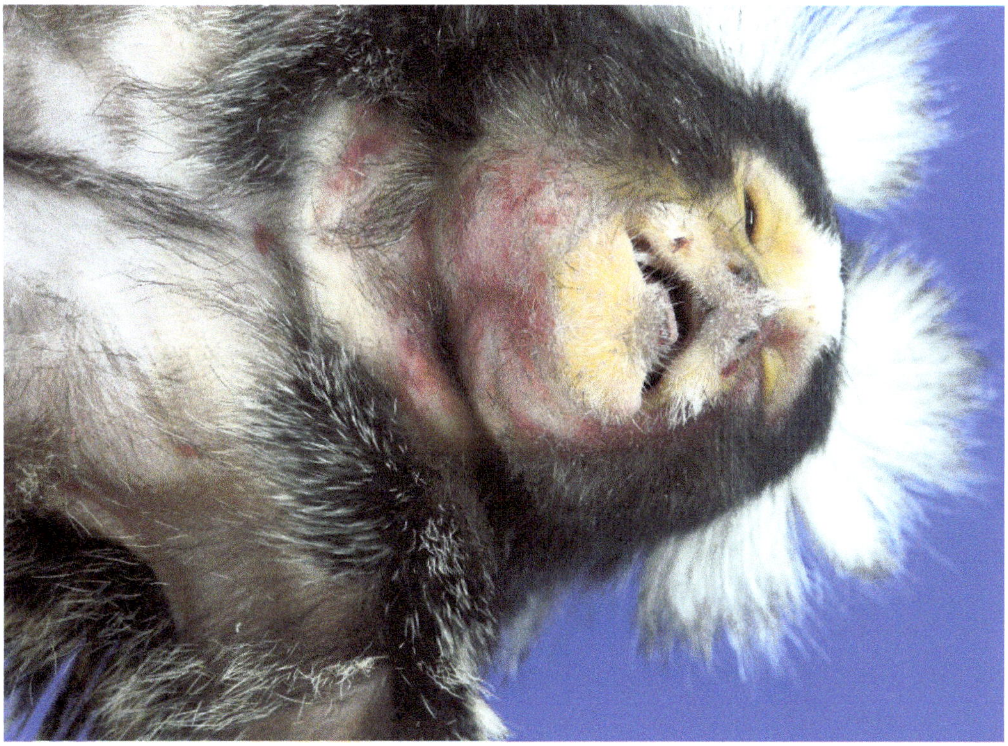

Figure 4. Calpox virus infected saddle back tamarin, skin. High-grade, focal, vesicular dermatitis with intracytoplasmatic eosinophilic inclusion bodies, ballooning degeneration and hemorrhage.

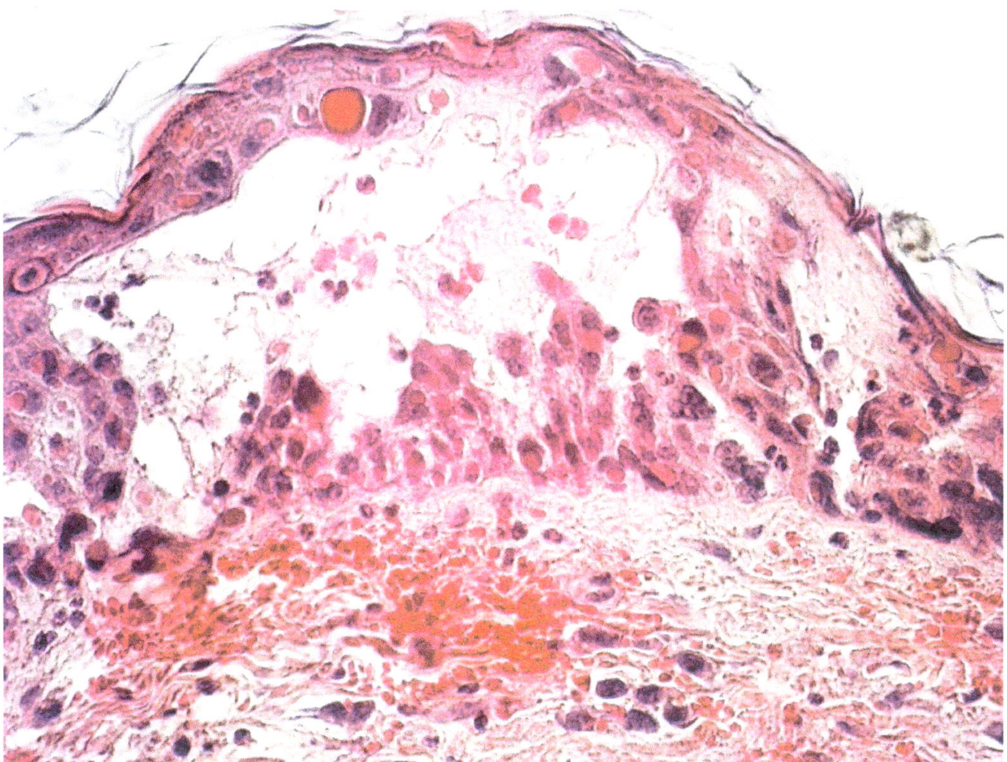

Recently, Johnson and colleagues inoculated fourteen cynomolgus macaques intravenously with different doses of CPXV (5×10^7–5×10^4 PFU) [99]. Nine of fourteen animals developed typical pox skin lesions. Further findings were hemorrhage in lymph nodes, multifocal petechial hemorrhages in the gastrointestinal tract, on heart, lung, kidneys, urinary bladder, and brain. This indicates a hemorrhagic disease course. All monkeys revealed interstitial pneumonia, interstitial nephritis, and hepatitis, and died within 12 days. The researchers conclude that this animal model may serve as a model for hemorrhagic smallpox, which is more feasible than the VARV using model of Jahrling [68].

Song and colleagues tried to find an early biological marker for prognosis of poxvirus infection, as clinical symptoms are not always reliable. Therefore, they infected nine cynomolgus macaques of both sexes intravenously with CPXV of different doses and monitored pox-antigen presence in immune cells by intracellular staining. They found that monocytes and granulocytes are the mainly affected cell population and that the presence of poxvirus antigen in the cells is closely connected to disease course and time of death. Based on these results, they suggest that the technique of monitoring pox-antigen staining in immune cells can be applied in human poxvirus infections to predict disease course and to value the efficacy of new antiviral therapeutics and vaccines [100].

Summary Cowpox

The number of diagnosed CPXV infections is increasing due to the cessation of vaccination against smallpox. Therefore, more research is needed to get a deeper insight into pathogenesis of CPXV infections and to develop antiviral drugs. NHP cowpox models can also be used as a model for hemorrhagic smallpox and have the advantage that CPXV does not need as high biosafety levels as MPXV or VARV and is therefore easier to work with. Cynomolgus macaques have been infected intravenously and intrabronchially with CPXV to study pathogenesis. Common marmosets have been infected intravenously and intranasally. The latter route of infection resembles the natural infection route of smallpox and is therefore a suitable model for the validation of therapeutics and vaccines. Compared to other NHP, common marmosets have several advantages: Their small size allows an easy handling and housing and an inexpensive keeping. Furthermore, they have a high reproduction rate. A disadvantage is that some critical reagents are not available yet for this species.

5. Conclusions

The main cause of NHP studies is to develop models to test new antiviral therapeutics and vaccines and to get a deeper insight into pathogenesis of OPXV infections. To sum up, there exists no NHP model that perfectly represents human disease (see Figure 5). Each model has its advantages and disadvantages. Concerning smallpox research, cynomolgus macaques infected with MPXV are, thus far, the best model for human smallpox [70]. Models, which use VARV, have the advantage that the original causative agent for human smallpox is used—but handling VARV is dangerous and can only be done in two laboratories worldwide.

In the last decades, promising new animal models have been developed, but none of them is good enough to safely predict a response to new therapeutics or vaccines in humans. Thus, there is a need for more research in this area. The next years will lead to interesting new findings concerning OPXV pathogenesis and development of new compounds driven by concerns of bioterrorism and increasing zoonotic potential of OPXV.

Figure 5. Comparison of disease courses in different orthopoxvirus models.

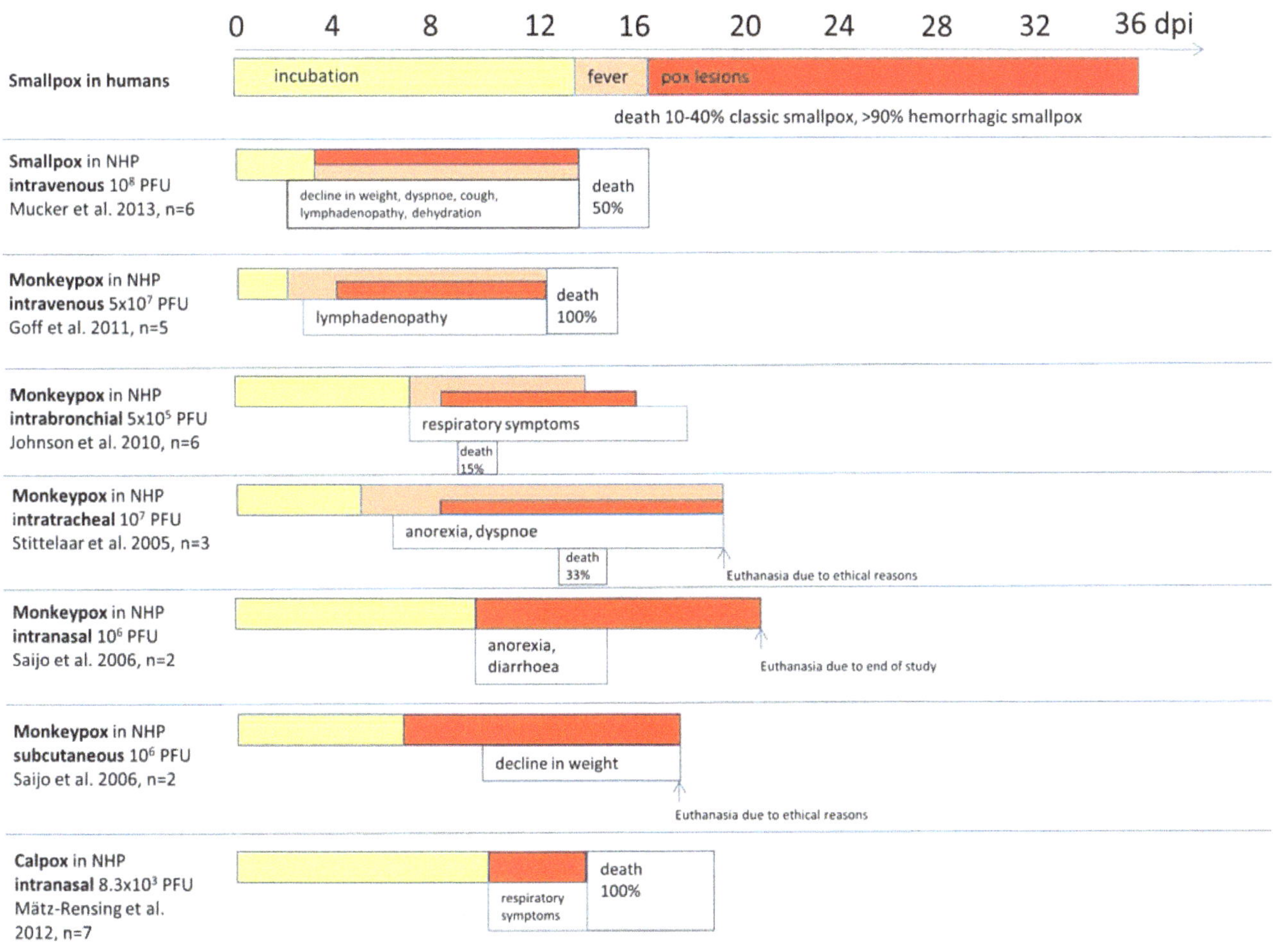

Table 1. Orthopoxvirus models in non-human primates.

Species	Route of Infection	Virus	Dose	Purpose of Study	Reference
M.f. and M.m.	i.m.	MPXV	10^5 PFU	pathogenesis	[33]
P.c.	i.m.	MPXV Copenhagen	$10^{6.5}$–$10^{7.5}$ $TCID_{50}$	pathogenesis	[34]
P.c.	via skin scarification	MPXV	10^7 $TCID_{50}$	pathogenesis	[35]
M.f.	i.v.	MPXV Zaire 79	5×10^7 PFU	Tecovirimat efficacy study	[20]
M.f.	i.v.	MPXV Zaire 79	5×10^7 PFU	Tecovirimat efficacy study	[37]
M.f.	i.v.	MPXV-GFP Zaire 79	5×10^7 PFU	pathogenesis	[38]
M.m.	i.v.	MPXV Zaire 79	5×10^8 PFU	DNA vaccine study	[39]
M.m.	i.v.	MPXV Zaire 79	2×10^7 PFU	MVA/gene based vaccine study	[40]
M.m.	i.v.	MPXV Zaire 79	1.5–2.5 $\times 10^6$ PFU	pathogenesis	[41]
M.f.	i.v. and i.b.	MPXV Zaire 79	5×10^6–5×10^7 PFU	pathogenesis	[42]
M.f.	i.v.	MPXV Zaire 79	5×10^7 PFU	Dryvax/MVA vaccine study	[43]
M.m.	i.v.	MPXV Zaire 79	5×10^7 PFU	Vaccine study in SIV-infected macaques	[44]

Table 1. *Cont.*

Species	Route of Infection	Virus	Dose	Purpose of Study	Reference
M.m.	i.v.	MPXV Zaire 79	5×10^7 PFU	MVA/NYVAC/ Dry-vax vaccine study	[45]
M.m.	i.v.	MPXV Zaire 79	5×10^7 PFU	Subunit recombinant vaccine study	[46]
M.f.	i.v.	MPXV Zaire 79	5×10^7 PFU	Il-15/Wyeth vaccine study	[47]
M.f.	i.t.	MPXV MSF #6	10^6–10^7 PFU in 5 mL	MVA vaccine study	[49]
M.f.	i.t.	MPXV MSF #6	10^7 PFU in 5 mL	Comparison post-exposure vaccination with antiviral therapeutics	[50]
M.f.	via head-only exposure chamber	MPXV Zaire 79	10^4–10^5 PFU	pathogenesis	[51]
M.f.	via head-only exposure chamber	MPXV Zaire 79	4.3×10^4–1.1×10^6 PFU	pathogenesis	[21]
M.f.	via head-only exposure system	MPXV Zaire 79	2.5×10^4–9.3×10^5 PFU	pathogenesis	[52]
M.f.	via Henderson- apparatus and modified anesthesia mask	MPXV Zaire 79	2.1×10^5–3.1×10^5 PFU	Imvamune, Acam2000 vaccine study	[53]
M.f.	bronchoscope and liquid MicroSprayer aerosolizer	MPXV Zaire	3.42×10^6–3.53×10^7 PFU	pathogenesis	[36]
M.m.	i.b.	MPXV Zaire and D14L KO MPXV	2×10^5 PFU	pathogenesis	[54]
M.f.	i.v. and i.b.	MPXV Zaire 79	i.v.: 5×10^7–5×10^4 PFU i.b.: 5×10^6–5×10^4 PFU	pathogenesis	[55]
M.m.	i.b.	MPXV Zaire 79	2×10^5 PFU	pathogenesis	[56]
M.f.	i.n. and subcutaneous	MPXV Liberia and Zaire-559	1×10^6 PFU	LC16m8 vaccine study	[57]
M.f.	i.n. and subcutaneous	MPXV Liberia and Zaire-559	1×10^6 PFU	pathogenesis	[58]
M.m.	via Henderson apparatus	VARV Higgins	?	pathogenesis	[64,66]
M.f.	aerosol	VARV	$>10^8$ PFU	pathogenesis	[67]
M.f.	aerosol and/or i.v.	VARV Harper and India 7124	10^6–10^9 PFU	pathogenesis	[68]
M.f.	aerosol and/or i.v.	VARV Harper and India 7124	Aerosol: 5×10^8 PFU i.v.: 10^9 PFU	pathogenesis	[62]
M.f.	i.v.	VARV Harper	10^8–10^9 PFU	pathogenesis	[69]
M.f.	i.v.	VARV Harper	1×10^8 PFU	ST-246 efficacy study	[20]
M.f.	i.v.	VARV Harper	1×10^8 PFU	ST-246 efficyacy study	[70]
C.j.	i.v. and i.n.	calpox	i.v.: 1.25×10^7–1×10^4 PFU i.n.: 5×10^2–3.5×10^5 PFU	pathogenesis	[93,94]
M.f.	i.b.	CPXV	5×10^7–5×10^4 PFU	pathogenesis	[98]
M.f.	i.v.	CPXV Brighton Red	5×10^7–5×10^5 PFU	pathogenesis	[99]
M.f.	i.v.	CPXV Brighton	5×10^2–5×10^4 PFU	pathogenesis	[100]

M.f.: Macaca fascicularis; M.m.: Macaca mulatta; P.c.: Papio cynocephalus; C.j.: Callithrix jacchus; i.v.: intravenous; i.n.: intranasal; i.b.: intrabronchial; i.t.: intratracheal; PFU: plaque-forming units.

Acknowledgments

We would like to thank Christiane Stahl-Hennig (German Primate Center) and Heinz Ellerbrok (Robert-Koch-Institute) for their collaboration.

Conflicts of Interest

The authors declare no conflict of interest.

References

1. Fenner, F.; Henderson, D.A.; Arita, I.; Jezek, Z.; Ladnyi, I.D. *Variola* virus and other orthopoxviruses. In *Smallpox and Its Eradication*; WHO: Geneva, Switzerland, 1988.
2. Shchelkunov, S.N. An increasing danger of zoonotic orthopoxvirus infections. *PLoS Pathog.* **2013**, *9*, doi:10.1371/journal.ppat.1003756.
3. Nitsche, A. Untersuchungen zur Diagnostik und Risikobewertung von Emerging und Re-Emerging Orthopockenviren in Deutschland. Habilitation Thesis, Robert Koch-Institute, Berlin, Germany, 2010.
4. Cardeti, G.; Brozzi, A.; Eleni, C.; Polici, N.; D'Alterio, G.; Carletti, F.; Scicluna, M.T.; Castilletti, C.; Capobianchi, M.R.; di Caro, A.; *et al.* Cowpox virus in llama, italy. *Emerg. Infect. Dis.* **2011**, *17*, 1513–1515.
5. Bonnekoh, B.; Falk, K.; Reckling, K.F.; Kenklies, S.; Nitsche, A.; Ghebremedhin, B.; Pokrywka, A.; Franke, I.; Thriene, B.; König, W.; *et al.* Cowpox infection transmitted from a domestic cat. *J. Dtsch. Dermatol. Ges.* **2008**, *6*, 210–213.
6. Baxby, D. Cowpox: Increased incidence or interest? *Lancet* **1994**, *343*, 543.
7. Dabrowski, P.W.; Radonic, A.; Kurth, A.; Nitsche, A. Genome-wide comparison of cowpox viruses reveals a new clade related to *variola* virus. *PLoS ONE* **2013**, *8*, doi:10.1371/journal.pone.0079953.
8. Rimoin, A.W.; Mulembakani, P.M.; Johnston, S.C.; Lloyd Smith, J.O.; Kisalu, N.K.; Kinkela, T.L.; Blumberg, S.; Thomassen, H.A.; Pike, B.L.; Fair, J.N.; *et al.* Major increase in human monkeypox incidence 30 years after smallpox vaccination campaigns cease in the democratic republic of congo. *Proc. Natl. Acad. Sci. USA* **2010**, *107*, 16262–16267.
9. Breman, J.G.; Henderson, D.A. Poxvirus dilemmas-monkeypox, smallpox, and biologic terrorism. *N. Engl. J. Med.* **1998**, *339*, 556–559.
10. Jahrling, P.B.; Fritz, E.A.; Hensley, L.E. Countermeasures to the bioterrorist threat of smallpox. *Curr. Mol. Med.* **2005**, *5*, 817–826.
11. Anderson, P.D.; Bokor, G. Bioterrorism: Pathogens as weapons. *J. Pharm. Pract.* **2012**, *25*, 521–529.
12. Hutson, C.L.; Damon, I.K. Monkeypox virus infections in small animal models for evaluation of anti-poxvirus agents. *Viruses* **2010**, *2*, 2763–2776.
13. Safronetz, D.; Geisbert, T.W.; Feldmann, H. Animal models for highly pathogenic emerging viruses. *Curr. Opin. Virol.* **2013**, *3*, 205–209.

14. Jordan, R.; Hruby, D. Smallpox antiviral drug development: Satisfying the animal efficacy rule. *Expert Rev. Anti-Infect. Ther.* **2006**, *4*, 277–289.
15. Parker, S.; Buller, R.M. A review of experimental and natural infections of animals with monkeypox virus between 1958 and 2012. *Future Virol.* **2013**, *8*, 129–157.
16. Chapman, J.L.; Nichols, D.K.; Martinez, M.J.; Raymond, J.W. Animal models of orthopoxvirus infection. *Vet. Pathol.* **2010**, *47*, 852–870.
17. Smee, D.F.; Sidwell, R.W. A review of compounds exhibiting anti-orthopoxvirus activity in animal models. *Antivir. Res.* **2003**, *57*, 41–52.
18. Smee, D.F. Progress in the discovery of compounds inhibiting orthopoxviruses in animal models. *Antivir. Chem. Chemother.* **2008**, *19*, 115–124.
19. Smee, D.F. Orthopoxvirus inhibitors that are active in animal models: An update from 2008 to 2012. *Future Virol.* **2013**, *8*, 891–901.
20. Huggins, J.; Goff, A.; Hensley, L.; Mucker, E.; Shamblin, J.; Wlazlowski, C.; Johnson, W.; Chapman, J.; Larsen, T.; Twenhafel, N.; *et al.* Nonhuman primates are protected from smallpox virus or monkeypox virus challenges by the antiviral drug st-246. *Antimicrob. Agents Chemother.* **2009**, *53*, 2620–2625.
21. Nalca, A.; Livingston, V.A.; Garza, N.L.; Zumbrun, E.E.; Frick, O.M.; Chapman, J.L.; Hartings, J.M. Experimental infection of cynomolgus macaques (*Macaca fascicularis*) with aerosolized monkeypox virus. *PLoS ONE* **2010**, *5*, doi:10.1371/journal.pone.0012880.
22. Jezek, Z.; Szczeniowski, M.; Paluku, K.M.; Mutombo, M. Human monkeypox: Clinical features of 282 patients. *J. Infect. Dis.* **1987**, *156*, 293–298.
23. Reynolds, M.G.; Carroll, D.S.; Karem, K.L. Factors affecting the likelihood of monkeypox's emergence and spread in the post-smallpox era. *Curr. Opin. Virol.* **2012**, *2*, 335–343.
24. McCollum, A.M.; Damon, I.K. Human monkeypox. *Clin. Infect. Dis.* **2014**, *58*, 260–267.
25. Damon, I.K. Status of human monkeypox: Clinical disease, epidemiology and research. *Vaccine* **2011**, *29* (Suppl. 4), D54–D59.
26. Von Magnus, P.; Anderson, E.; Petersen, K.; Birch-Anderson, A. A pox-like disease in cynomolgus monkeys. *Acta Pathol. Microbiol. Scand.* **1959**, *46*, 156–176.
27. Prier, J.E.; Sauer, R.M. A pox disease of monkeys. *Ann. N. Y. Acad. Sci.* **1960**, *85*, 951–959.
28. Khodakevich, L.; Jezek, Z.; Kinzanzka, K. Isolation of monkeypox virus from wild squirrel infected in nature. *Lancet* **1986**, *1*, 98–99.
29. DiGiulio, D.B.; Eckburg, P.B. Monkeypox in the western hemisphere. *N. Engl. J. Med.* **2004**, *350*, 1790–1791; author reply 1790–1791.
30. Reed, K.D.; Melski, J.W.; Graham, M.B.; Regnery, R.L.; Sotir, M.J.; Wegner, M.V.; Kazmierczak, J.J.; Stratman, E.J.; Li, Y.; Fairley, J.A.; *et al.* The detection of monkeypox in humans in the western hemisphere. *N. Engl. J. Med.* **2004**, *350*, 342–350.
31. Centers for Disease, Control and Prevention. Update: Multistate outbreak of monkeypox—Illinois, Indiana, Kansas, Missouri, Ohio, and Wisconsin, 2003. *MMWR. Morb. Mortal. Wkly. Rep.* **2003**, *52*, 642–646.
32. Parker, S.; Nuara, A.; Buller, R.M.; Schultz, D.A. Human monkeypox: An emerging zoonotic disease. *Future Microbiol.* **2007**, *2*, 17–34.

33. Wenner, H.A.; Bolano, C.R.; Cho, C.T.; Kamitsuka, P.S. Studies on the pathogenesis of monkey pox. 3. Histopathological lesions and sites of immunofluorescence. *Arch. Gesamte Virusforsch.* **1969**, *27*, 179–197.
34. Heberling, R.L.; Kalter, S.S. Induction, course, and transmissibility of monkeypox in the baboon (*Papio cynocephalus*). *J. Infect. Dis.* **1971**, *124*, 33–38.
35. Heberling, R.L.; Kalter, S.S.; Rodriguez, A.R. Poxvirus infection of the baboon (*Papio cynocephalus*). *Bull. World Health Organ.* **1976**, *54*, 285–294.
36. Goff, A.J.; Chapman, J.; Foster, C.; Wlazlowski, C.; Shamblin, J.; Lin, K.; Kreiselmeier, N.; Mucker, E.; Paragas, J.; Lawler, J.; *et al.* A novel respiratory model of infection with monkeypox virus in cynomolgus macaques. *J. Virol.* **2011**, *85*, 4898–4909.
37. Jordan, R.; Goff, A.; Frimm, A.; Corrado, M.L.; Hensley, L.E.; Byrd, C.M.; Mucker, E.; Shamblin, J.; Bolken, T.C.; Wlazlowski, C.; *et al.* St-246 antiviral efficacy in a nonhuman primate monkeypox model: Determination of the minimal effective dose and human dose justification. *Antimicrob. Agents Chemother.* **2009**, *53*, 1817–1822.
38. Goff, A.; Mucker, E.; Raymond, J.; Fisher, R.; Bray, M.; Hensley, L.; Paragas, J. Infection of cynomolgus macaques with a recombinant monkeypox virus encoding green fluorescent protein. *Arch. Virol.* **2011**, *156*, 1877–1881.
39. Hooper, J.W.; Thompson, E.; Wilhelmsen, C.; Zimmerman, M.; Ichou, M.A.; Steffen, S.E.; Schmaljohn, C.S.; Schmaljohn, A.L.; Jahrling, P.B. Smallpox DNA vaccine protects nonhuman primates against lethal monkeypox. *J. Virol.* **2004**, *78*, 4433–4443.
40. Golden, J.W.; Josleyn, M.; Mucker, E.M.; Hung, C.F.; Loudon, P.T.; Wu, T.C.; Hooper, J.W. Side-by-side comparison of gene-based smallpox vaccine with MVA in nonhuman primates. *PLoS ONE* **2012**, *7*, doi:10.1371/journal.pone.0042353.
41. Song, H.; Josleyn, N.; Janosko, K.; Skinner, J.; Reeves, R.K.; Cohen, M.; Jett, C.; Johnson, R.; Blaney, J.E.; Bollinger, L.; *et al.* Monkeypox virus infection of rhesus macaques induces massive expansion of natural killer cells but suppresses natural killer cell functions. *PLoS ONE* **2013**, *8*, doi:10.1371/journal.pone.0077804.
42. Dyall, J.; Johnson, R.F.; Chen, D.Y.; Huzella, L.; Ragland, D.R.; Mollura, D.J.; Byrum, R.; Reba, R.C.; Jennings, G.; Jahrling, P.B.; *et al.* Evaluation of monkeypox disease progression by molecular imaging. *J. Infect. Dis.* **2011**, *204*, 1902–1911.
43. Earl, P.L.; Americo, J.L.; Wyatt, L.S.; Espenshade, O.; Bassler, J.; Gong, K.; Lin, S.; Peters, E.; Rhodes, L., Jr.; Spano, Y.E.; *et al.* Rapid protection in a monkeypox model by a single injection of a replication-deficient vaccinia virus. *Proc. Natl. Acad. Sci. USA* **2008**, *105*, 10889–10894.
44. Edghill-Smith, Y.; Bray, M.; Whitehouse, C.A.; Miller, D.; Mucker, E.; Manischewitz, J.; King, L.R.; Robert-Guroff, M.; Hryniewicz, A.; Venzon, D.; *et al.* Smallpox vaccine does not protect macaques with AIDS from a lethal monkeypox virus challenge. *J. Infect. Dis.* **2005**, *191*, 372–381.
45. Edghill-Smith, Y.; Golding, H.; Manischewitz, J.; King, L.R.; Scott, D.; Bray, M.; Nalca, A.; Hooper, J.W.; Whitehouse, C.A.; Schmitz, J.E.; *et al.* Smallpox vaccine-induced antibodies are necessary and sufficient for protection against monkeypox virus. *Nat. Med.* **2005**, *11*, 740–747.

46. Heraud, J.M.; Edghill-Smith, Y.; Ayala, V.; Kalisz, I.; Parrino, J.; Kalyanaraman, V.S.; Manischewitz, J.; King, L.R.; Hryniewicz, A.; Trindade, C.J.; *et al.* Subunit recombinant vaccine protects against monkeypox. *J. Immunol.* **2006**, *177*, 2552–2564.
47. Zielinski, R.J.; Smedley, J.V.; Perera, P.Y.; Silvera, P.M.; Waldmann, T.A.; Capala, J.; Perera, L.P. Smallpox vaccine with integrated il-15 demonstrates enhanced *in vivo* viral clearance in immunodeficient mice and confers long term protection against a lethal monkeypox challenge in cynomolgus monkeys. *Vaccine* **2010**, *28*, 7081–7091.
48. Arita, I.; Jezek, Z.; Khodakevich, L.; Ruti, K. Human monkeypox: A newly emerged orthopoxvirus zoonosis in the tropical rain forests of africa. *Am. J. Trop. Med. Hyg.* **1985**, *34*, 781–789.
49. Stittelaar, K.J.; van Amerongen, G.; Kondova, I.; Kuiken, T.; van Lavieren, R.F.; Pistoor, F.H.; Niesters, H.G.; van Doornum, G.; van der Zeijst, B.A.; Mateo, L.; *et al.* Modified vaccinia virus ankara protects macaques against respiratory challenge with monkeypox virus. *J. Virol.* **2005**, *79*, 7845–7851.
50. Stittelaar, K.J.; Neyts, J.; Naesens, L.; van Amerongen, G.; van Lavieren, R.F.; Holy, A.; de Clercq, E.; Niesters, H.G.; Fries, E.; Maas, C.; *et al.* Antiviral treatment is more effective than smallpox vaccination upon lethal monkeypox virus infection. *Nature* **2006**, *439*, 745–748.
51. Zaucha, G.M.; Jahrling, P.B.; Geisbert, T.W.; Swearengen, J.R.; Hensley, L. The pathology of experimental aerosolized monkeypox virus infection in cynomolgus monkeys (*Macaca fascicularis*). *Lab. Investig.* **2001**, *81*, 1581–1600.
52. Barnewall, R.E.; Fisher, D.A.; Robertson, A.B.; Vales, P.A.; Knostman, K.A.; Bigger, J.E. Inhalational monkeypox virus infection in cynomolgus macaques. *Front. Cell. Infect. Microbiol.* **2012**, *2*, 117.
53. Hatch, G.J.; Graham, V.A.; Bewley, K.R.; Tree, J.A.; Dennis, M.; Taylor, I.; Funnell, S.G.; Bate, S.R.; Steeds, K.; Tipton, T.; *et al.* Assessment of the protective effect of Imvamune and Acam2000 vaccines against aerosolized monkeypox virus in cynomolgus macaques. *J. Virol.* **2013**, *87*, 7805–7815.
54. Estep, R.D.; Messaoudi, I.; O’Connor, M.A.; Li, H.; Sprague, J.; Barron, A.; Engelmann, F.; Yen, B.; Powers, M.F.; Jones, J.M.; *et al.* Deletion of the monkeypox virus inhibitor of complement enzymes locus impacts the adaptive immune response to monkeypox virus in a nonhuman primate model of infection. *J. Virol.* **2011**, *85*, 9527–9542.
55. Johnson, R.F.; Dyall, J.; Ragland, D.R.; Huzella, L.; Byrum, R.; Jett, C.; St Claire, M.; Smith, A.L.; Paragas, J.; Blaney, J.E.; *et al.* Comparative analysis of monkeypox virus infection of cynomolgus macaques by the intravenous or intrabronchial inoculation route. *J. Virol.* **2011**, *85*, 2112–2125.
56. Brown, J.N.; Estep, R.D.; Lopez-Ferrer, D.; Brewer, H.M.; Clauss, T.R.; Manes, N.P.; O’Connor, M.; Li, H.; Adkins, J.N.; Wong, S.W.; *et al.* Characterization of macaque pulmonary fluid proteome during monkeypox infection: Dynamics of host response. *Mol. Cell. Proteomics* **2010**, *9*, 2760–2771.

57. Saijo, M.; Ami, Y.; Suzaki, Y.; Nagata, N.; Iwata, N.; Hasegawa, H.; Ogata, M.; Fukushi, S.; Mizutani, T.; Sata, T.; *et al.* Lc16m8, a highly attenuated vaccinia virus vaccine lacking expression of the membrane protein b5r, protects monkeys from monkeypox. *J. Virol.* **2006**, *80*, 5179–5188.
58. Saijo, M.; Ami, Y.; Suzaki, Y.; Nagata, N.; Iwata, N.; Hasegawa, H.; Iizuka, I.; Shiota, T.; Sakai, K.; Ogata, M.; *et al.* Virulence and pathophysiology of the congo basin and west african strains of monkeypox virus in non-human primates. *J. Gen. Virol.* **2009**, *90*, 2266–2271.
59. Olsen, R.G.; Blakeslee, J.R.; Mathes, L.; Nakano, J.H. Preparation and evaluation of a noninfectious monkey pox virus vaccine. *J. Clin. Microbiol.* **1977**, *6*, 50–54.
60. Sauer, R.M.; Prier, J.E.; Buchanan, R.S.; Creamer, A.A.; Fegley, H.C. Studies on a pox disease of monkeys. I. Pathology. *Am. J. Vet. Res.* **1960**, *21*, 377–380.
61. Cann, J.A.; Jahrling, P.B.; Hensley, L.E.; Wahl-Jensen, V. Comparative pathology of smallpox and monkeypox in man and macaques. *J. Comp. Pathol.* **2013**, *148*, 6–21.
62. Rubins, K.H.; Hensley, L.E.; Jahrling, P.B.; Whitney, A.R.; Geisbert, T.W.; Huggins, J.W.; Owen, A.; Leduc, J.W.; Brown, P.O.; Relman, D.A. The host response to smallpox: Analysis of the gene expression program in peripheral blood cells in a nonhuman primate model. *Proc. Natl. Acad. Sci. USA* **2004**, *101*, 15190–15195.
63. Brinckerhoff, W.R.; Tyzzer, E.E. Studies upon experimental *variola* in monkeys (*Macacus cynomologus* and *Macaca nemestrinus*) and in the orang utan (*Simia satyrus*): Part II. *J. Med. Res.* **1906**, *14*, 263–320.
64. Hahon, N.; Wilson, B.J. Pathogenesis of *variola* in Macaca irus monkeys. *Am. J. Hyg.* **1960**, *71*, 69–80.
65. Westwood, J.C.; Boulter, E.A.; Bowen, E.T.; Maber, H.B. Experimental respiratory infection with poxviruses. I. Clinical virological and epidemiological studies. *Br. J. Exp. Pathol.* **1966**, *47*, 453–465.
66. Lancaster, M.C.; Boulter, E.A.; Westwood, J.C.; Randles, J. Experimental respiratory infection with poxviruses. Pathological studies. *Br. J. Exp. Pathol.* **1966**, *47*, 466–471.
67. LeDuc, J.W.; Jahrling, P.B. Strengthening national preparedness for smallpox: An update. *Emerg. Infect. Dis.* **2001**, *7*, 155–157.
68. Jahrling, P.B.; Hensley, L.E.; Martinez, M.J.; Leduc, J.W.; Rubins, K.H.; Relman, D.A.; Huggins, J.W. Exploring the potential of *variola* virus infection of cynomolgus macaques as a model for human smallpox. *Proc. Natl. Acad. Sci. USA* **2004**, *101*, 15196–15200.
69. Wahl-Jensen, V.; Cann, J.A.; Rubins, K.H.; Huggins, J.W.; Fisher, R.W.; Johnson, A.J.; de Kok-Mercado, F.; Larsen, T.; Raymond, J.L.; Hensley, L.E.; *et al.* Progression of pathogenic events in cynomolgus macaques infected with *variola* virus. *PLoS ONE* **2011**, *6*, doi:10.1371/journal.pone.0024832.
70. Mucker, E.M.; Goff, A.J.; Shamblin, J.D.; Grosenbach, D.W.; Damon, I.K.; Mehal, J.M.; Holman, R.C.; Carroll, D.; Gallardo, N.; Olson, V.A.; *et al.* Efficacy of Tecovirimat (ST-246) in nonhuman primates infected with *variola* virus (smallpox). *Antimicrob. Agents Chemother.* **2013**, *57*, 6246–6253.
71. Alzhanova, D.; Fruh, K. Modulation of the host immune response by cowpox virus. *Microbes Infect.* **2010**, *12*, 900–909.

72. Wolfs, T.F.; Wagenaar, J.A.; Niesters, H.G.; Osterhaus, A.D. Rat-to-human transmission of cowpox infection. *Emerg. Infect. Dis.* **2002**, *8*, 1495–1496.
73. Postma, B.H.; Diepersloot, R.J.; Niessen, G.J.; Droog, R.P. Cowpox-virus-like infection associated with rat bite. *Lancet* **1991**, *337*, 733–734.
74. Becker, C.; Kurth, A.; Hessler, F.; Kramp, H.; Gokel, M.; Hoffmann, R.; Kuczka, A.; Nitsche, A. Cowpox virus infection in pet rat owners: Not always immediately recognized. *Dtsch. Ärztebl. Int.* **2009**, *106*, 329–334.
75. Campe, H.; Zimmermann, P.; Glos, K.; Bayer, M.; Bergemann, H.; Dreweck, C.; Graf, P.; Weber, B.K.; Meyer, H.; Büttner, M.; *et al.* Cowpox virus transmission from pet rats to humans, germany. *Emerg. Infect. Dis.* **2009**, *15*, 777–780.
76. Baxby, D.; Bennett, M.; Getty, B. Human cowpox 1969–93: A review based on 54 cases. *Br. J. Dermatol.* **1994**, *131*, 598–607.
77. Schwarzer, H.; Kurth, A.; Hermel, M.; Plange, N. Severe ulcerative keratitis in ocular cowpox infection. *Graefe's Arch. Clin. Exp. Ophthalmol.* **2013**, *251*, 1451–1452.
78. Hall, C.J.; Stevens, J.D. Ocular cowpox. *Lancet* **1987**, *1*, 111.
79. Dugmore, W.N.; Dabir, Z.M. Cowpox virus. *Br. J. Ophthalmol.* **1992**, *76*, 510.
80. Blackford, S.; Roberts, D.L.; Thomas, P.D. Cowpox infection causing a generalized eruption in a patient with atopic dermatitis. *Br. J. Ophthalmol.* **1993**, *129*, 628–629.
81. Eis-Hubinger, A.M.; Gerritzen, A.; Schneweis, K.E.; Pfeiff, B.; Pullmann, H.; Mayr, A.; Czerny, C.P. Fatal cowpox-like virus infection transmitted by cat. *Lancet* **1990**, *336*, 880.
82. Pelkonen, P.M.; Tarvainen, K.; Hynninen, A.; Kallio, E.R.; Henttonen, K.; Palva, A.; Vaheri, A.; Vapalahti, O. Cowpox with severe generalized eruption, Finland. *Emerg. Infect. Dis.* **2003**, *9*, 1458–1461.
83. Czerny, C.P.; Eis-Hübinger, A.M.; Mayr, A.; Schneweis, K.E.; Pfeiff, B. Animal poxviruses transmitted from cat to man: Current event with lethal end. *Zentralbl. Veterinärmed. B* **1991**, *38*, 421–431.
84. Klingebiel, T.; Vallbracht, A.; Doller, G.; Stierhof, Y.D.; Gerth, H.J.; Glashauser, E.; Herzau, V. A severe human cowpox infection in south germany. *Pediatr. Infect. Dis. J.* **1988**, *7*, 883–885.
85. Baxby, D. Is cowpox misnamed? A review of 10 human cases. *Br. Med. J.* **1977**, *1*, 1379–1381.
86. Essbauer, S.; Pfeffer, M.; Meyer, H. Zoonotic poxviruses. *Vet. Microbiol.* **2010**, *140*, 229–236.
87. Kinnunen, P.M.; Henttonen, H.; Hoffmann, B.; Kallio, E.R.; Korthase, C.; Laakkonen, J.; Niemimaa, J.; Palva, A.; Schlegel, M.; Ali, H.S.; *et al.* Orthopox virus infections in eurasian wild rodents. *Vector Borne Zoonotic Dis.* **2011**, *11*, 1133–1140.
88. Coras, B.; Essbauer, S.; Pfeffer, M.; Meyer, H.; Schroder, J.; Stolz, W.; Landthaler, M.; Vogt, T. Cowpox and a cat. *Lancet* **2005**, *365*, 446.
89. Kurth, A.; Wibbelt, G.; Gerber, H.P.; Petschaelis, A.; Pauli, G.; Nitsche, A. Rat-to-elephant-to-human transmission of cowpox virus. *Emerg. Infect. Dis.* **2008**, *14*, 670–671.
90. Wisser, J.; Pilaski, J.; Strauss, G.; Meyer, H.; Burck, G.; Truyen, U.; Rudolph, M.; Frölich, K. Cowpox virus infection causing stillbirth in an asian elephant (*Elephas maximus*). *Vet. Rec.* **2001**, *149*, 244–246.

91. Martina, B.E.; van Doornum, G.; Dorrestein, G.M.; Niesters, H.G.; Stittelaar, K.J.; Wolters, M.A.; van Bolhuis, H.G.; Osterhaus, A.D. Cowpox virus transmission from rats to monkeys, The Netherlands. *Emerg. Infect. Dis.* **2006**, *12*, 1005–1007.
92. Mätz-Rensing, K.; Ellerbrok, H.; Ehlers, B.; Pauli, G.; Floto, A.; Alex, M.; Czerny, C.P.; Kaup, F.J. Fatal poxvirus outbreak in a colony of new world monkeys. *Vet. Pathol.* **2006**, *43*, 212–218.
93. Kramski, M.; Mätz-Rensing, K.; Stahl-Hennig, C.; Kaup, F.J.; Nitsche, A.; Pauli, G.; Ellerbrok, H. A novel highly reproducible and lethal nonhuman primate model for orthopox virus infection. *PLoS ONE* **2010**, *5*, doi:10.1371/journal.pone.0010412.
94. Mätz-Rensing, K.; Stahl-Hennig, C.; Kramski, M.; Pauli, G.; Ellerbrok, H.; Kaup, F.J. The pathology of experimental poxvirus infection in common marmosets (*Callithrix jacchus*): Further characterization of a new primate model for orthopoxvirus infections. *J. Comp. Pathol.* **2012**, *146*, 230–242.
95. Abbott, D.H.; Barnett, D.K.; Colman, R.J.; Yamamoto, M.E.; Schultz-Darken, N.J. Aspects of common marmorset basic biology and life history important for biomedical research. *Comp. Med.* **2003**, *53*, 339–350.
96. Vorou, R.M.; Papavassiliou, V.G.; Pierroutsakos, I.N. Cowpox virus infection: An emerging health threat. *Curr. Opin. Infect. Dis.* **2008**, *21*, 153–156.
97. Seet, B.T.; Johnston, J.B.; Brunetti, C.R.; Barrett, J.W.; Everett, H.; Cameron, C.; Sypula, J.; Nazarian, S.H.; Lucas, A.; McFadden, G. Poxviruses and immune evasion. *Annu. Rev. Immunol.* **2003**, *21*, 377–423.
98. Smith, A.L.; St Claire, M.; Yellayi, S.; Bollinger, L.; Jahrling, P.B.; Paragas, J.; Blaney, J.E.; Johnson, R.F. Intrabronchial inoculation of cynomolgus macaques with cowpox virus. *J. Gen. Virol.* **2012**, *93*, 159–164.
99. Johnson, R.F.; Yellayi, S.; Cann, J.A.; Johnson, A.; Smith, A.L.; Paragas, J.; Jahrling, P.B.; Blaney, J.E. Cowpox virus infection of cynomolgus macaques as a model of hemorrhagic smallpox. *Virology* **2011**, *418*, 102–112.
100. Song, H.; Janosko, K.; Johnson, R.F.; Qin, J.; Josleyn, N.; Jett, C.; Byrum, R.; St Claire, M.; Dyall, J.; Blaney, J.E.; *et al.* Poxvirus antigen staining of immune cells as a biomarker to predict disease outcome in monkeypox and cowpox virus infection in non-human primates. *PLoS ONE* **2013**, *8*, doi:10.1371/journal.pone.0060533.

5

Medical Management of Cyclosporine-Induced Gingival Overgrowth Using Oral Azithromycin in Six Dogs

Alison Diesel [1,*] and Karen Moriello [2]

[1] Department of Small Animal Clinical Sciences, College of Veterinary Medicine and Biomedical Sciences, Texas A&M University, College Station, TX 77843, USA

[2] Department of Medical Sciences, School of Veterinary Medicine, 2015 Linden Drive West, University of Wisconsin, Madison, WI 53706, USA; E-Mail: moriellk@svm.vetmed.wisc.edu

* Author to whom correspondence should be addressed; E-Mail: adiesel@cvm.tamu.edu;

Academic Editors: Duncan Ferguson and Margarethe Hoenig

Abstract: Gingival overgrowth is an uncommon adverse effect of cyclosporine administration in veterinary species. In people, gingival overgrowth is a common complication of cyclosporine administration for immunosuppression, generally following transplant procedures. Azithromycin has been used successfully for managing gingival overgrowth in human transplant patients when cyclosporine administration cannot be reduced or discontinued. This case series describes six dogs being administered cyclosporine for various dermatologic diseases that developed gingival overgrowth. The dogs were prescribed systemic azithromycin, with or without concurrent dose reduction of cyclosporine. Oral administration of 6.6–10.8 mg/kg of azithromycin once daily for 4–14 weeks was effective for complete clinical resolution of gingival overgrowth. In most cases, gingival overgrowth did not recur even with continued cyclosporine administration long-term. Adverse events of long-term azithromycin administration did not occur in any of the dogs. This series highlights a potentially beneficial medical treatment option for gingival overgrowth even when cyclosporine dose reduction is not possible or elected, without the need for surgical resection of proliferative gingival tissue.

Keywords: cyclosporine; gingival overgrowth; azithromycin; dog

---

1. Introduction

Cyclosporine is an immunosuppressive medication used to treat a variety of dermatological diseases in veterinary medication. This calcinurin inhibitor works by binding cyclophilin in the cytoplasm of primarily T cells which thereby inhibits activation. This results in decreased production of various inflammatory cytokines including interleukin (IL)-2, 3, 4 and tumor necrosis factor alpha. The drug was originally designed for use in human transplant patients and has been used since the 1970s [1]. Human formulations have been used in veterinary medicine since the 1980s [2], however it wasn't until 2003 that the first veterinary approved product (Atopica®, Novartis Animal Health) was available. The modified form is absorbed more effectively and predictably in small animals leading to enhanced bioavailability [3]. Although the most common adverse effects reported in veterinary patients are gastrointestinal issues (vomiting, diarrhea, nausea, anorexia), numerous other complications with cyclosporine therapy have been noted [3].

Gingival overgrowth is a well-documented side effect of cyclosporine administration in both dogs and people [3–8]. The exact incidence of occurrence is unknown, but is thought to affect approximately 2%–3% of canine patients treated for atopic dermatitis with the medication [3,9]. At higher dose levels, incidence has been reported as high as 75% [6]. Duration of therapy, genetics, and breed factors have also been purported to play a role in development of cyclosporine-induced gingival overgrowth. Other than cosmetic concerns, gingival overgrowth can result in the formation of dental pseudopockets resulting in plaque accumulation and potential tooth detachment [10]. Additionally, pain and difficulty chewing along with gingival bleeding have also been noted in canine patients [6]. Historically, cyclosporine dose reduction and/or surgical resection of excess gingival tissue have been considered to be the best option for management of gingival overgrowth in canine patients.

In people, gingival overgrowth is a common complication of cyclosporine administration for immunosuppression, generally following transplant procedures. Azithromycin has been used successfully in managing gingival overgrowth in humans when cyclosporine administration cannot be reduced or discontinued [11,12]. This macrolide (azalid family) antibiotic is thought to reduce gingival overgrowth by means of antimicrobial effects, reduction of inflammation, and possible disruption of protein synthesis by fibroblasts [13]. A single study exists in the veterinary literature evaluating the use of azithromycin (both as an oral capsule and toothpaste form) for management of cyclosporine-induced gingival overgrowth in dogs [14]. In this prospective study, only a single parameter (gingival sulcus depth) was improved with a four week administration of azithromycin, however a single dog did experience complete resolution of gingival overgrowth during the study time period (eight weeks).

The purpose of this retrospective case series is to review the records of dogs that had been treated with oral azithromycin (Zithromax®; Pfizer, New York, NY, USA) for cyclosporine-induced gingival overgrowth prior to the publication of the more recent prospective study. All cases of cyclosporine-induced gingival overgrowth seen by the authors over a five year time frame were included in the review. As much of the evidence regarding this option was previously anecdotal, additional cases were used to further evaluate the potential benefit of this alternative medical therapy over surgical correction, particularly in cases where cyclosporine administration was continued long-term for disease management.

2. Case Series

2.1. Case #1

A four-year, 26.4 kg female spayed golden retriever dog was presented for atopic dermatitis. Her primary care veterinarian had initiated therapy with modified cyclosporine (human generic) 3.8 mg/kg once daily and concurrent ketoconazole 3.8 mg/kg once daily approximately nine months prior to presentation on referral. The dog presented after owners noted severe halitosis, excessive drooling, "disappearance of her teeth", and gingival bleeding. The dog's appetite was not affected. Oral examination revealed marked gingival overgrowth with gingivitis affecting the entire oral cavity. Gingival tissue had proliferated to cover incisors, premolars and molars over all dental arcades (Figure 1a,b).

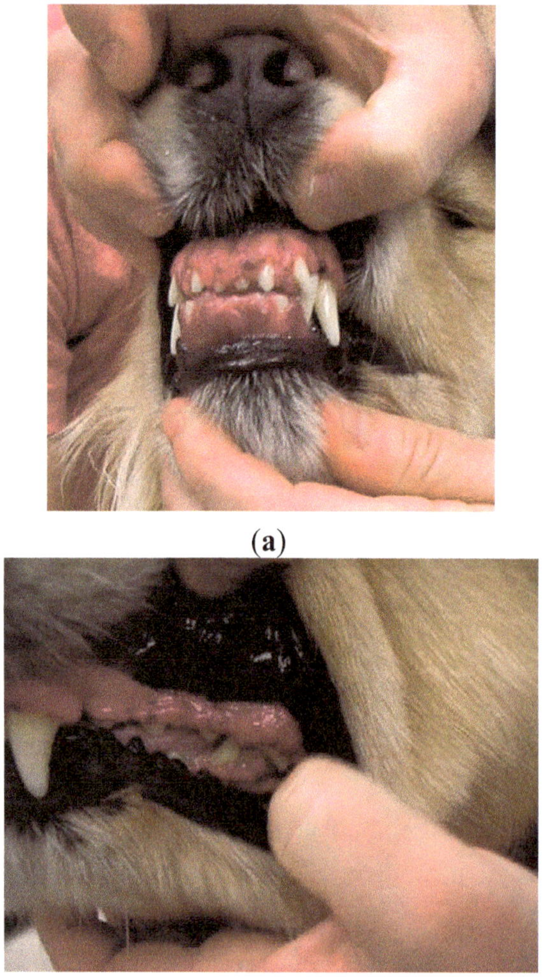

(a)

(b)

Figure 1. Case #1—Severe gingival overgrowth over the upper and lower incisors (**a**); and premolars and molars (**b**) prior to initiating azithromycin therapy.

Intradermal allergy testing was pursued and allergen-specific immunotherapy (ASIT; injectable) was formulated; however due to marked improvement in the dog's pruritus, the owner requested to continue cyclosporine administration pending ASIT benefits. Both cyclosporine and ketoconazole were changed to alternate day administration. In addition, azithromycin was initiated at 9.6 mg/kg orally once daily.

At week 4, there was marked improvement in gingival overgrowth as evidenced by less gingival hyperemia and increased visibility of teeth on all arcades (photographed to document visual changes at each visit); however persistent evidence of excessive gingival tissue over the molars was seen. All treatments were continued unchanged. At week 10, gingival overgrowth was still improving. Lower incisors were visible and only mild excessive gingival tissue over upper molars was noted. Azithromycin was continued for an additional 4 weeks at which time full clinical resolution of gingival overgrowth was noted; the dog received a total of 14 weeks of azithromycin therapy. The dog was followed for over six years; gingival overgrowth has not recurred with continued cyclosporine administration (no further dose adjustments) (Figure 2a,b).

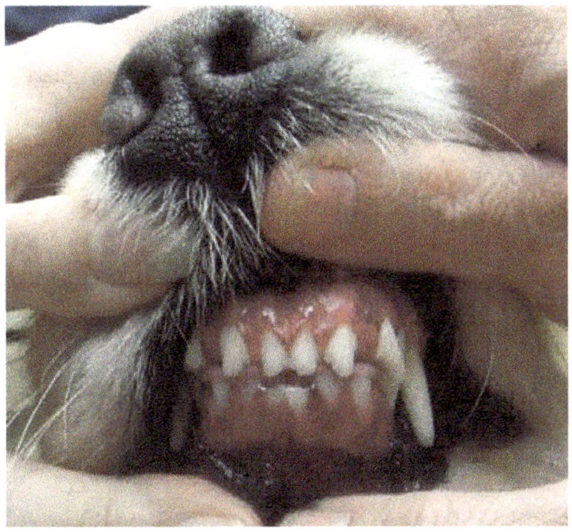

(a)

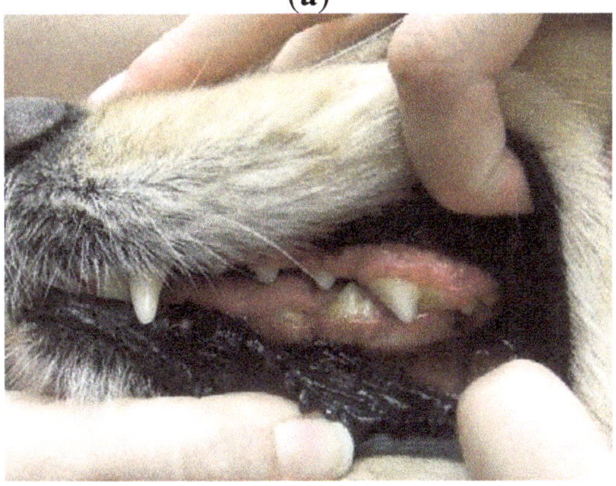

(b)

Figure 2. Same dog as in Figure 1(a,b), showing complete clinical remission of gingival overgrowth following 14 weeks of continued azithromycin administration.

2.2. Case #2

A 2.5 year, 13.6 kg male castrated Pembroke Welsh corgi dog presented for a follow up examination of atopic dermatitis which had not responded to ASIT after one year of administration. The dog responded favorably to prednisone 0.2–0.4 mg/kg every other day; however the owner was concerned with long-term side effects of continued corticosteroid administration. Modified cyclosporine (human generic) therapy was initiated at a dose of 5.5 mg/kg once daily.

At a nine month follow up examination, moderate gingival overgrowth was noted over all dental arcades, particularly the molars. The owners had not noted this adverse effect however, as the dog did not show any evidence of oral discomfort. Cyclosporine was reduced to 3.7 mg/kg once daily and azithromycin was initiated at 9.3 mg/kg orally once daily. After 12 weeks of azithromycin administration, complete clinical resolution of gingival overgrowth was noted. Cyclosporine administration was continued at the current dose.

Approximately one year later, the dog presented for an annual examination. Mild-moderate gingival overgrowth was again noted over all arcades; excessive gingival tissue extended to almost completely cover the molars and premolars. Azithromycin therapy was repeated; the dog however had lost weight (2 kg) over the last year resulting in an oral azithromycin dose of 10.8 mg/kg once daily. The cyclosporine dose remained the same. Complete clinical resolution of gingival overgrowth was noted after 8 weeks. Recurrence was not noted with continued cyclosporine administration (dose unchanged) over a course of over four years.

2.3. Case #3

A three year, 40 kg male castrated German shepherd dog was presented for presumed atopic dermatitis. At the time, corticosteroid administration could not be withdrawn to pursue intradermal allergy testing due to the severity of the dog's pruritus. Modified cyclosporine (human generic) 5 mg/kg once daily was prescribed. After six weeks of administration, the owners were able to reduce the dose to 2.5 mg/kg once daily to achieve the same clinical effect. Due to marked improvement in the dog's comfort, the owners elected not to pursue additional allergy testing or allergen specific immunotherapy.

At one year follow-up examination, the dog was reported to be comfortable while receiving cyclosporine 2.5 mg/kg daily. The previous month however, the dog's primary care veterinarian had noted moderate gingival overgrowth (biopsy confirmed gingival hyperplasia) when the dog was presented for evaluation of oral bleeding when chewing on toys. On examination, there was moderate gingival overgrowth over all dental arcades with pronounced excessive tissue over premolars and molars. Azithromycin 6.6 mg/kg once daily was prescribed with continued cyclosporine administration (dose unchanged). Moderate improvement in gingival overgrowth was noted by week 4 and complete clinical resolution by week 6. Recurrence was not noted one year later with continued cyclosporine administration.

2.4. Case #4

An eight year, 28 kg castrated male Labrador retriever dog was presented for a follow up examination of atopic dermatitis. The dog had failed to respond to ASIT, and the pruritus was being managed with modified cyclosporine (Atopica®, Novartis Animal Health) 5.3 mg/kg on alternate days for greater than two years. On examination, moderate gingival overgrowth was present along the upper molars and premolars. Azithromycin was prescribed 8.9 mg/kg orally once daily. Complete clinical resolution of gingival overgrowth was appreciated after 6 weeks. Even with continued cyclosporine administration (dose unchanged), recurrence was not seen for over three years.

2.5. Case #5

A nine year, 14.1 kg male castrated Boston terrier dog was presented for a follow up examination of atopic dermatitis. After failing to respond to ASIT, the dog had been managed with cyclosporine

(Atopica®, Novartis Animal Health) administration. Initial dosing of 5 mg/kg once daily had been reduced to 1.8 mg/kg once daily for one year. During that time however, the dog developed severe gingival overgrowth (biopsy confirmed gingival hyperplasia) and the primary care veterinarian performed surgical resection. Moderate gingival overgrowth remained after surgery, impairing the dog's ability to eat comfortably. When the dog presented for re-evaluation of allergy management on referral, azithromycin was prescribed 8.9 mg/kg once daily; complete clinical resolution was noted by week 7. Recurrence was not noted even with continued cyclosporine administration (dose unchanged) for over a year. Eventually however the owner discontinued cyclosporine administration after initiation of sublingual immunotherapy successfully managed the dog's pruritus from atopic dermatitis.

2.6. Case #6

A nine year, 32 kg male castrated German shepherd dog was presented for evaluation of a perianal fistula. On examination, a single 1cm diameter draining tract was found which extended into the perianal tissue. No communication with the rectum or anal glands was noted. Modified cyclosporine (human generic) 4.6 mg/kg twice daily and ketoconazole 6.3 mg/kg once daily were administered concurrently; dramatic improvement in the clinical appearance was noted within 1–2 weeks of initiation of therapy.

At week 6, there was marked clinical improvement of perianal fistula, however the dog had developed a focal firm swelling of gingival tissue at the rostral maxilla. Biopsy confirmed gingival hyperplasia. Due to the clinical improvement in perianal fistula, the cyclosporine dose was reduced to 4.6 mg/kg once daily with continued concurrent ketoconazole administration. Azithromycin was prescribed 7.8 mg/kg orally once daily. After 4 weeks of therapy, gingival overgrowth showed complete clinical resolution. Dose reduction was continued for cyclosporine until the perianal fistula completely healed, however the lesion eventually returned. Re-initiation of cyclosporine therapy 4.6 mg/kg daily again resulted in resolution of perianal fistula without recurrence of gingival overgrowth for over one year.

3. Results and Discussion

The signalment and case specific details are summarized in Table 1. This case series describes canine patients successfully treated for cyclosporine-induced gingival overgrowth with systemic azithromycin administration without the need for surgical resection; the duration of azithromycin therapy was variable ranging from 4 to 14 weeks. In most cases, gingival overgrowth occurred at cyclosporine doses below what is typically used for induction of management of atopic dermatitis (e.g., 5 mg/kg/day), confirming the fact that gingival overgrowth can occur even at low doses in some dogs. All dogs experienced complete clinical remission long-term, documented with prolonged follow-up. Although valid concern exists regarding the use of antibiotics for anti-inflammatory purposes as a contributing factor to the development of bacterial antibiotic resistance, risk is relatively low due to maintained remission long-term without the need for continued antimicrobial therapy.

Table 1. Signalment and summary of case specific details.

Case Number	Age, Sex, Breed	Underlying Disease	Duration of CsA Therapy at Diagnosis (Months)	Dose of CsA at Diagnosis (mg/kg)	Changes in CsA Dose Post Diagnosis	Concurrent Drugs During Treatment	Azithromycin Dose	Weeks to Clinical Remission	Follow-Up	Relapse
1	FS, 4 year, golden retriever	AD	9	3.8 q24h	Changed interval to q48 h	Ketoconazole 3.8 mg/kg/day	9.6 mg/kg/day	14 weeks	6 year	No
2	MC, 2.5 year, Pembroke Welsh corgi	AD, failed ASIT	9	5.5 q24h; 4.3 q24h (at time of GO recurrence)	Decrease to 3.7 mg/kg/day; None	None	9.3 mg/kg/day; 10.8 mg/kg/day	12 weeks; 8weeks	4 year	Yes at 1 year, remission induced within 8 weeks of retreatment
3	MC, 3 year, German shepherd	AD	12	2.5 q24h	None	None	6.6 mg/kg/day	6 weeks	1 year	No
4	MC, 8 year Labrador retriever	AD, failed ASIT	24	5.3 q48h	None	None	8.9 mg/kg/day	6 weeks	3 year	No
5	MC, 9 year Boston terrier	AD, failed ASIT	12	1.8 q24h	None	None	8.9 mg/kg/day	7 weeks	1 year; CsA eventually discontinued due to favorable response to SLIT	No
6	MC, 9 year, German shepherd	Perianal Fistula	1.5	4.6 q12h	Decrease CsA to once a day	Ketoconazole 6.3 mg/kg/day	7.8 mg/kg/day	4 weeks	1 year	No

Abbreviations: AD = atopic dermatitis; ASIT = allergen-specific immunotherapy (injectable); CsA = cyclosporine; GO = gingival overgrowth; SLIT = sublingual immunotherapy.

Gingival overgrowth is a reported rare adverse effect of cyclosporine administration in veterinary species. Several reports have noted this adverse finding; however gingival overgrowth was generally reported at dosages much higher than those used for dermatologic conditions (*i.e.*, anywhere from 15–30 mg/kg) [3]. Onset and occurrence of gingival overgrowth may be associated with elevated cyclosporine levels in the blood; trough levels maintained above 400–700 ng/mL for at least 32 weeks resulted in marked gingival overgrowth in a canine renal transplant model [6]. In most cases, cyclosporine levels are not measured when treating veterinary dermatological diseases; rather, clinical improvement is used as therapeutic monitoring. None of the reported cases in this series had cyclosporine drug concentrations evaluated. It would be interesting however to determine whether patients that develop gingival overgrowth secondary to cyclosporine administration also have documented elevations in serum cyclosporine concentrations, even when administered low doses of the medication.

In people, gingival overgrowth is a well-documented complication of organ transplant patients being administered cyclosporine as part of anti-rejection therapy. Studies indicate that 21%–35% of renal transplant patients are affected [7]. Various antibiotics have been used for treatment of gingival overgrowth in people, particularly those of the azalid family. Azithromycin administration at 500 mg per day for three consecutive days has shown particularly successful results in reduction of gingival overgrowth; this is the most commonly prescribed therapeutic regime in people [11]. Although the exact reason for clinical benefit is uncertain, beneficial response may be due in part to the ability of azithromycin to block cyclosporine-induced cell proliferation and collagen synthesis while activating matrix metalloproteinase-2 in gingival fibroblasts, thereby reducing hyperplastic lesions [15]. Down-regulation of transforming growth factors (TGF) may also contribute to decreased overgrowth [16]; several studies have documented increased levels of TGFβ110 and TGFβ211 in patients with cyclosporine-induced gingival overgrowth. Additionally, the antimicrobial effects and decreased inflammation secondary to concurrent infection likely plays a role in clinical improvement. The mechanism of development of cyclosporine-associated gingival overgrowth however has not been well documented in dogs.

Long-term administration of azithromycin did not cause any adverse effects in any of the dogs treated. In people, there has not been evidence to show that azithromycin inhibits the cytochrome P450 enzyme system [17], although a single case report has noted a potential interaction leading to elevated cyclosporine blood levels in a man administered intravenous azithromycin [18]. Evidence is unclear however whether azithromycin or another concurrently administered medication led to elevated cyclosporine blood levels in this patient. It is clear that other macrolide antibiotics (e.g., erythromycin, clarithromycin) can competitively bind the cytochrome P450 enzyme resulting in increased circulating serum cyclosporine concentration, however this does not appear to be the case with the azalid subclass (e.g., azithromycin). Never the less, given the possibility of interaction of these two medications (albeit rather unlikely), side effects of increased cyclosporine concentrations should be monitored in dogs receiving the medications concurrently.

Significant clinical improvement of gingival overgrowth was noted in all patients within the first four weeks of therapy, however complete clinical resolution of gingival overgrowth necessitated from 4 to 14 weeks of continued azithromycin treatment. All dogs however experienced complete clinical resolution of gingival overgrowth within the time frame noted. This is in contrast to what has recently been reported in the prospective study [14]. In the eight dogs that received oral azithromycin, only one had complete resolution gingival overgrowth during the four week treatment period. In addition, only two other dogs had >50% reduction in their global dental scores. In this current case series, azithromycin treatment was continued until complete clinical resolution of gingival overgrowth. Doses ranged from 6.6 mg/kg to 10.8 mg/kg orally once daily; the target dose was approximately 10 mg/kg. In most dogs, resolution of gingival overgrowth was a permanent effect without recurrence noted, even with continued administration of cyclosporine.

Findings of this case series should be taken in light of potential confounding factors. Notably, in some patients, the cyclosporine dose was decreased along with concurrent administration of azithromycin. Which intervention led to the greatest clinical benefit in regards to gingival overgrowth resolution is uncertain in these cases. In other cases however, there was a clear benefit of azithromycin administration for cyclosporine-induced gingival overgrowth. In four of six cases the cyclosporine dose was unchanged (Case 2 on relapse, 3, 4, and 5). Together, these current findings and those of the prospective study [14], offer a medical treatment option or adjunct therapy to surgery for gingival overgrowth in dogs receiving cyclosporine when the drug cannot be reduced/discontinued. Further evaluation of optimal duration of azithromycin therapy, as well as the formulation used (oral tablet, compounded capsule, toothpaste), is warranted.

4. Conclusions

This series highlights a potentially beneficial medical treatment option for gingival overgrowth even when cyclosporine dose reduction is not possible or elected, without the need for surgical resection of proliferative gingival tissue.

Acknowledgments

Case #1 was presented as a poster at the North American Veterinary Dermatology Forum, Denver, Colorado, 9–12 April 2008.

Author Contributions

Both authors were responsible for clinical examination and treatment recommendations for patients discussed in this series.

Conflicts of Interest

The authors declare no conflict of interest.

References

1. Cosimi, A.B.; Shield, C.F.; Peters, C.; Burton, R.C.; Scott, G.; Russell, P.S. Prolongation of allograft survival by cyclosporine A. *Surg. Forum* **1979**, *30*, 287–289.
2. McMaster, P.; Procyshyn, A.; Calne, R.Y.; Valdes, R.; Rolles, K.; Smith, D.J. Prolongation of canine pancreas allograft survival with cyclosporine A: Preliminary report. *Br. Med. J.* **1980**, *280*, 444–445.
3. Robson, D. Review of pharmacokinetics, interactions and adverse reactions of cyclosporine in people, dogs, and cats. *Vet. Rec.* **2003**, *152*, 739–748.

4. Seibel, W.; Yahia, N.A.; McCleary, L.B.; Lesko, L.J.; Hassell, T.M. Cyclosporine-induced gingival overgrowth in beagle dogs. *J. Oral Pathol. Med.* **1989**, *18*, 240–245.
5. Radowicz, S.N.; Power, H.T. Long-term use of cyclosporine in the treatment of canine atopic dermatitis. *Vet. Dermatol.* **2005**, *16*, 81–86.
6. Nam, H.S.; McAnulty, J.F.; Kwak, H.H.; Yoon, B.I.; Hyun, C.; Kim, W.H.; Woo, H.M. Gingival overgrowth in dogs associated with clinically relevant cyclosporine blood levels: Observations in a canine renal transplantation model. *Vet. Surg.* **2008**, *37*, 247–253.
7. Pernu, H.E.; Pernu, L.M.; Knuuttila, M.L.; Huttunen, K.R. Gingival overgrowth among renal transplant recipients and uremic patients. *Nephrol. Dial. Transplant.* **1993**, *8*, 1254–1258.
8. Pernu, H.E.; Pernu, L.M.; Huttunen, K.R.; Nieminen, P.A.; Knuuttila, M.L. Gingival overgrowth among renal transplant recipients related to immunosuppressive medication and possible local background factors. *J. Periodontol.* **1992**, *63*, 548–553.
9. Steffan, J.; Alexander, D.; Brovedani, F.; Fisch, R.D. Comparison of cyclosporine A with methylprednisolone for treatment of canine atopic dermatitis: A parallel, blinded, randomized controlled trial. *Vet. Dermatol.* **2003**, *14*, 11–22.
10. Lewis, J.R.; Reiter, A.M. Management of generalized gingival enlargement in a dog—Case report and literature review. *J. Vet. Dent.* **2005**, *22*, 160–169.
11. Hirsch, R.; Deng, H.; Laohachai, M.N. Azithromycin in periodontal treatment: More than an antibiotic. *J. Periodontal Res.* **2012**, *47*, 137–148.
12. Tokgöz, B.; Sari, H.I.; Yildiz, O.; Aslan, S.; Sipahioğlu, M.; Okten, T.; Oymak, O.; Utaş, C. Effects of azithromycin on cyclosporine-induced gingival hyperplasia in renal transplant patients. *Transplant. Proc.* **2004**, *36*, 2699–2702.
13. Gladue, R.P.; Snider, M.E. Intracellular accumulation of azithromycin by cultured human fibroblasts. *Antimicrob. Agents Chemother.* **1990**, *34*, 1056–1060.
14. Rosenberg, A.; Rosenkrantz, W.; Griffin, C.; Angus, J.; Keys, D. Evaluation of azithromycin in systemic and toothpaste forms for the treatment of ciclosporin-associated gingival hyperplasia in dogs. *Vet. Dermatol.* **2013**, *24*, 337–345.
15. Kim, J.Y.; Park, S.H.; Cho, K.S.; Kim, H.J.; Lee, C.K.; Park, K.K.; Choi, S.H.; Chung, W.Y. Mechanism of azithromycin treatment on gingival overgrowth. *J. Dent. Res.* **2008**, *87*, 1075–1079.
16. Condé, S.A.; Bastos, M.G.; Vieira, B.J.; Aarestrup, F.M. Down-regulation of transforming growth factor beta-2 expression is associated with the reduction of cyclosporine induced gingival overgrowth in rats treated with roxithromycin: An experimental study. *BMC Oral Health* **2009**, *9*, 33–41.
17. Pai, M.P.; Graci, D.M.; Amsden, G.W. Macrolide drug interactions: An update. *Ann. Pharmacother.* **2000**, *34*, 495–513.
18. Page, R.L., II; Ruscin, J.M.; Fish, D.; Lapointe, M. Possible interaction between intravenous azithromycin and oral cyclosporine. *Pharmacotherapy* **2001**, *21*, 1436–1443.

6

Preliminary Metabolism of Lomustine in Dogs and Comparative Cytotoxicity of Lomustine and Its Major Metabolites in Canine Cells

Thushara Chakkath [1], Sidonie N. Lavergne [1], Timothy M. Fan [2], David Bunick [1] and Levent Dirikolu [1,*]

[1] Department of Comparative Biosciences, College of Veterinary Medicine, University of Illinois, Urbana, IL 61802, USA; E-Mails: chakkat1@illinois.edu (T.C.); sidolavergne@hotmail.com (S.L.); dbunick@illinois.edu (D.B.)

[2] Department of Veterinary Clinical Medicine, College of Veterinary Medicine, University of Illinois, Urbana, IL 61802, USA; E-Mail: t-fan@illinois.edu

* Author to whom correspondence should be addressed; E-Mail: dirikolu@illinois.edu;

Abstract: The nitrosourea drug lomustine is used clinically for treating a wide variety of malignancies, most commonly brain tumors and lymphoma. Lomustine undergoes hydrolysis *in vivo* to form isomeric metabolites, primarily trans-4-hydroxylomustine (trans-4) and cis-4-hydroxylomustine (cis-4) in various animal species including humans. Despite its widespread usage to treat canine lymphoma, the metabolism of lomustine has not been studied in dogs. It is reported that 4'-hydroxylation products of lomustine (trans-4 and cis-4) have enhanced alkylating activity and reduced toxic effects relative to lomustine, resulting in a better therapeutic index of each of the metabolites relative to the parent compound. Our results show that the metabolic profile of lomustine in dogs is similar to that in humans with trans-4 being the major metabolite and cis-4 as the minor metabolite. Comparative cytotoxicity studies of lomustine and its trans-4 and cis-4 metabolites in canine lymphoma cell lines 17–71 and GL-1 show that there is no difference in the cytotoxicity of the three compounds. In addition, a concentration and time-dependent cell killing was seen in both of these cell lines. Also, primary canine cells like peripheral blood mononuclear cells (PBMC) from lymphoma dogs did not show any sensitivity towards lomustine and its metabolites.

Keywords: Lomustine; trans-4-hydroxylomustine; cis-4-hydroxylomustine; lymphoma; cytotoxicity

---

Abbreviations

PBMC	Peripheral blood mononuclear cells
RBC	Red blood cells
VC	Vehicle Control
PAC-1	Procaspase-3 activating compound

1. Introduction

Lymphoma is one of the most common hematopoietic neoplasm seen in dogs, accounting for 7–24% of all cancers diagnosed in canines [1]. Multicentric lymphoma is the most common anatomic form accounting for over 80% of all diagnosed cases [2]. A common manifestation of multicentric lymphoma is the development of non-painful generalized lymphadenopathy with peripheral lymph nodes often bilaterally and symmetrically enlarged [3]. The treatment approach for canine lymphoma is determined by the stage of the disease. The current standard of care for dogs with lymphoma involves the use of multiagent chemotherapy, which achieves response rates of 65% to 96% and first-remission durations of 6 to 9 months [4]. There are various multiagent chemotherapy protocols such as different variations of 'CHOP' (cyclophosphamide, doxorubicin, vincristine, prednisolone). Despite favorable treatment outcomes initially, the majority of dogs will experience relapse, necessitating the reinstitution of additional chemotherapies for the management of refractory disease. Second remission is harder to achieve and may be of shorter duration [5]. Some relapsed dogs become refractory to the initial treatment and hence may require a different chemotherapeutic agent/rescue therapy to achieve second remission. For rescue therapy, again a multiagent protocol is followed; however, a single agent therapy may be preferred for clients with financial or logistical restrictions. Also cross-resistance between chemotherapeutic agents can decrease the efficacy of rescue protocols. Alkylating agents seldom show cross-resistance and are quite effective in achieving clinical remission [6]. Alkylating agents include chemotherapeutic drug classes such as nitrosoureas, nitrogen mustards, and alkyl sulfonates, and they function by attaching an alkyl group to the DNA.

The nitrosourea drug, lomustine (CCNU, CeeNU, $C_9H_{16}ClN_3O_3$, 1-(2-chloroethyl)-3-cyclohexyl-1-nitrosourea), is used clinically for treating a wide variety of human malignancies, most commonly brain tumors and lymphoma [7,8]. In veterinary medicine, lomustine has been successfully used primarily for the treatment of resistant lymphoma [5,9,10], but also for the treatment of mast cell tumors [11], intracranial meningioma [12], epitheliotropic lymphoma [13], and histiocytic sarcoma [14] in dogs either alone or in combination with other chemotherapeutic agents. There are several studies in the literature indicating good efficacy of lomustine in combination with other chemotherapeutic agents such as L-asparaginase, doxorubicin, *etc.* for the treatment of resistant canine lymphoma [5,9,10]. However, its potential as a single agent for first line therapy or to treat relapsed canine lymphoma is less promising. Lomustine as a single agent may be preferred when treatment costs prohibit exploring other options or when a multidrug treatment is not tolerated by the patient due to extreme side effects.

In a clinical setting, lomustine is usually administered to dogs orally at 50–90 mg/m^2 every three weeks [5,10,15]. Lomustine is a highly lipophilic nitrosourea compound, which undergoes hydrolysis *in vivo* to form isomeric metabolites, primarily trans-4-hydroxylomustine (trans-4) and cis-4-hydroxylomustine (cis-4) (Figure 1) in various animal species including humans [16–18]. The comparative biological effects of lomustine and its metabolites were studied in mice. The single dose lethal dose $(LD)_{10}$ (dose causing death of 10% of the mice when administered intraperitoneally) and single dose effective dose $(ED)_{50}$ (dose producing 45 day survival in 50% of the mice after intraperitoneal implantation of 10^5 L1210 cells) were compared to determine the therapeutic index for each compound [19]. The metabolites showed an approximately two-fold greater therapeutic index compared to the parent drug. It was therefore suggested that hydroxylation at the 4'-position of the cyclohexyl ring of lomustine, confers both isomers (cis-4 and trans-4) of the metabolite with enhanced alkylating activity and reduced toxic effects relative to lomustine, resulting in better therapeutic index of each of the metabolites relative to the parent compound [19].

Figure 1. Chemical structure of lomustine (**a**), trans-4-hydroxylomustine (**b**) and cis-4-hydroxylomustine (**c**).

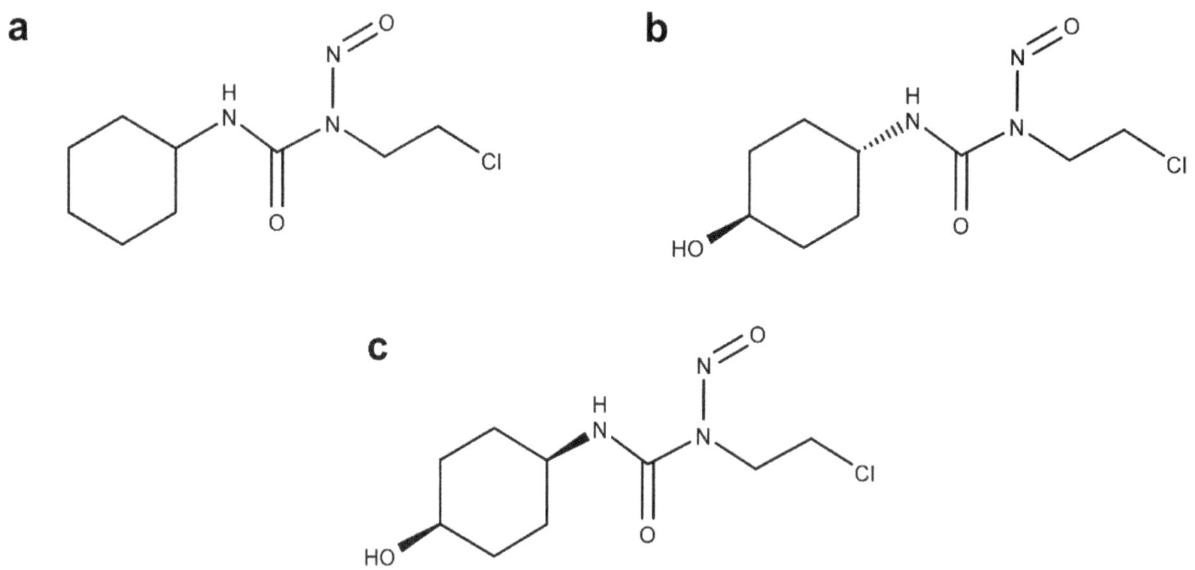

Hence it is plausible that the metabolites of lomustine could be better options for chemotherapy than the parent drug, with greater efficacy and a more favorable side effect profile. In addition to the above metabolites, minor metabolites are also formed due to hydroxylation at the second and third position of the cyclohexyl ring [16,19,20]. The primary objectives of this study were: (1) to determine the preliminary metabolism characteristics of lomustine in dogs; (2) to evaluate the comparative cytotoxicity of lomustine and its trans-4 and cis-4 metabolites in canine lymphoma cell lines 17–71 and GL-1 and also in peripheral blood mononuclear cells (PBMC) from lymphoma dogs.

2. Materials and Methods

2.1. Animals and Sample Collections

The *in vivo* metabolism characteristics of lomustine were studied in two healthy research hounds. The dogs received 1.7 mg/kg (53.6 mg/m^2) oral administration of commercially available lomustine capsules, and blood samples were collected at 15, 30, 45 min, 1, 2, 4, 6, 8 and 12 h after drug administration. Samples were placed in EDTA microcentrifuge tubes and kept on ice until centrifugation (10 min 5,000 g). Additionally, lomustine was also administered to a dog with lymphoma. The dog was presented at the veterinary teaching hospital and was newly diagnosed for lymphoma. No signs of any concurrent illness were noted in the dog. Lomustine and its metabolites were analyzed in the plasma samples immediately using the high performance liquid chromatography (HPLC) method described below. All study procedures were approved by the university's Institutional Animal Care and Use Committee.

2.2. Analytical Detection of Lomustine and Its Monohydroxylated Metabolites

The samples were analyzed using a peer-reviewed and published analytical method described elsewhere [21]. Briefly, a standard solution of 1 mg lomustine (Sigma-Aldrich Co., St. Louis, MO, USA), trans-4 and cis-4 was prepared in 1 mL HPLC grade ice-cold methanol. Standards were prepared by the addition of a specified amount of lomustine, trans-4, and cis-4 in ice-cold methanol to blank canine plasma samples, 0.5 mL each, over a range from 25 to 5,000 ng/mL. Phenytoin (Sigma-Aldrich Co., St. Louis, MO, USA) was used as an internal standard. Clean 16 × 150 mm screw-cap culture tubes with polytetrafluoroethylene cap liners (Fisher Scientific, Pittsburg, PA, USA) were silanized with trimethylchlorosilane (TMCS) before use by rinsing them first with methanol (MX0488-1, EMD Chemicals, Gibbstown, NJ, USA), followed by a 5% solution of TMCS in hexane (Fisher Scientific, Pittsburg, PA, USA). This step was followed by rinsing with methanol (MX0488-1, EMD Chemicals, Gibbstown, NJ, USA) twice. The silanized tubes were allowed to air-dry at room temperature. The analytical method used was as follows: Plasma samples (0.5 mL) were pipetted into 15-mL screw-cap tubes. Twenty microliters of 100 ng/μL internal standard were added to each tube, followed by 2 mL of dichloromethane. The tubes were then vortex mixed for a few seconds, then centrifuged at 2,000 rpm for 15 min. The top aqueous layer was discarded off and the organic layer was transferred into clean tubes and dried under a stream of nitrogen at 20 °C in a water bath. The residue was reconstituted with 120 μL of ice-cold methanol, vortex mixed briefly, and then transferred to an autosampler vial equipped with a 300 μL spring-loaded insert. All samples were analyzed within 24 h post-extraction.

The HPLC procedure was adapted from that described elsewhere [18]. The instrument employed was HP 1100 HPLC system with quaternary solvent delivery pumps, vacuum degasser, thermostated column compartment, 1100 series photodiode array detector, and 1100 series autosampler (Agilent Technologies, Santa Clara, CA, USA). The column was an Inertsil ODS, 5 μm particle size, 4.6 mm × 250 mm column size. The mobile phase consisted of 34% acetonitrile in water (Solvent A), 44% acetonitrile in water (Solvent B), and 64% acetonitrile in water (Solvent C) run with a flow rate of 0.8 mL/min. Samples were eluted by running two-step linear gradient commencing at the time of injection, with an initial condition of solvent A and proceeding to solvent B within 6 min, and then to solvent C within 8 min with a total running time of 30 min. Acetonitrile (A998-4) (Fisher Scientific, Pittsburg, PA, USA) and methanol (MX0488-1, EMD Chemicals, Gibbstown, NJ, USA) were HPLC grade. The diode array detector was set up for single wavelength acquisition at 254 nm with a 12 nm span. Injections were made with a 20 µl sample loop [21].

2.3. RBC Partitioning of Lomustine and Its Metabolites

Certain drugs that have greater lipophilicity may penetrate red blood cells (RBCs) where it can be stored temporarily and this may bring down the plasma concentration of the drugs. Hence studying the RBC partitioning of drugs can help to select the appropriate matrix among whole blood, plasma or serum for assaying pharmacokinetic behavior of the drug [22]. For this study, commercially purchased canine whole blood in EDTA (The Veterinarians' Blood Bank) was used. Two sets of blood samples (four samples in each set, 1 mL/sample) were spiked with lomustine, trans-4 and cis-4 at the concentration of 500 ng/mL. After incubating the samples at 37 °C for 1 h, one set of blood samples was directly analyzed for drug concentration and in the other set, the plasma was separated and the drug concentration was measured in plasma.

The concentration in RBCs was calculated as:

$$C_{RBC} = \frac{[(C_{blood} - C_{plasma}) \times (1 - \text{Hematocrit})]}{\text{Hematocrit}}$$

where C_{blood} and C_{plasma} are the concentrations of the drug in blood and plasma, respectively.

Further, the extent of partitioning of the drugs was measured by the following formula:

$$K_{e/p} = \frac{\text{Concentration of drug in RBC}}{\text{Concentration of drug in plasma}}$$

2.4. Cytotoxicity of Lomustine and Its Metabolites in Canine Lymphoma Cell Lines and PBMC

The canine lymphoma cell lines 17–71 [23,24] and GL-1 [25] and PBMC obtained from lymphoma dogs were used for this assay.

2.4.1. PBMC Isolation

Blood samples were collected from three lymphoma dogs that were brought to the veterinary teaching hospital. The dogs were newly diagnosed cases of lymphoma and did not have any concurrent illnesses. Four milliliters of whole blood were collected into one 5 mL heparinized tubes. The procedure for isolation of PBMC from lymphoma dogs was as described by Lavergne *et al.* [26]. Tubes were placed on ice immediately, and PBMC were isolated using density centrifugation. Blood was kept on ice, and cell isolation was begun within 30 min of venipuncture. Whole blood was diluted with two volumes of prewarmed (37 °C) HBSS with 5 mM EDTA. This was carefully overlaid on 5 mL of prewarmed (37 °C) Lymphocyte Separation Media (Cellgro). After centrifugation, the buffy coat was harvested and washed with three to four volumes of Hank's balanced salt solution (HBSS) with 5 mM EDTA. Lysing buffer (2 mL; 15.5 mM NH_4Cl, 10 mM $KHCO_3$, 1 mM EDTA, pH 7.4) was added to pelleted cells to lyse the residual erythrocytes. After washing with HBSS with 5 mM EDTA, cells were re-suspended in PBS and an aliquot was used to quantitate viable cells using Trypan blue dye exclusion.

2.4.2. Cytotoxicity Assays

Cytotoxicity was evaluated after 48 h by XTT cell proliferation assay and Annexin-PI assay (flow cytometry). The cell lines 17–71 and GL-1 were grown and maintained at 37 °C in 5% CO_2, and cultures were passaged as necessary to maintain high cell viability (above 90%) in culture media Dulbecco's modified eagle's medium (DMEM) supplemented with 10% fetal bovine serum (FBS), 1% penicillin/streptomycin. The PBMC were maintained in culture media RPMI-1640 supplemented with 10% FBS, 1% penicillin/streptomycin. The cell viability was assessed by Trypan blue dye exclusion test. For the XTT assay, the cells were plated in 96 well plates at a density of 20,000 cells per well. The cells were exposed to fresh media (DMEM supplemented with 10% FBS, 1% penicillin/streptomycin for the cell lines and RPMI-1640 supplemented with 10% FBS, 1% penicillin/streptomycin for PBMC) containing varying concentrations of lomustine, trans-4, or cis-4 metabolites (300, 1,000, 3,000, and 10,000 ng/mL). Staurosporine (1 μM for 24 h) was used as positive control for apoptosis in GL-1 cells and PBMC while PAC-1 (procaspase-3 activating compound, 10 μM for 48 h) was used as positive controls for apoptosis in 17–71 cells. The positive controls were chosen based on initial experimentation. Staurosporine produced more than 60% apoptosis in GL-1 cells, however it was not as effective (<30% apoptosis) in 17–71 cells. Additionally, a previously published study by Lucas *et al.* [27] had shown that 17–71 cells were sensitive to PAC-1 (>70% apoptosis) but the GL-1 cells were not as susceptible (<40% apoptosis). The vehicle control (VC) was 0.1% methanol corresponding to the concentration of methanol present in each of the drug treated samples. Forty-eight hours after drug exposure, the cytotoxicity was measured using XTT Cell Proliferation Assay Kit (Promega, Madison, WI, USA). For the Annexin/PI assay, 100,000 cells were plated per well in a 12-well plate. The drug treatment protocol was similar to that in the XTT assay. In addition to the apoptosis controls, a necrosis control was also used which was Triton-X (0.03% for 10 min). At the end of 48 h of incubation, the cells were stained using the Annexin V-FITC Apoptosis detection Kit (BD Biosciences, San Jose, CA, USA) and analyzed by flow cytometry. The experiments were done three separate times in the lymphoma cell lines with two technical replicates used for each assay. The experiment was done on PBMC obtained from three lymphoma dogs (n = 3) with two technical replicates for each assay.

2.5. Time Dependent Cytotoxicity of Lomustine and Its Metabolites

In this experiment, the cytotoxicity of lomustine, trans-4 and cis-4 was measured in canine cell lines 17–71 and GL-1 at 48, 96, and 144 h after drug exposure in order to see if there was a time dependent cytotoxic effect of these drugs. The cells were treated with the drugs similarly as mentioned above, and apoptosis was measured by XTT and Annexin/PI assay at the end of 48, 96, and 144 h of incubation. During incubation, half the media in each well was aspirated every 48 h and replaced with an equal volume of fresh media (without drug) very carefully in order to not disturb the cells at the bottom. This was done in order to avoid acid build up in wells during the long incubation time especially in the vehicle control and at lower concentrations of the drugs where most of the cells would be viable.

2.6. Statistical Analysis

Statistical analysis was done using SPSS software. Descriptive statistics were produced for all continuous variables. Mean and standard deviation were calculated. Normality of data was assessed using the Shapiro-Wilks test. Paired t-tests were performed to evaluate differences between technical repeats of each drug and dose combination. Multiple one way ANOVA and Tukey's *post hoc* test were performed to evaluate the following within and between group differences: Between drugs within each dose in each cell type at each time point, between doses (concentrations) within each drug in each cell type at each time, between time points within dose in cell types for the each drug. The threshold for statistical significance was set at a p value of 0.05. For the canine lymphoma cell lines, two out of seventy two groups did not show normal distribution using Shapiro-Wilks test. However when these groups were further evaluated for normality using kurtosis, skewness, and Q-Q plots, the data showed normal distribution. Hence a parametric test was used to reduce the probability of type II error. *Power analysis:* Cytotoxicity data from two canine lymphoma cell lines were used to estimate sample size requirements for PBMC. Using the data from the 17–71 and GL-1 cell lines, based on *a priori* information of alpha = 0.05, power of 0.8 and an expected difference in mean of 3.77 (corresponding to the maximum standard deviation seen at any concentration), we would require 3 three samples. The lowest concentration of 300 ng/mL was excluded from the power analysis as no statistically significant cell killing was seen in either of the cell lines with any of the drugs at that concentration.

3. Results

Lomustine was not detected in plasma samples of the three dogs following oral administration of the drug. Figure 2a shows that trans-4 is the major metabolite of lomustine and the maximum concentration was about 325 ng/mL detected 1 h after drug administration for both the research hounds. The maximum concentration of cis-4 in the three dogs was around 40–65 ng/mL (Figure 2b).

Figure 2. Plasma concentration of trans-4-hydroxylomustine (**a**) and cis-4-hydroxylomustine (**b**) following single 1.7 mg/kg oral administration of lomustine in three dogs.

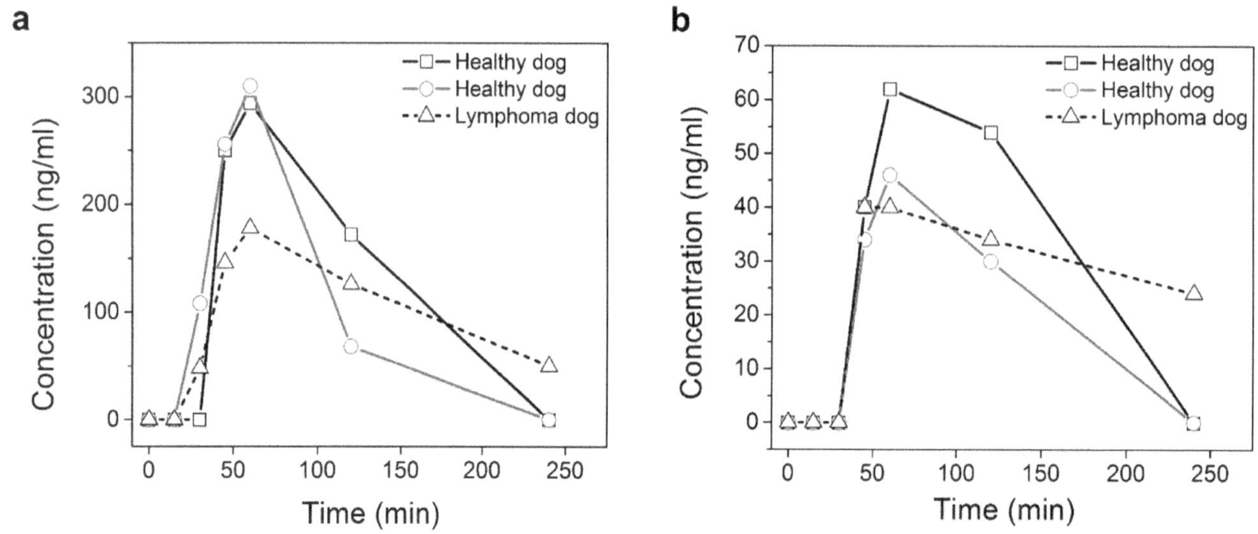

The results show that there is a minor partitioning of these drugs into/onto RBC (Table 1). About 9–15% of the drug was found to be in the RBC compartment. For our metabolism studies, drug concentrations were measured in plasma and not whole blood. This small difference in the drug levels in plasma and whole blood could have led to a slight underestimation of the actual drug concentrations in blood.

Table 1. *In vitro* concentrations of lomustine, trans-4-hydroxylomustine and cis-4-hydroxylomustine (ng/mL) in whole blood, plasma and red blood cells.

Drug	Plasma mean ± SD	Whole blood mean ± SD	RBC± SD	$K_{e/p}$
Lomustine	287.18 ± 27.42	309.87 ± 14.03	37.49 ± 4.16	0.12
Trans-4-hydroxylomustine	256.42 ± 41.13	273.38 ± 16.11	27.71 ± 5.01	0.10
Cis-4-hydroxylomustine	228.98 ± 12.40	253.81 ± 15.90	40.75 ± 5.66	0.17

* All samples spiked at 500 ng/mL. Hematocrit for the blood sample was 0.38 (38%). $K_{e/p}$ is the red blood cell (RBC) partitioning coefficient (Ratio of concentration of drug in RBC to plasma).

The results obtained from the XTT assay (Figure 3) and annexin/PI assay (Figure 4) in the 48 h cytotoxicity study show that there is a statistically significant cell killing at 3,000 and 10,000 ng/mL concentrations, when comparing to control for lomustine, trans-4 and cis-4 metabolites in canine lymphoma cell lines 17–71. In the canine lymphoma cell line GL-1, in addition to the above concentrations, 1,000 ng/mL also showed significant cytotoxicity compared to the VC. After treating the cells with the highest drug concentration, 10,000 ng/mL, about 50% and 40% of the cells were still viable at 48 h in 17–71 and GL-1 cells, respectively (Figure 4). The results obtained from both XTT and Annexin/PI assay do not show any statistically significant difference in the cytotoxicity caused by lomustine, trans-4, and cis-4 in 17–71 and GL-1 cells at 48 h. Lomustine and its metabolites did not show any cell killing in the PBMC obtained from three lymphoma dogs at 48 h after exposure to lomustine, trans-4, and cis-4 (Figure 5). Our results show that terminally differentiated lymphocytes in circulation may not be as sensitive to alkylating agents as lomustine at 48 h. It is possible that PBMC may require a longer incubation time for the cytotoxicity of lomustine to become apparent.

In the time-dependent cytotoxicity study, all three compounds showed a greater degree of cell killing at 96 and 144 h as compared to 48 h, thus confirming the premise that cytotoxicity with these drugs is delayed in nature (Figure 6). However, no statistically significant difference was seen in the cytotoxicity among the three compounds. In the 17–71 cell, the 300 ng/mL samples did not show any cell killing or reduction in viability even at 144 h after drug treatment. The 3,000 and 10,000 ng/mL concentrations resulted in a comparable level of cell killing at 144 h. Also, using 10,000 ng/mL at 96 h data, more than 60% of the cells were non-viable. Due to this 'saturation' in cell killing, very little difference was seen in cytotoxicity at 144 h as compared to 96 h at 10,000 ng/mL. These results show that there is a delay in cell killing by lomustine and its metabolites, and hence measuring cell viability/apoptosis after 48 h of incubation may not be the best indicator of the cytotoxic potential of the compounds.

Figure 3. Graphs showing the results of XTT assay in 17–71 (**a**) and GL-1 (**b**) cells at 48 h. Vehicle control (VC) was 0.1% methanol. The results show the mean and standard deviation of three independent experiments (n = 3).

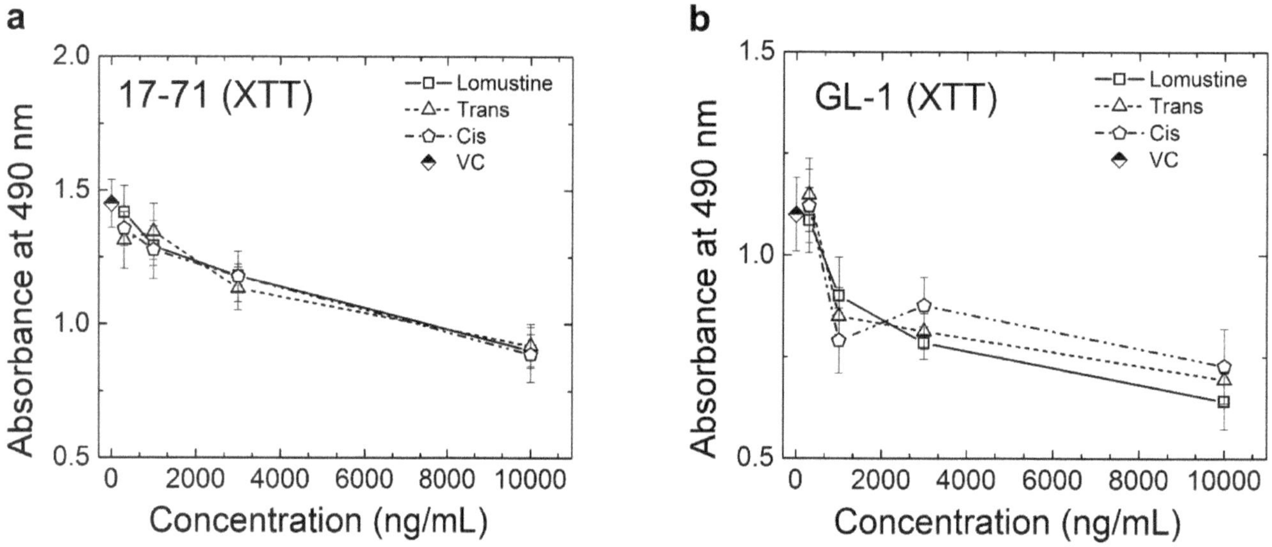

Figure 4. Graphs showing the percent viable cells obtained from Annexin/PI assay in 17–71 (**a**) and GL-1 (**b**) cells at 48 h. Vehicle control (VC) was 0.1% methanol. The results show the mean and standard deviation of three independent experiments (n = 3).

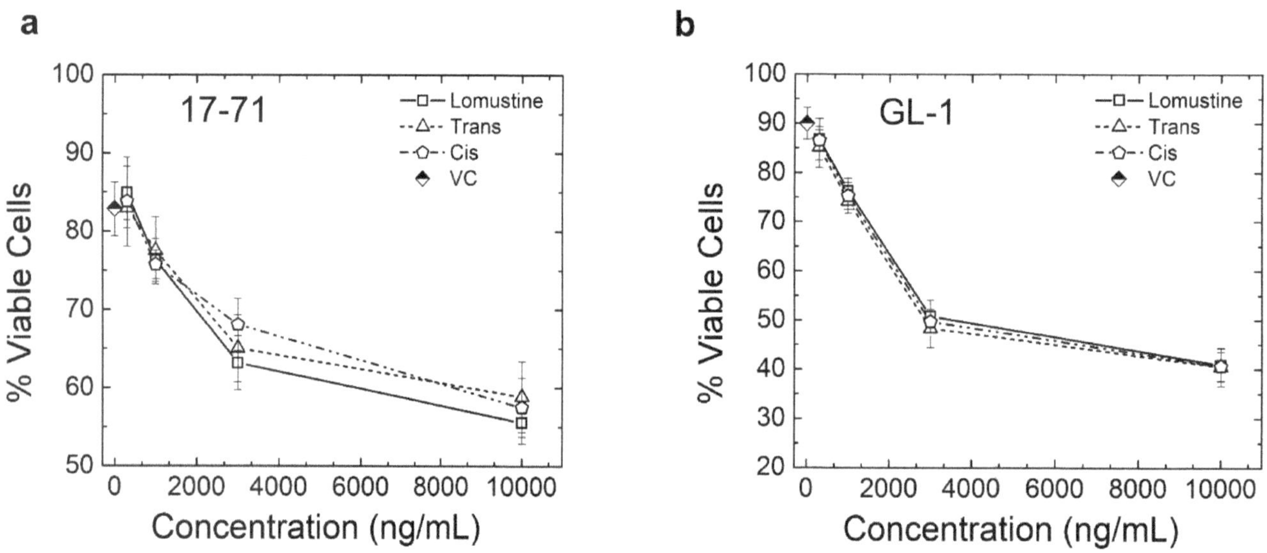

Figure 5. Graphs showing the results of XTT assay (**a**) and Annexin/PI assay (**b**) in peripheral blood mononuclear cells (PBMC) isolated from three lymphoma dogs. Vehicle control (VC) was 0.1% methanol. The graph shows the mean and standard deviation of results obtained from three dogs. No statistically significant difference was seen in any of the drug treated samples compared to VC.

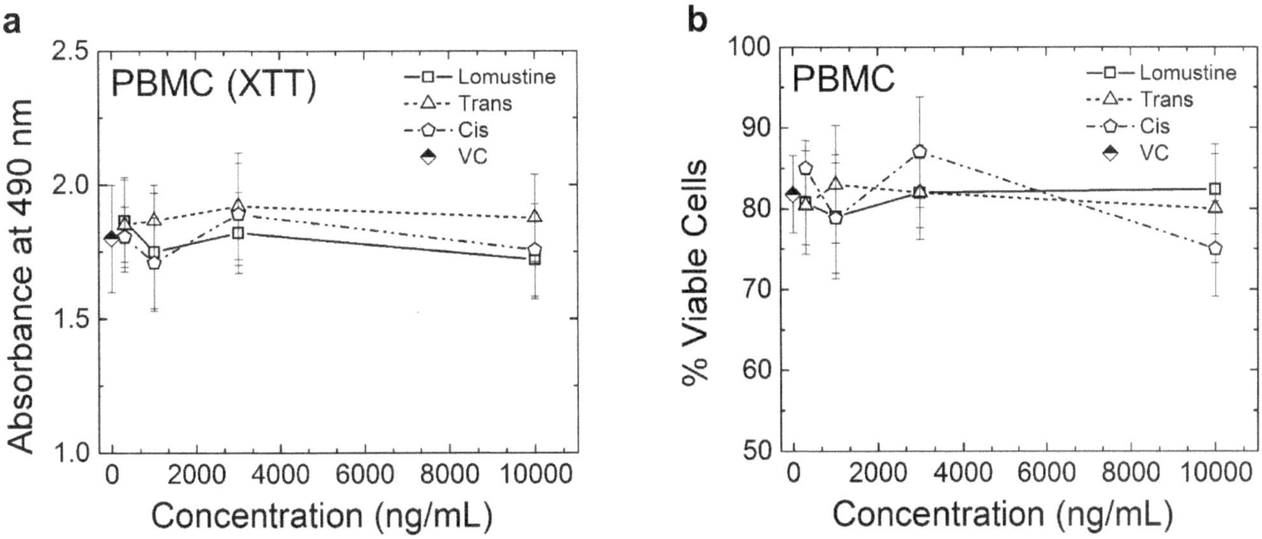

Figure 6. Graphs showing the results of Annexin/PI assay in 17–71 cells (**a**, **b** and **c**) and GL-1 cells (**d**, **e**, and **f**) at 48, 96 and 144 h after treatment with lomustine, trans- and cis-4-hydroxylomustine. Vehicle control (VC) was 0.1% methanol. The results show the mean and standard deviation of three independent experiments (n = 3).

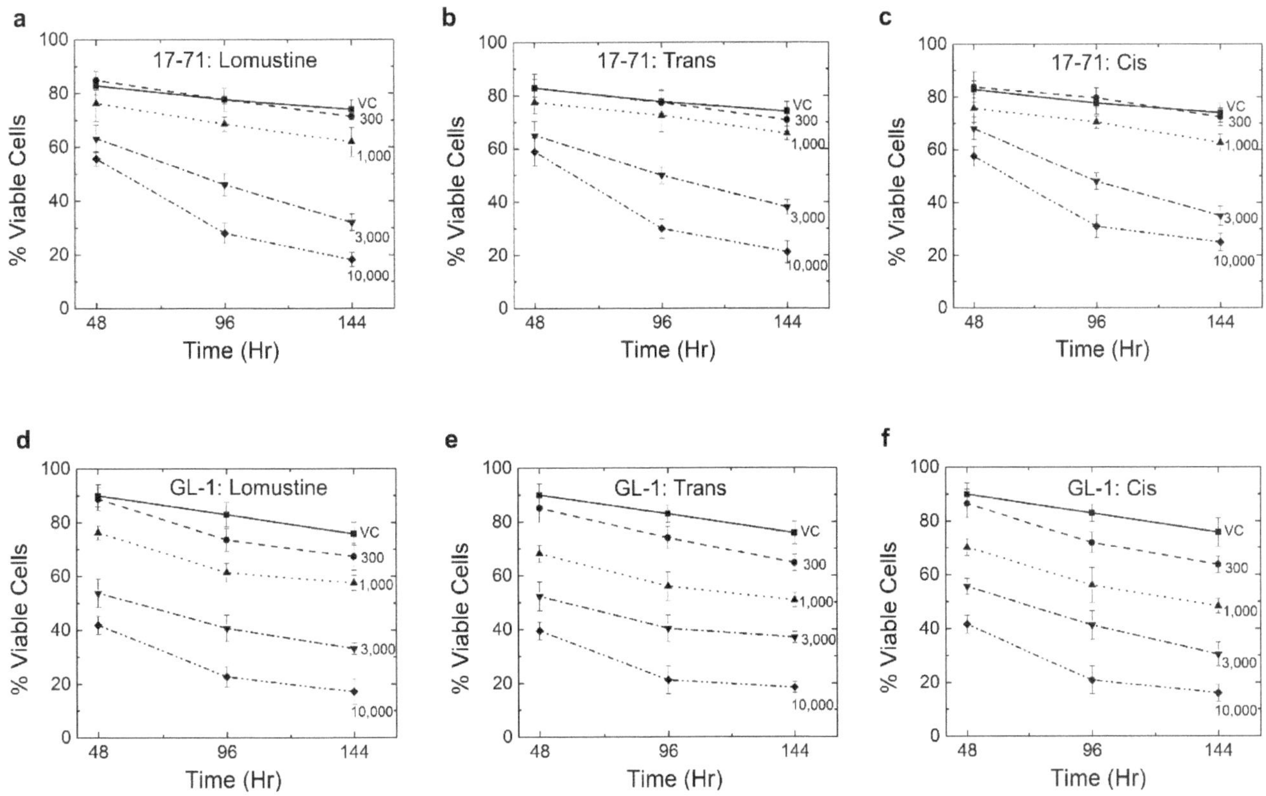

4. Discussion

Lomustine has been identified as a potentially important therapeutic agent for use in the treatment of various cancers in dogs; as such, we needed a sensitive and reliable analytical method to perform pharmacokinetic experiments with this agent in dogs. In particular, the method selected needed to be sufficiently sensitive to detect low concentrations of lomustine and its possible monohydroxylated metabolites in canine plasma from test animals.

The resultant HPLC method is a sensitive analytical method with the LOD of lomustine, cis-4 and trans-4 in plasma of about 10 ng/120 μL, 5 ng/120 μL, and 5 ng/120 μL, respectively, based on signal to noise ratio. Additionally, satisfactory recovery was obtained for lomustine and its monohydroxylated metabolites extracted from plasma samples. The developed extraction procedure is very simple (one step liquid/liquid extraction procedure) and suitable to analyze multiple samples in a short-time period. The CV for within-run and between-run samples were less than 15% for lomustine, trans-4, and cis-4, indicating good method precision [21].

The metabolic profile of oral lomustine in dogs established in our study is similar to that reported in humans and rats with trans-4 being the major metabolite followed by cis-4 and the complete absence of parent lomustine. However, since the study was only done in three dogs, these results have to be considered as preliminary. In our study, the dogs received lomustine at the dose of 1.7 mg/kg, and the two research hounds showed similar peak levels of trans-4 (about 325 ng/mL), but the level for the same in the lymphoma dog was lower. The peak cis-4 lomustine level was between 40–65 ng/mL. In a published study of four human patients that received lomustine at the dose of 4.1 mg/kg, parent lomustine was not detected in the blood. The average peak concentration of trans-4 was 530 ng/mL and that for cis-4 was 320 ng/mL [18]. In another study in human patients that used high dose lomustine (15 mg/kg), the peak plasma concentration detected ranged between 410–2,310 ng/mL for trans-4 and 180–1,820 ng/mL for cis-4 [17], a five- and 10-fold difference between the maximum concentrations observed among patients, respectively. This supports the premise that there is a large inter-individual difference in the metabolic profile of lomustine.

As parent lomustine was not detected in the blood at any time after administration of the drug, the RBC partitioning behavior of lomustine and its metabolites was investigated. The results showed that there is a minor partitioning of these drugs into RBC. However, RBC partitioning values were not high enough to explain why lomustine was not detected in our canine plasma samples. It is likely that, like in other animal species, the absence of lomustine in dogs' plasma is due to rapid "first pass" metabolism and not due to significant RBC partitioning.

As mentioned previously it has been reported that the major hydroxylated metabolites of lomustine may have enhanced alkylating activity and reduced toxic effects relative to parent lomustine [19]. In this study, we wanted to investigate whether the major hydroxylated metabolites showed potential as a more effective chemotherapeutic option than lomustine using *in vitro* studies. The metabolism studies discussed show that trans-4 and cis-4 are the major metabolites in dogs after oral treatment with lomustine, with trans-4 being in greater proportion.

The drug concentrations for the cytotoxicity study were derived from the metabolism studies in dogs where we found that the maximum plasma concentration of trans-4 was about 300 ng/mL and that for cis-4 was 50 ng/mL. Hence we used concentrations starting at 300 ng/mL up till 10,000 ng/mL as we did not know at what concentration the *in vitro* biological effects of the drugs would be seen. We found no significant difference in the cytotoxicity caused by lomustine and its trans-4 and cis-4 metabolites in both the canine lymphoma cell lines 17–71 and GL-1. At 48 h after treatment with 10,000 ng/mL lomustine or its metabolites, 40–50% of the cells were still viable. However, after 96 h of incubation this number had dropped to about 20% indicating a time-dependent effect of lomustine cytotoxicity. In the PBMC from three lymphoma dogs, none of the drugs showed any significant cell killing compared to the control at 48 h after lomustine treatment. In two of the dogs, there were no circulating lymphoma cells detected. Hence the cytotoxicity results in PBMC of those two patients should represent the sensitivity of "normal" lymphocytes to the three agents. However, the third lymphoma patient had a lot of circulating lymphoma cells (37% of all of the nucleated cells). Hence, for this patient, it is highly probable that when we screened the sensitivity of "normal lymphocytes", we were indeed also screening a good proportion of malignant lymphoma cells too. This would make interpretation of results from this patient more difficult and problematic. Interestingly, the *in vitro* inhibitory concentration $(IC)_{50}$ for lomustine mentioned in literature varies from 50–250 μM (11,650–58,400 ng/mL) [28–30]. These studies have utilized different cell lines and also used different techniques of detecting the cell killing. However, a time-dependent study of lomustine cytotoxicity has not been done before. Our findings suggest that apoptosis of cells after lomustine administration is not an immediate event but rather a delayed one. Also, the therapeutic concentration of lomustine measured in the three dogs (about 300 ng/mL) did not show any cytotoxic effect in the *in vitro* study with the canine cell lines even at 144 h (6 days) of incubation. One reason for this disparity could be that since lomustine is metabolized rapidly to form pharmacologically active metabolites and also spontaneously breaks down into reactive intermediates which ultimately cause the alkylation of DNA, measuring the parent compound alone may not indicate the extent of the cytotoxic effect of the drug. The anticancer effect of lomustine may be brought about by the combined action of lomustine and its active metabolites whose absolute quantification in blood is precluded by their rapid breakdown in physiological body conditions.

5. Conclusion

In conclusion, our previously published analytical method have shown that lomustine and its metabolites are highly unstable and that careful consideration must be given to the stability of these compounds while storing and using them for experimental purposes [21]. In addition, we have shown that the metabolism profile of lomustine in dogs is similar to that in humans. We also conclude that there is no difference between the cytotoxicity of lomustine, trans-4, and cis-4 in the two canine lymphoma cell lines 17–71 and GL-1 and that cell killing by all three compounds appears to be time-dependent. Finally, lomustine and its metabolites did not significantly reduced the viability of canine primary cells like PBMCs suggesting that a much longer exposure time or delay after exposure is required to significantly kill primary leukocytes in dogs.

Acknowledgement

This study was supported by the University of Illinois at Urbana-Champaign Research Board as the Arnold O. Beckman Research Award.

Authors Contributions

All the authors included in this study contributed to study design, data analysis, sample collection, and manuscript preparation.

Conflict of Interest

The authors declare no conflict of interest.

References

1. Vail, D.; MacEwen, E.; Young, K. Canine lymphoma and lymphoid leukemia. In *Small Animal Clinical Oncology*, 5th ed.; Withrow, S.J., Vail, D.M., Page, R., Eds.; Elsevier: Maryland Heights, MO, USA, 2012; p. 608.
2. Madewell, B.R.; Theilen, G.H. Haematopoietic neoplasms, sarcomas and related conditions (IV). In *Veterinary Cancer Medicine*, 2nd ed.; Theilen, G.H., Madewell, B.R., Eds.; Lea & Febiger: Philadelphia, PA, USA, 1987; pp. 392–407.
3. Meuten, D.J.; Jacobs, R.M.; Messick, J.B.; Valli, V.E. Tumors of the Hemolymphatic System. In *Tumors in Domestic Animals*, 4th ed.; Meuten, D.J., Ed.; Wiley-Blackwell: Ames, IA, USA, 2002; p. 138.
4. Morrison, W. *Lymphoma in Dogs and Cats*; Teton NewMedia: Jackson, WY, USA, 2004.
5. Moore, A.; London, C.; Wood, C.; Williams, L.; Cotter, S.; L'Heureux, D.; Frimberger, A. Lomustine (CCNU) for the treatment of resistant lymphoma in dogs. *J. Vet. Intern. Med.* **1999**, *13*, 395–398.
6. Tew, K.; Coluin, O.; Jones, R. Clinical and high-dose akylating agents. In *Cancer Chemotherapy and Biotherapy: Principles and Practice*, 4th ed.; Longo, D.L., Chabner, B.A., Eds.; Lippincott Willimas & Wilkins: Philadelphia, PA, USA, 2006; p. 283.
7. Mitchell, E.; Schein, P. Contributions of nitrosoureas to cancer-treatment. *Cancer Treat. Rep.* **1986**, *70*, 31–41.
8. Gerson, S.L.; Bulgar, A.D.; Weeks, L.D.; Chabner, B.A. Alkylating agents. In *Cancer Chemotherapy and Biotherapy*, 5th ed.; Chabner, B.A., Longo, D.L., Eds.; Lippincott-Raven: Philadelphia, PA, USA, 2011; p. 267.
9. Saba, C.F.; Thamm, D.H.; Vail, D.M. Combination chemotherapy with L-asparaginase, lomustine, and prednisone for relapsed or refractory canine lymphoma. *J. Vet. Intern. Med.* **2007**, *21*, 127–132.
10. Sauerbrey, M.L.; Mullins, M.N.; Bannink, E.O.; van Dorp, T.E.; Renate, K.J.; Obradovich, J.E. Lomustine and prednisone as a first-line treatment for dogs with multicentric lymphoma: 17 cases (2004–2005). *J. Am. Vet. Med. Assoc.* **2007**, *230*, 1866–1869.
11. Rassnick, K.; Moore, A.; Williams, L.; London, C.; Kintzer, P.; Engler, S.; Cotter, S. Treatment of canine mast cell tumors with CCNU (lomustine). *J. Vet. Intern. Med.* **1999**, *13*, 601–605.
12. Jung, D.; Kim, H.; Park, C.; Kim, J.; Kang, B.; Lim, C.; Park, H. Long-term chemotherapy with lomustine of intracranial meningioma occurring in a miniature schnauzer. *J. Vet. Med. Sci.* **2006**, *68*, 383–386.

13. Williams, L.; Rassnick, K.; Power, H.; Lana, S.; Morrison-Collister, K.; Hansen, K.; Johnson, J. CCNU in the treatment of canine epitheliotropic lymphoma. *J. Vet. Intern. Med.* **2006**, *20*, 136–143.
14. Skorupski, K.A.; Clifford, C.A.; Paoloni, M.C.; Lara-Garcia, A.; Barber, L.; Kent, M.S.; Sorenmo, K.U. CCNU for the treatment of dogs with histiocytic sarcoma. *J. Vet. Intern. Med.* **2007**, *21*, 121–126.
15. Kristal, O.; Rassnick, K.; Gliatto, J.; Northrup, N.; Chretin, J.; Morrison-Collister, K.; Moore, A. Hepatotoxicity associated with CCNU (lomustine) chemotherapy in dogs. *J. Vet. Intern. Med.* **2004**, *18*, 75–80.
16. Hilton, J.; Walker, M. Hydroxylation of 1-(2-chloroethyl)-3-cyclohexyl-1-nitrosourea. *Biochem. Pharmacol.* **1975**, *24*, 2153–2158.
17. Kastrissios, H.; Chao, N.; Blaschke, T. Pharmacokinetics of high dose oral CCNU in bone marrow transplant patients. *Cancer Chemother. Pharmacol.* **1996**, *38*, 425–430.
18. Lee, F.; Workman, P.; Roberts, J.; Bleehen, N. Clinical pharmacokinetics of oral CCNU (lomustine). *Cancer Chemother. Pharmacol.* **1985**, *14*, 125–131.
19. Wheeler, G.; Johnston, T.; Bowdon, B.; McCaleb, G.; Hill, D.; Montgomery, J. Comparison of the properties of metabolites of CCNU. *Biochem. Pharmacol.* **1977**, *26*, 2331–2336.
20. Reed, D.J. Synthesis and characterization of nitrosoureas. In *Drugs and the Pharmaceutical Sciences, Anticancer and Interferon Agents: Synthesis and Properties*; Ottenbrite, R.M., Butler, G.B., Eds.; Marcel Dekker, Inc.: New York, NY, USA, 1984; Volume 24, pp. 177–202.
21. Dirikolu, L.; Chakkath, T.; Fan, T.; Mente, M. Synthesis of trans- and cis-4'- hydroxylomustin and development of validated analytical method for lomustine, trans- and cis-4'-hydroxylomustine in canine plasma. *J. Anal. Toxicol.* **2009**, 33, 595–603.
22. Hinderling, P.H. Red blood cells: A neglected compartment in pharmacokinetics and pharmacodynamics. *Pharmacol. Rev.* **1997**, *49*, 279–295.
23. Steplewski, Z.; Jeglum, K.A.; Rosales, C.; Weintraub, N. Canine lymphoma-associated antigens defined by murine monoclonal antibodies. *Cancer Immunol. Immunotherapy* 1**987**, *24*, 197–201.
24. Suter, S.E.; Chein, M.B.; Messling, V.; Yip, B.; Cattaneo, R.; Vernau, W.; Bruce, R.; Madewell, B.R.; London, C.A. *In vitro* canine distemper virus infection of canine lymphoid cells: A prelude to oncolytic therapy for lymphoma. *Clin. Cancer Res.* **2005**, *11*, 1579–1587.
25. Nakaichi, M.; Taura, Y.; Kanki, M.; Mamba, K.; Momoi, Y.; Tsujimoto, H.; Nakama, S. Establishment and characterization of a new canine B-cell leukemia cell line. *J. Vet. Med. Sci.* **1996**, *58*, 469–471.
26. Lavergne, S.; Kurian, J.; Bajad, S.; Maki, J.; Yoder, A.; Guzinski, M.; Trepanier, L. Roles of endogenous ascorbate and glutathione in the cellular reduction and cytotoxicity of sulfamethoxazole-nitroso. *Toxicology* **2006**, *222*, 25–36.
27. Lucas, P.W.; Schmit, J.M.; Peterson, Q.P.; West, D.C.; Hsu, D.C.; Novotny, C.J.; Dirikolu, L.; Deorge, D.R.; Garrett, L.D.; Hergenrother, P.J; Fan, T.M. Pharmacokinetics and derivation of an anticancer dosing regimen for PAC-1 in healthy dogs. *Invest. New Drugs* **2011**, *29*, 901–911.
28. Astier, A.; Ferrer, M.; Gibaud, S. Enhancement by 1-(2-chloroethyl)-3-cyclohexyl-1-nitrosourea (CCNU) of the cytotoxic properties of 1-β-d-arabinofuranosylcytosine (Ara-C) on human promyelocytic leukemia cell line HL-60. *EJHP Sci.* **2005**, *11*, 62–67.

29. Shinwari, Z.; Manogaran, P.S.; Alrokayan, S.A.; Al-Hussein, K.A.; Aboussekhra, A. Vincristine and lomustine induce apoptosis and p21(WAF1) up-regulation in medulloblastoma and normal human epithelial and fibroblast cells. *J. Neuro-Oncol.* **2008**, *87*, 123–132.
30. Wilkoff, L.J.; Dulmadge, E.A. Sensitivity of proliferating cultured murine pancreatic tumor cells to selected antitumor agents. *J. Nat. Cancer Instit.* **1986**, *77*, 1163–1169.

7

Effect of Transportation and Pre-Slaughter Handling on Welfare and Meat Quality of Cattle: Case Study of Kumasi Abattoir, Ghana

Samuel Frimpong [1], Girma Gebresenbet [2,*], Emmanuel Bobobee [1,3], Elias D. Aklaku [1] and Ibrahim Hamdu [1]

[1] Department of Agricultural Engineering, Kwame Nkrumah University of Science and Technology, Kumasi, PMB, Ghana; E-Mails: smlfrimpong@gmail.com (S.F.); edaklaku@yahoo.com (E.D.A.); hamdu2000@gmail.com (I.H.)

[2] Department of Energy and Technology, Swedish University of Agricultural Sciences, Uppsala, 750 07, Sweden

3 Institute for Agricultural Engineering, Agricultural Research Council, Private Bag X519, Silverton, Pretoria, 0127, South Africa; E-Mail: BobobeeE@arc.agric.za

* Author to whom correspondence should be addressed; E-Mail: Girma.Gebresenbet@slu.se;

Abstract: This study was conducted at the Kumasi Abattoir Company Limited (K.A.C.L) in Ghana to assess the effect of pre-slaughter handling on welfare and meat quality of cattle. Behaviour measurements were done on 200 cattle pre-slaughter and the methods by which the cattle were handled were recorded to evaluate the effect of pre-slaughter handling on their welfare. Ultimate pH_{24} and percent cooking loss were measured on 50 poorly-handled cattle pre-slaughter. The cattle were poorly-handled because they were beaten and, whipped. Based on pH_{24}, meat quality was assessed as normal (pH from 5.5–5.8), moderate dark, firm and dry (DFD) ($5.8 \leq pH \leq 6.2$), and DFD (pH from 6.2–6.7). Five hundred carcasses were visually observed for bruising in them and the number of non-ambulatory cattle slaughtered in a week was recorded. The relationship between pH_{24} value and cooking loss in meat from the 50 poorly-handled cattle was investigated. Behaviours exhibited by poorly-handled cattle pre-slaughter included raising of their tail, kicking, lying down and refusing to move, jumping, vocalising, panting, and charging at handlers. Also lashes/whips, pulling of animals' tails, stamping on their tails, and hitting them with sticks, stones and ropes were among the prominent methods by which the cattle were handled. Mean pH_{24} and mean percent cooking loss were significant ($p < 0.05$) at 6.22 ± 0.10 and 22.51 ± 3.25, respectively, for poorly-handled cattle. There was a strong negative correlation between pH_{24} and percent cooking loss in poorly-handled cattle ($r = -0.77$). Out of the 500 carcasses assessed for bruising, 18% had no bruises, 60% had slight bruises while 22% had severe bruises. Ninety (90) non-ambulatory cattle were slaughtered within seven (7) days, representing 7.1% of the total number of cattle slaughtered within that period. The results indicated that handling of cattle pre-slaughter have effects on their meat quality and welfare. Eighty-two percent of the bruised carcass and 7.1% of non-ambulatory animals indicated poor meat quality. Meat quality assessment indicated that most of the meat had dark, firm and dry (DFD) tendency. The water holding capacity of the meat sampled in this study (by means of cooking loss) indicated that the meat quality was compromised.

Keywords: welfare; transport; meat quality; non-ambulatory

---

1. Introduction

Pre-slaughter transport and handling of animals are accompanied by many stressful events, which affect animal welfare and meat quality [1–3]. Pre-slaughter handling involves a number of critical points which include loading of animals at the farm, transport from farm to abattoir, unloading of animals at the abattoir, and slaughter [2]. A study by Gebresenbet *et al.* [2] revealed that loading and unloading are among the main activities that cause an increase in heart rate of cattle. Stress is an invariable consequence of transporting animals destined for slaughter from the farm to the abattoir [3–5]. However, stress during transport can be minimized by improving facilities, vehicle designed, and handling methods. As is also widely known, pre-slaughter stress commences during loading of animals onto a vehicle that sends them to abattoirs [4]. Transport time is also known to have an impact on transported animals. A study by Gebresenbet *et al.* [2] showed that concentration of plasma cortisol (stress hormone) decreased with an increase in transport time while lactate and creatine kinase (CK) increased significantly ($p < 0.001$) after 6 h of transport time.

During transport and handling, animals are sometimes faced with unfavourable conditions, which compromise their welfare and meat quality [5,6] such as food and water deprivation, unfavourable temperature or ventilation, aggressions and physical shocks which cause hunger and thirst, heat stress and pain [7]. To some extent, mortality of animals during transport may be an indication of their welfare and transport conditions [8,9]. People occasionally hit animals and cause great pain and injury mostly because they consider the animals as commodities and not as sentient beings that feel pain and stress, or because of lack of knowledge about animals and their welfare [10].

Inappropriate handling, improper use of sticks by handlers, violent impact of the animals against facilities or impact with other animals are potential bruising events [11]. Handling animals without the practice of using sticks results in better welfare and less risk of poor carcass quality [8]. Poor handling or a physical blow that leads to bruising or other animal injury can lead to parts of the carcass being condemned or the meat being dark [12]. Such meat, they say, does not appeal to consumers and spoils quickly. A study in Canada [13] revealed that 15% of the cattle showed severe bruising while 78% of the carcasses exhibited bruising of some sort. Indicators of an animal having difficulty coping with handling or transport are changes in behaviour, which show that some aspect of the situation is aversive [14].

Assessment of culled cattle in holding pens at 21 slaughter facilities in the United States recorded an overall incidence of 1.1% non-ambulatory cattle [13]. Estimated number of starved cattle slaughtered at federally inspected facilities showed that the incidence of non-ambulatory cattle was between 0.7% and 1.1% [15]. The same study [16] recorded an aggregated sum of beef and dairy cattle that could not stand and walk in the years 2003 and 2004 to be 0.04% and 0.38%, respectively. According to [16], causes of non-ambulatory cattle differ by region, herd size and herd management. Main causes of non-ambulatory conditions in cattle are injuries related to dystocia, fractures, muscle and ligament damage, infectious diseases such as toxic mastitis, lymphoma, peritonitis, and metabolic disorders such as acidosis [16].

The abattoir system in the developed world is quite different from that in the developing world. While the abattoir system in the developed world provides services that are geared towards meat quality, the abattoir system in the developing world typically may not always consider animal welfare and meat quality issues [17,18]. Cattle destined for slaughter at the Kumasi Abattoir are transported from Burkina Faso (800–1000 km), Mali (1500–2500 km), Niger (1800–2500 km), Yeji (180–250 km) in Brong Ahafo and the three northern regions of Ghana [17]. The animals are bought from individual farms, small and big markets and are sent to a collection centre before onward transportation to Kumasi. At the farm, the animals are treated humanely as they are precious assets to the family that owns them. As soon as they are bought from the farm, they are treated as a commodity. During loading and unloading, the animals are subjected to lashes (whips) with sticks and ropes that compromise their welfare and meat quality. Some of these events were observed during the study.

The vehicles used to transport the animals are mostly unsuitable for such a purpose and this could induce stress on the animals. The vehicles do not have loading ramps and majority of them are not suitable for animal transport because, for instance, they do not have top covers to protect the animals from the vagaries of the weather. Many animals are often crammed into vehicles without due consideration of appropriate loading densities. This brings about bruises, downed or crippled or non-ambulatory animals and damage to animal hides. During transportation, the animals are exposed to extremes of temperature, rain and humidity because they are not offered any form of protection against the weather. The vehicles used are mostly not designed for animal transport. Most of the vehicles have exposed tops making the animals liable to extremes of the weather. The movement of the animals from the cattle market at the abattoir premises to the lairage and subsequently into the abattoir is often marked by inappropriate handling. They were stoned, beaten with sticks and ropes and other inhumane treatments. Lairage times vary and while some animals spend less than five (5) min in the lairage, others are moved straight from the cattle market into the abattoir for slaughter. There is insufficient knowledge among stakeholders that bad handling of animals can impinge on their welfare and meat quality. This knowledge gap led to the present study.

Objective

The aim of the study was to investigate the effect of transport and pre-slaughter handling on welfare and meat quality of cattle.

2. Methodology

2.1. The Study Area

The Kumasi Abattoir Company Limited (K.A.C.L) was established in 1997 with grants from the Government of Ghana and the Canadian International Development Agency (CIDA) and commenced its operations in 1998. The Abattoir is located at a suburb called *Kaase* in Kumasi. Kumasi Abattoir is located on latitude 6°43'55"N, longitude 1°31'28"W and at an altitude of 274 m. There is a cattle market at the Abattoir premises about 150 m away from the Abattoir. At the cattle market, there are kraals which are used to house the animals while they are being sold. There is a holding pen for the cattle which are destined for slaughter. The holding pen which is about 10 m away from the slaughterhouse is used to keep cattle overnight until the next morning when they are slaughtered. There is a lairage which is supposed to be used to rest animals for some time before slaughter. There is a defunct waste treatment plant and an abandoned fish pond about 100 m away from the slaughterhouse.

The company slaughters cattle, pigs, sheep and goats for processing and packaging for the targeted Ghanaian market. The company has 151 regular employees and 15 casual employees. The original daily slaughtering capacity of the Abattoir was 200 cattle, 100 pigs, and 250 sheep and goats. The production facility has been redesigned to enable the company to slaughter an additional 200 cattle daily. This was achieved by converting one of the slaughter lines meant for the slaughter of sheep and goats into another cattle line and developing a singeing platform with the support of the Kwame Nkrumah University of Science and Technology (KNUST) to take care of the singeing of sheep and goat carcasses [19].

2.2. Data Collection

In this study, the bases of sampling were interviews, field measurements, and observations of activities during animal transport and slaughter operations. For better planning of field work and proper design of questionnaires, preceding exploratory visits and interviews with key people at the Abattoir were made.

2.3. Interview of Stakeholders

Face-to-face interviews were conducted of dealers (merchants), middlemen (landlords), and butchers to investigate how transport and pre-slaughter could affect welfare and meat quality of cattle. The dealers' work is to go to the points of purchase, buy animals and transport them to the Abattoir. The middlemen's work is to receive and sell the animals brought to the Abattoir by the dealers, while the butchers' work is to buy, slaughter the animals, and sell the meat.

2.4. Measurement of Cattle Behaviours and Methods of Handling

A pre-feasibility study was done to observe and record the behaviour of the animals as they were being moved by cattle handlers from the cattle market until they were slaughtered in the abattoir. To record behaviour of the animals, a video film was shot at random on 200 animals. Ten animals were sampled each day for 20 days. The selection of the different behavioural observations was partly based on literature and partly on preceding exploratory work. Behaviours and handling methods observed and recorded are shown in Table 1.

Table 1. Definitions of observed behaviours.

Behaviour	Definition
Easily pulled	The number of animals allowing themselves to be moved from the Cattle Market into the Abattoir by cattle handlers.
Beatings (whips)	Animals which failed to move voluntarily were whipped/ lashed by cattle handlers with ropes and sticks or clubs until they moved.
Charging at handlers	Sometimes as the animals were being moved by cattle handlers, they charged at the handlers.
Defecation and urinating	Due to inappropriate handling by cattle handlers, animals mostly defecated and or urinated.
Ear erection	Some animals due to agitation and stress, raised their ears while they were being moved by cattle handlers into the Abattoir.
Foaming	Some animals foamed at the mouth due to stress from handling by cattle handlers as they were moved into the Abattoir.
Forcing animals to fall down	When some animals got to the entrance of the lairage or the entrance of the Abattoir, they resisted entry and the cattle handlers had to physically restrain those animals and force them to fall down before dragging them into the Abattoir for slaughter.
Head swings	Some animals swung their heads from one side to the other as an indication of being traumatised while they were being moved into the Abattoir.
Horn pulling	Sometimes some animals which failed to move voluntarily as they were sent into the Abattoir had to be held by the horn by cattle handlers and pulled.
Jumping	Sometimes some animals while in their natural environments, exhibit play behaviours such as jumping but when they are inhumanely handled, they jump as well in distress.
Kicking	Animals which were traumatised and were temperamental, tried to kick the cattle handlers with their hind legs while they were being moved into the Abattoir for slaughter.
Crippled during handling	Animals which became lame and could not continue walking due to inappropriate handling by cattle handlers as they were being moved into the Abattoir were counted and recorded.
Leg pulling	Some animals instead of being pulled by ropes attached to their horns were pulled by ropes attached to their leg(s) because those animals stopped, lay down and would not move.
Lying down and refusing to move	Sometimes some of the animals lay down and refused to move during handling.
Moving without pulling	Some animals moved voluntarily into the Abattoir without being pulled by cattle handlers.
Panting	At certain times, some of the animals panted for breath while being moved by cattle handlers into the Abattoir due to stress from inappropriate handling.
Raising of tail	Some animals due to agitation raised their tails while they were being moved by cattle handlers into the Abattoir.

Table 1. *Cont.*

Behaviour	Definition
Resistance to be lazooed	Before each animal was moved into the Abattoir for slaughter, it was tied by the horns with a rope. Some animals resisted these restrictions by running away from the cattle handlers.
Resistance to be pulled	Some of the animals resisted pulling by cattle handlers from the cattle market into the Abattoir.
Retreating	Due to fear and inappropriate handling by cattle handlers, some animals moved backwards while they were being moved into the Abattoir for slaughter.
Running	Some animals ran when being moved by cattle handlers into the Abattoir.
Slapping	Sometimes the cattle handlers had to use their bare hands to slap recalcitrant animals which offered some resistance to pulling.
Sniffing	Due to fear and inappropriate handling by cattle handlers, some animals sniffed while they were being moved into the Abattoir for slaughter.
Stoning	Hitting animals with stones when animals failed to move voluntarily
Stretching	Some animals stretched their bodies by extending their forelegs forward and their hind legs backwards and arched their bodies due to stress from inappropriate handling by cattle handlers.
Stamping of feet	Due to fear and inappropriate handling by cowboys, some animals remained stationary and kept stamping their feet on the ground while they were being moved into the Abattoir for slaughter.
Tail pulling/twisting and, Stumping on tail	Animals which lay down and refused to stand up while they were being sent into the Abattoir had to have their tails pulled, twisted or stamped upon by the cattle handlers before they stood up and began to move.
Vocalisations	At certain times, some of the animals vocalised not because they were badly handled or stressed (vocalisation level 1) while others vocalised because they were inappropriately handled by cattle handlers (vocalisation level 2).

2.5. Measurement of pH of Meat from Poorly-Handled Cattle

By visual observation, meat from 50 poorly-handled cattle was sampled for determination of pH value. Fifty meat samples were excised from the left *longissimus muscle* between the 11th and 12th ribs of each of 50 cattle postmortem. Ten meat samples were taken each day for 5 days. Each sample was taken immediately after slaughter, placed in an air tight bag (a sandwich sealer), and put into an ice chest [20]. Ice blocks were placed on the meat samples and then sent to the Biochemistry Laboratory at the Kwame Nkrumah University of Science and Technology for pH readings to be taken. Transportation of the samples to the laboratory took about 30 min. Two (2 g) of each sample was taken and homogenised in 20 mL of distilled water (1:10 ratio) [21]. The spear tip electrode (Model: PE- 06HD, OCS GMBH/TOP MESSTECHNIK, Deutschland) of a pH metre (Model:PH-212, OCS GMBH/TOP MESSTECHNIK, Deutschland) was dipped into the mixture to read the pH. For each sample, pH was determined at various time intervals of 0 (immediately after slaughter), 6, 18, and 24 h after slaughter. Sections of each excised meat sample were kept refrigerated at +4 °C for determination of pH at the specified times.

2.6. Measurement of Cooking Loss of Meat from Poorly-Handled Cattle

Samples were taken from longissimus in the same way as elaborated under Section 2.5. At the laboratory, 15 g each of the fresh meat samples was weighed, put back into the self-sealing air tight bags and cooked for 35 min in a hot water bath (Büchi Waterbath B-480, Switzerland) at 75 °C. After cooking, the samples were cooled to room temperature in a bucket containing ice.

Each of the samples was re-weighed after cooling to room temperature and cooking loss was calculated as the weight lost during cooking divided by fresh sample weight and expressed as a percentage. Determination of cooking loss was adopted from [22] with some modifications. The modifications were made because the fresh samples had to be transported over a distance (about 30 min), from the Abattoir to the laboratory where the cooking loss determination apparatus was set up.

2.7. Measurement of Carcass Bruising

To investigate carcass bruising, 500 carcasses were evaluated at random for bruises according to the Finnish Meat Research Institute's carcass-evaluation system [23]. Three evaluation categories used in this system were: "none", denoting a clean non-bruised surface; "slight" denoting a reddish area with damage on the surface and "severe", meaning the bruise is reddish, deep and bleeding damage can be observed on the surface.

2.8. Measurement of Proportion of Non-Ambulatory Cattle

Cattle that were non-ambulatory and were drawn by cart to the abattoir to be slaughtered were counted for a period of one week of 7 days. The researcher sat at the gate of the cattle market and counted the number of non-ambulatory animals drawn by cart into the abattoir. The proportion of non-ambulatory animals was calculated as the ratio of the total number of non-ambulatory animals drawn by cart to the total number of animals moved from the cattle market into the abattoir for slaughter expressed as a percentage.

2.9. Data Analysis

Data analyses of the face-to-face interviews and the correlation co-efficients for percent cooking loss and ultimate pH were done with the Statistical Package for the Social Sciences (SPSS Version 16). Microsoft Office Excel 2007 was used to generate the charts for the pre-slaughter handling methods of animals and the behaviours expressed by those stressed animals. Excel was also used to generate the charts showing percent normal, moderate DFD, and DFD meat, ultimate pH of meat against time postmortem, and the charts showing the relationships between percent cooking loss and ultimate pH.

3. Results

3.1. Interview Results

The dealers were asked whether animals were whipped/lashed during loading and unloading and 88% answered in the affirmative while 12% answered otherwise. Eighty-two percent (82%) reported they did not use rest stops for the animals while being sent to Kumasi. All the dealers interviewed

(100%) reported they did not protect their animals from bad weather. Eighteen percent (18%) of the dealers said they fed and watered their animals during transport to Kumasi while 82% of them reported they did not feed and water their animals during transport to Kumasi.

Ninety-seven percent (96.9%) of the middlemen interviewed reported receiving crippled or non-ambulatory animals. All the middlemen (100%) who said they received non-ambulatory animals said those animals were put up for sale. Ninety-one percent (90.6%) of the landlords interviewed reported receiving dead animals from dealers. On the issue of sickness of animals while being sold, 71.9% ($n = 23$) of the interviewed middlemen confirmed such incidences while 28.1% ($n = 9$) did not report any such incidences. Also, all the middlemen interviewed reported that while the animals were being sold, no form of protection against bad weather was provided for them. Ninety-four percent (93.8%) of the middlemen said animals put up for sale were fed and watered while 6.2% ($n = 2$) of them said no feed or water was provided for such animals.

Fifty-six percent (55.8%) of the butchers interviewed said they did not provide their animals feed and water before slaughter while the rest provided them feed and water before slaughter. On the issue of purchase of non-ambulatory animals, 60.5% of the butchers said they purchased non-ambulatory animals while the rest did not purchase such animals. Also, 58.1% purchased sick animals while the rest did not. All the butchers said cattle handlers were responsible for moving animals destined for slaughter from the cattle market into the abattoir and 100% of the butchers reported that they were responsible for paying the cattle handlers for services rendered.

3.2. Behaviours Shown by Cattle and Pre-Slaughter Handling Methods

Prominent among the behaviours regularly exhibited by the cattle during handling were raising of tail, kicking, lying down and refusing to move and jumping (Figure 1).

Among the inhumane methods of handling by cattle handlers, whips ranked highest followed by tail pulling, stamping on the tail of the cattle, stoning, slapping of the cattle with bare hands, forcing animal to fall down, leg pulling, and horn pulling (Figure 2).

3.3. Meat Quality

According to [24], the pH range of normal meat from an animal which is not stressed is 5.4–5.7. DFD meat will have a much higher pH of 5.9–6.5, with some meat being as high as a pH of 6.8. However, the cause of DFD is not primarily due to stress.

The percentage cooking loss of meat samples from the cattle that were subjected to poor handling ranged from 19.10–34.70 with a mean of 22.51 ± 3.25. From Figure 3, the ultimate pH of meat from the poorly-handled cattle averaged (6.22 ± 0.10, $p \leq 0.05$).

Of the 50 cattle that were poorly-handled, none had normal meat (pH from 5.5–5.8) in relation to ultimate pH, 14% had moderate DFD ($5.8 \leq \text{pH} \leq 6.2$) tendency, while 86% had DFD (from 6.2–6.7) meat (Figure 4).

The correlation analysis and the fitted equation (Figure 5) show that meat from the cattle that were subjected to poor handling, percentage cooking loss increased as ultimate pH decreased (a strong negative correlation, $r = -0.77$, $p \leq 0.05$).

Figure 1. Frequency of occurrence of regularly-occurring behaviours exhibited by cattle (n = 200) as they were moved from the cattle market into the abattoir.

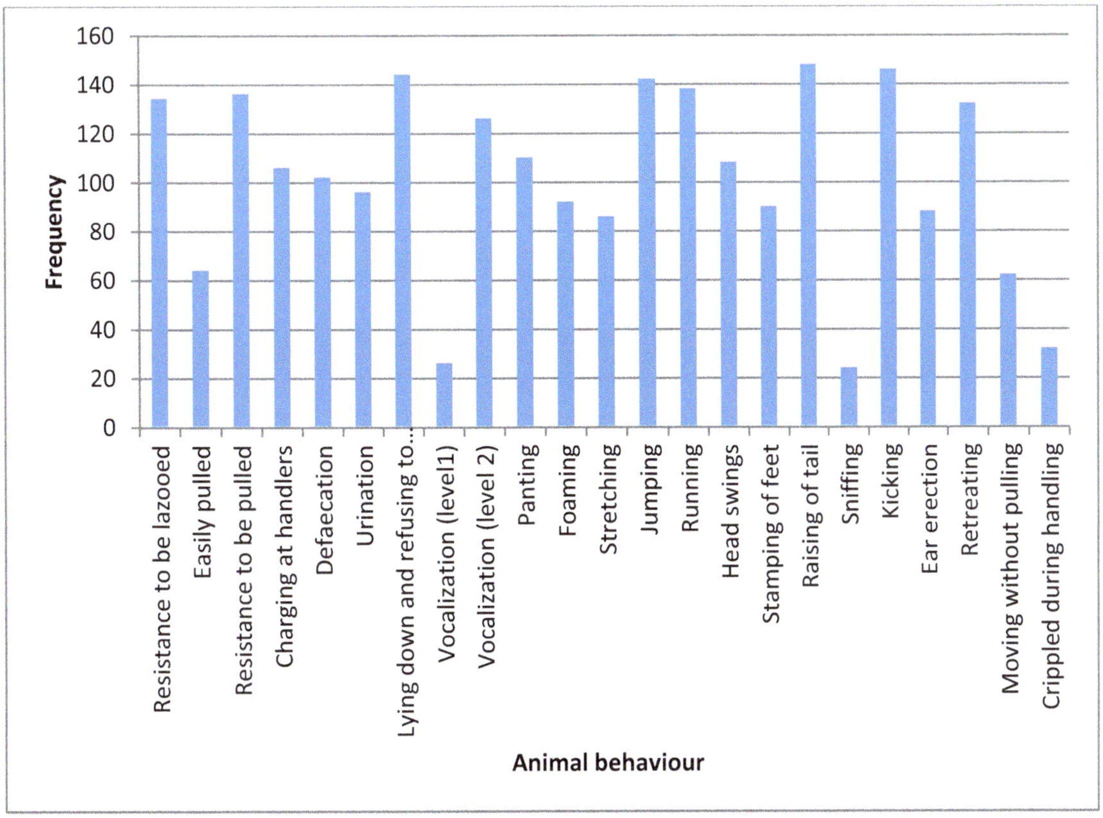

Figure 2. Frequency of occurrence of ways of handling cattle (n = 200) as they were being moved from the cattle market into the abattoir.

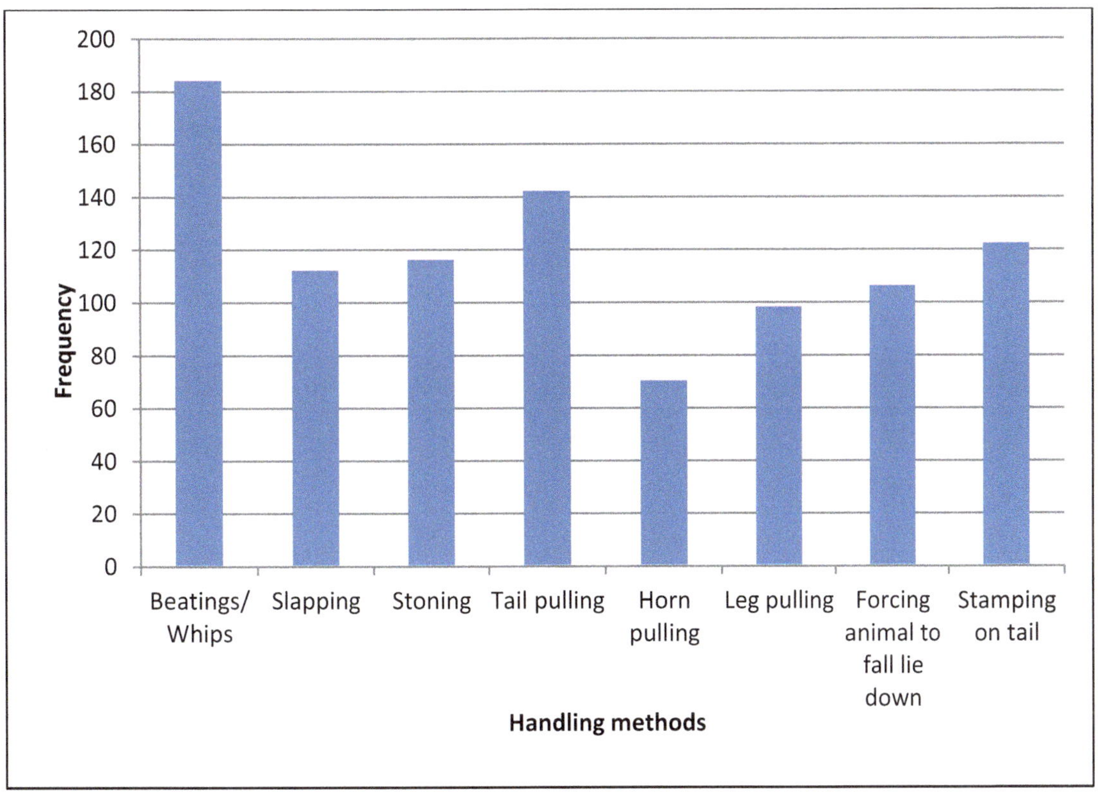

Figure 3. Mean pH of meat against time postmortem for poorly-handled cattle (PHC), non-ambulatory cattle (NAC), bruised carcasses (BRC), and unbruised carcasses (UBRC).

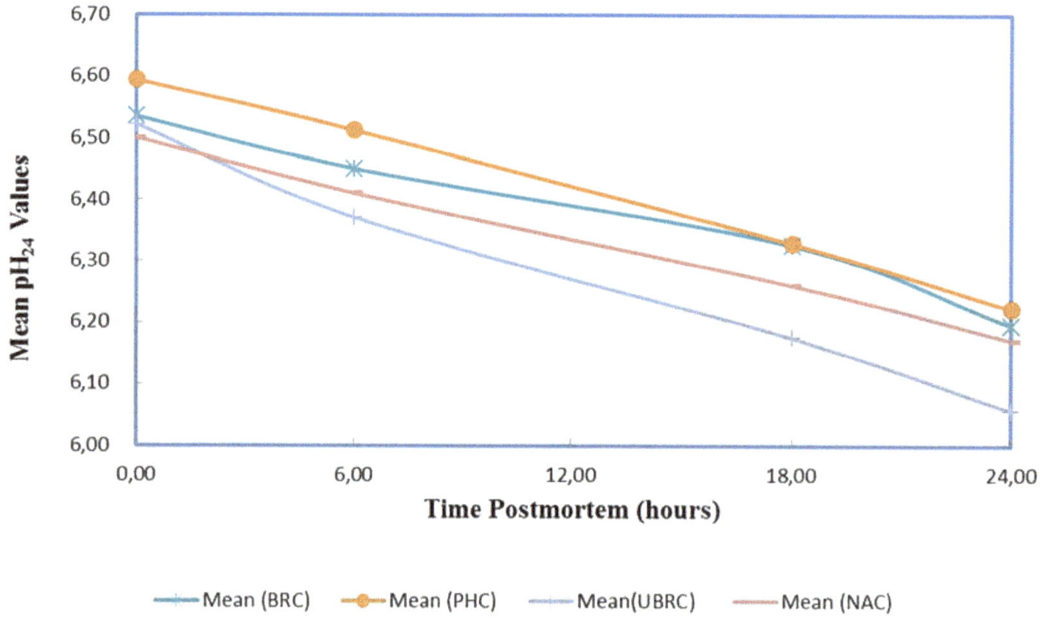

Figure 4. Percent normal, moderate DFD, and DFD meat from poorly-handled cattle.

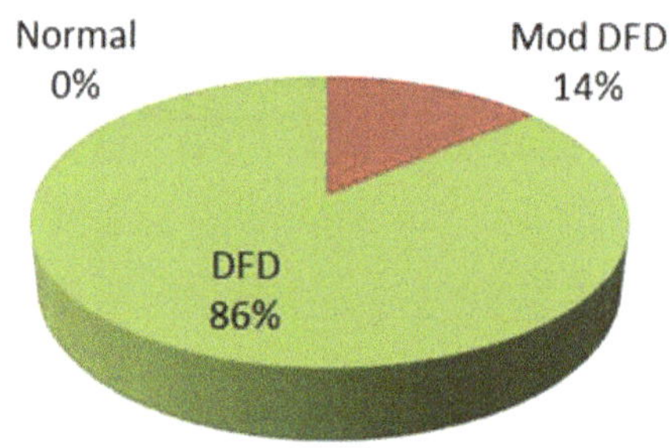

Figure 5. Linear correlation of percent cooking loss and ultimate pH (pH_{24}) of poorly-handled cattle.

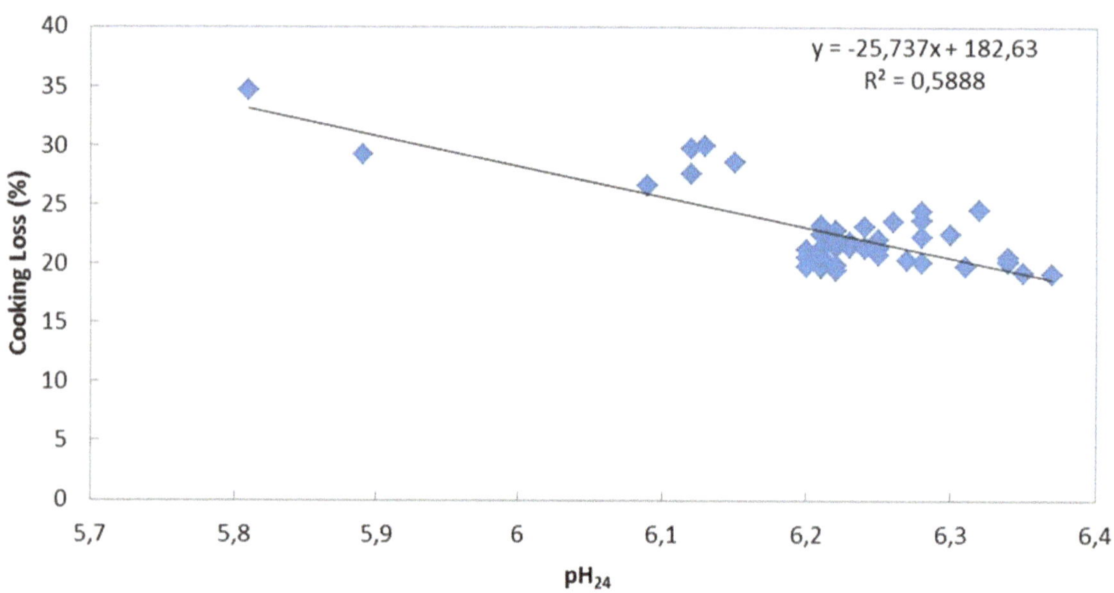

Of the 500 carcasses that were visually observed for bruises (Table 2), 18% had no bruises, 60% showed slight bruises while 22% showed severe bruises. The numbers that showed no bruises ranged from 5–13 carcasses per day with a mean of 8.9 ± 2.60, those which showed slight bruises ranged from 21–37 carcasses per day with a mean of 30.3 ± 4.62.while those that showed severe bruises ranged from 5–17 carcasses per day with a mean of 10.8 ± 4.02. In total, 82.2% (n = 411) of the carcasses observed were bruised (Figure 6).

Table 2. Bruising in carcasses (n = 500).

Bruising Category	Minimum No. of Carcasses/Day	Maximum No. of Carcasses/Day	Mean ± SD	n	Percentage of Carcasses (%)
None [1]	5	13	8.9 ± 2.60	89	17.8
Slight [2]	21	37	30.3 ± 4.62	303	60.6
Severe [3]	5	17	10.8 ± 4.02	108	21.6

[1] clean non-bruised surface of carcass; [2] reddish area with damage on the surface of carcass; [3] bruise is reddish, deep and bleeding damage can be observed on the surface of carcass.

Figure 6. Meat bruise of a carcass at Kumasi Abattoir.

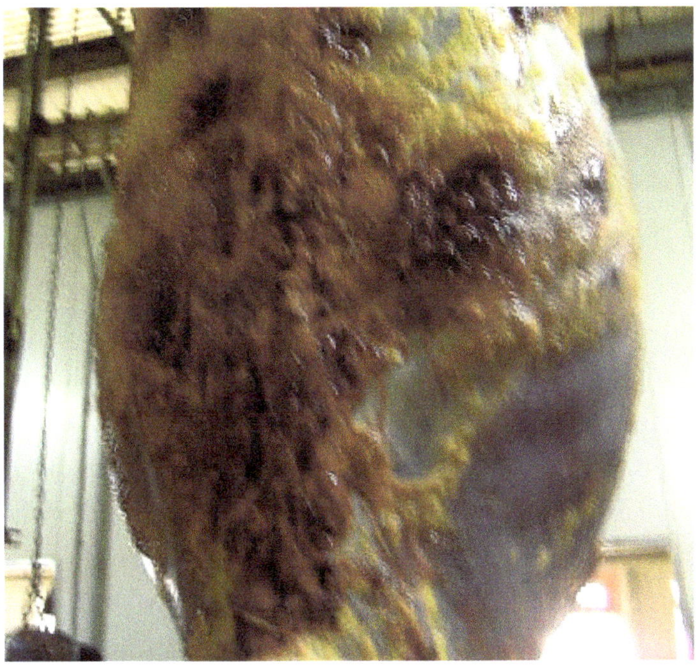

3.4. Non-Ambulatory Cattle

For a period of 7 days, 90 non-ambulatory cattle were sent by carts into the abattoir for slaughter among a total slaughtered animals of 1260. This represents 7.1% of the total number of animals slaughtered within that period. The number of non-ambulatory cattle ranged from 8–21 per day with a mean of 12.86 ± 5.08.

4. Discussion

4.1. Interview of Stakeholders

The dealers were asked whether animals were whipped/lashed during loading and unloading and majority answered in the affirmative. Whipping animals is known to have welfare and economic implications because when the animals are lashed it can lead to bruises, which may have to be trimmed. These trimmings may reduce the quality of the carcass as well as profits gained [25]. Most of the dealers reported they did not use rest stops for the animals sent to Kumasi. The chain of events associated with marketing may be prolonged if animals are sold through live auctions, as is the case of Kumasi Abattoir, rather than directly from farm to slaughter plant [26]. This practice puts physical fatigue on the animals, which are transported from long distances to Kumasi. According to [11], physical stress by hunger, fatigue, and lesions, besides the physiological stress, can lead to depletion of muscle glycogen reserves and lead to the incidence of DFD meat. All the dealers interviewed reported they did not protect their animals from bad weather. Less than 20% of the dealers said they fed and watered their animals transported to Kumasi. According to [4], during transport and handling, animals are faced with unfavourable conditions that compromise their welfare and meat quality. These include food and water deprivation, unfavourable temperature or ventilation, aggressions and physical shocks which cause hunger and thirst, heat stress and pain [6].

Almost all of the middlemen interviewed reported of incidences of receiving crippled or non-ambulatory animals. All the landlords who said they received non-ambulatory animals said those animals were put up for sale. The fact that most of the middlemen confirmed that they received non-ambulatory animals may show that the animals were often overcrowded and when one falls due to poor driving coupled with poor road networks, it finds it difficult to get up again. Majority of the middlemen interviewed reported receiving dead animals from dealers sometimes. Since most of the middlemen confirmed that they received dead animals on arrival, it may indicate that the welfare of the animals was compromised during transportation to the abattoir. According to [8, 9], to some extent, mortality of animals during transport may be an indication of their welfare and transport conditions. On the issue of sickness of animals sold, approximately 72% of the interviewed middlemen confirmed such incidences. The fact that some of the animals displayed for sale fell sick or died, could be attributed to their exposure to the harsh weather without being offered any protection in such weather. Also, all the middlemen interviewed reported that while the animals were being sold, no form of protection against bad weather was provided for them. A great majority of the middlemen said animals put up for sale were fed and watered.

More than half of the butchers interviewed said they did not provide their animals feed and water before slaughter while the rest provided them feed and water before slaughter. On the issue of purchase of non-ambulatory animals, 60.5% of the butchers said they purchased non-ambulatory animals while the rest did not purchase such animals. Also, 58.1% purchased sick animals while the rest did not. This proves that most of the butchers are willing to buy animals without much worry about the health status of the animals. All the butchers said cattle handlers were responsible for moving animals destined for slaughter from the cattle market into the abattoir.

4.2. Behaviours Shown by Cattle and Pre-Slaughter Handling Methods

Among the methods of handling by cattle handlers, whips ranked highest followed by tail pulling, stamping on the tail of the cattle, stoning, slapping the animals with bare hands, forcing animal to fall down, leg pulling, and horn pulling (Figure 2). The methods of handling were ranked by frequency of occurrence. These maltreatments could be associated with the high proportion of bruised carcasses (82.2%) in this study. According to [11], inappropriate handling, improper use of sticks by handlers violent impact of the animals against facilities or impact with other animals are potential bruising events. In a study by [12], it was reported that poor handling or a physical blow that leads to bruising or other animal injury can lead to parts of the carcass being condemned or the meat being dark. Such meat, they say, does not appeal to consumers and spoils quickly.

The most frequently occurring behaviours (Figure 1) exhibited by the cattle while being moved by cattle handlers from the cattle market to the abattoir were raising of tail, kicking, lying down and refusing to move, jumping, running, resistance to being pulled, resistance to being lazooed, retreating, vocalisation (level 2), panting, head swings, charging at handlers, defecation, urinating, foaming at the mouth, stamping of feet repeatedly on the ground, and stretching. According to [14], feedlot and slaughter-plant managers have reported that animals that rear-kick, struggle, and run into objects are not easy to handle and have more dark-cutters. The most obvious indicators that an animal is having difficulty coping with handling or transport are changes in behaviour which show that some aspect of the situation is aversive. The animal may stop moving forward, freeze, back off, rapidly move away, vocalise or show other behaviours including lying down [26]. Handling animals without the practice of using sticks results in better welfare and less risk of poor carcass quality [8]. The cattle in this study were difficult to handle by cattle handlers because they (the cattle) were sent into the abattoir in isolation (individually) from their groups but cattle are known to be herd animals so when one gets nearer to them, they instinctively want to rejoin their herd mates [27]. The handlers had no basic training in animal handling which also made it difficult to handle the cattle.

According to [28], if animal handlers learnt the basics of animal behaviour, their ability to move animals in a safer, more efficient and less stressful manner would improve. According to the dealers and middlemen, while cattle were being loaded and unloaded, they were whipped with sticks. This is a bad handling practice which might have contributed to the difficulty in moving the cattle from the cattle market to the abattoir. This is because cattle have long memories so their previous experiences will affect their stress reaction to handling. Roughly handled cattle will be more stressed and difficult to handle in the future [27].

4.3. Meat Quality

As long as there is adequate glycogen present at slaughter, the pH of cattle will fall to within the normal range of 5.4–5.7 [29]. If there is not enough glycogen (due to stress or poor nutrition) then pH will remain above the acceptable limit of pH 5.7 and the meat is likely to be dark in colour, with poor keeping quality [30]. As muscle is converted to meat, a host of metabolic and structural changes occur. In the immediate postmortem period, as the muscle attempts to maintain homeostasis, muscle glycogen is metabolised through anaerobic glycolysis, thus phosphorylating ADP to ATP. Anaerobic glycolysis generates lactate that builds up, lowering the intracellular pH, so that by 24 h postmortem the pH has fallen to an ultimate pH value of about 5.4–5.7 [29]. In a study in summer on pigs by [31], pigs that were transported for longer times had higher pH_{24} (5.99 ± 0.29 for 12 h; 5.79 ± 0.18 for 8 h; and 5.65 ± 0.17 for 4 h of travel According to [23], the pH range of normal meat from an animal which is not stressed is 5.4–5.7. DFD meat will have a much higher pH of 5.9–6.5, with some meat having as high a pH as 6.8. Previous studies have found out that dark-cutting meat is more prevalent in cattle, which become agitated or excited immediately before slaughter [1, 32] stated that meat from such cattle are darker, drier and firmer and has a shorter shelf life. All the meat sampled in this study were poor in quality based on pH_{24} (Figure 4), due to stress of the cattle from factors such as poor pre-slaughter handling, feed and water deprivation, mixing of unfamiliar animals, exposure to poor weather, and long distances the animals mostly travel.

Water-holding capacity has been significantly correlated with muscle pH, exhibiting that lower cook losses are associated with higher muscle pH and better protein functionality [33]. Higher muscle pH values are farther from the isoelectric point of the contractile proteins; as a result, the proteins are more functional, resulting in lower cook losses [33]. The correlation analyses in this present study are in agreement with these assertions. In a study on turkeys [34], ultimate pH was found to be negatively correlated with cooking loss ($r = -0.52$) which is in agreement with what was reported in this study though beef and turkey meat are different.

4.4. Carcass Bruising

In a study on the relationship between pre-slaughter and bull carcass bruising, bruised carcasses constituted 66.9% [35]. This was less than what was observed in the present study because cattle in this study mostly suffered inhumane handling prior to slaughter. They reported that slightly bruised bull carcasses constituted 54.9% as against 12.0% in severely bruised bull carcasses. Although the amounts of slight and severe bruising in this study were more than those reported by [35], the trend is the same, with more slight bruises observed than severe bruises. In a study by [36], cattle from a feedlot where handlers handled them roughly had 15.5% bruising. A Canadian study [37] revealed that 15% of the cattle showed severe bruising while 78% of the carcasses exhibited bruising of some sort. These results are not in agreement with those of the present study.

4.5. Non-Ambulatory Cattle

In an assessment of culled cattle in holding pens at 21 slaughter facilities in the United States, approximate overall incidence of non-ambulatory cattle of 1.1% was recorded [38]. Estimates of the number of starved cattle slaughtered at federally inspected facilities showed that the incidence of non-ambulatory cattle was between 0.7% and 1.1%. The aggregated sum of beef and dairy cattle that could not stand and walk in the years 2003 and 2004 were 0.04% and 0.38%, respectively [15]. What was recorded in this study exceeds what were observed in the above assessments. According to [36], causes of downed or non-ambulatory cattle probably differ by region, herd size and herd management. The major kinds of causes for non-ambulatory cattle are injuries related to dystocia, other injuries such as fractures, muscle and ligament damage, infectious diseases such as toxic mastitis, lymphoma, peritonitis, and metabolic disorders such as acidosis. According to Carolyn *et al.* [16], if the non-ambulatory animal is suffering and the pain or distress cannot be controlled or is not likely to be controlled quickly, the animal should be euthanised. However, during this study, non-ambulatory cattle which were in pain were not slaughtered without being euthanized.

5. Conclusions and Recommendations

The main conclusions from the present study are that:

- The indications of compromised welfare of the cattle as deduced from the interviews conducted in this study were feed and water deprivation by some dealers and middlemen, avoidance of the use of animal rest stops by some dealers, overcrowding in vehicles, no protection against bad weather, and maltreatment of animals by handlers.
- The prominent methods of handling by cattle handlers which put stress on the animals were lashes/whips, pulling the tails of the animals, stamping on their tails, and hitting them with stones. As a result of these inhumane ways of handling the animals, they exhibited some behaviours to show that they were stressed. Prominent among those behaviours were raising of their tails, kicking, lying down and refusing to move, jumping, running, resistance to be lazooed and pulled, retreating, vocalisation (level 2), panting, head swings, charging at handlers, defecation, urination, and foaming at the mouth.
- Poor handling of cattle prior to slaughter might led to a high incidence of DFD meat (6.22 ± 0.10) and a low mean value of percent cooking loss (22.5 ± 3.25). This proves that poor handling of cattle immediately before slaughter had an effect on meat quality in terms of ultimate pH and percent cooking loss.
- In poorly-handled cattle, cooking loss increased as ultimate pH decreased (that is, an inverse relationship as can be seen from the correlation co-efficient).
- For a period of 7 days, 90 non-ambulatory cattle were sent by carts into the abattoir for slaughter among a total slaughtered animals of 1260. This represents 7.1% of the total number of animals slaughtered within that period. This to some extent is an indication of compromised welfare of cattle pre-slaughter. This study is useful in exposing the sufferings that slaughter animals suffer in the hands of handlers from some farms through transport to the abattoir in Kumasi.
- It is recommended that the preliminary results from this study concerning the compromised welfare situation of slaughter animals during transport, at lairage, and slaughter should be brought to the attention of stakeholders in the business. Further studies are recommended, for instance, to obtain more reliable scientific evidence to help guide legislation on animal welfare in Ghana.

Acknowledgments

The authors acknowledge the financial supports from the Agricultural Engineering Department of the Kwame Nkrumah University of Science and Technology, Kumasi, Ghana, and the Department of Energy and Technology, Swedish University of Agricultural Sciences, Uppsala, Sweden. We are indebted to the numerous cattle dealers and butchers at the Kumasi abattoir for their co-operation during the study. Finally, we appreciate the efforts of the anonymous reviewers of this paper for their constructive criticisms

Author Contributions

All the authors plan the experiments. Data collection was done by Frimpong and Hamdu. Data, analysis and manuscript writing was done by Frimpong, Bobobee and Gebresenbet with revisions from the other authors.

Conflicts of Interest

The authors declare no conflict of interest.

References

1. Ljungberg, D.; Gebresenbet, G.; Aradom, S. Logistics chain of animal transport and abattoir operations. *Biosyst. Eng.* **2007**, *96*, 267–277.
2. Gebresenbet, G.; Wikner, I.; Bobobee, E.Y.H.; Maria, G.; Villarroel, M. Effect of Transport Time and Handling on Physiological Responses of Cattle. *J. Agric. Sci. Technol. A* **2012**, *2*, 800–814.
3. Ferguson, D.; Warner, R. Have we underestimated the impact of pre-slaughter stress on meat quality in ruminants? *Meat Sci.* **2008**, *80*, 12–19.
4. Gregory, N. Animal welfare at markets and during transport and slaughter. *Meat Sci.* **2008**, *80*, 2–11.
5. Gebresenbet, G.; Ljunberg, D.; Geers, R.; van de Water, G. Effective logistics to improve animal welfare in the production chain, with special emphasis on farm-abattoir system. *Int. Soc. Anim. Hyg.* **2004**, *1*, 37–38.
6. Sossidou, E.; Broom, D.M.; Cziszter, L.T.; Geers, R.; Gebresenbet, G.; Szücs, E. Welfare of Long Distance Transportation of Cattle. *Lucrări Ştiintifice Zootehnie Şi Biotehnologii* **2009**, *42*, 603–613.
7. Deiss, V.; Temple, D.; Ligout, S.; Racine, C.; Bouix, J.; Terlouw, C.; Boissy, A. Can emotional reactivity predict stress responses at slaughter in sheep? *Appl. Anim. Behav. Sci.* **2009**, *119*, 193–202.
8. Malena, M.; Voslářova, E.; Tomanová, P.; Lepková, R.; Bedáňová, I.; Večerek, V. Influence of travel distance and season upon transport-induced mortality in fattened cattle. *Acta Vet. Brno* **2006**, *75*, 619–624.
9. Warriss, P.D. The welfare of slaughter pigs during transport. *Anim. Welf.* **1998**, *7*, 365–381.
10. Broom, D.M. The effects of land transport on animal welfare. *Rev. Sci. Tech.* **2005**, *24*, 683–691.
11. Warriss, P.D. The handling of cattle pre-slaughter and its effects on carcass and meat quality. *Appl. Anim. Behav. Sci.* **1990**, *28*, 171–186.
12. Costa, L.N.; Lo Fiego, D.P.; Tassone, F.; Russo, V. The relationship between carcass bruising in bulls and behaviour observed during pre-slaughter phases. *Vet. Res. Commun.* **2006**, *30* (Suppl. 1), 379–381.
13. van Donkergoed, J.; Jewison, G.; Mann, M.; Cherry, B.; Altwasser, B.; Lower, R.; Wiggins, K.; Dejonte, R.; Thorlakson, B.; Moss, E.; *et al*. Canadian Beef Quality Audit. *Can. J. Anim. Sci.* **1997**, *38*, 217–225.

14. Chambers, P.G.; Grandin, T. Guidelines for Humane Handling, Transport and Slaughter of Livestock from the Food and Agriculture Organisation of the United Nations Regional Office for Asia and the Pacific, 2001. Available online: http://www.aphca.org/publications/files/2001-04_low.pdf (accessed on 7 July 2009).
15. Cox, V.S.; Marsh, W.E.; Steurnagel, G.R. Downer cow occurrence in Minnesota dairy herds. *Prev. Vet. Med.* **1986**, *4*, 249–260.
16. Carolyn, L.S.; Payne, M.A.; Berry, S.L.; Reynolds, J.P. A review of the causes, prevention, and welfare of nonambulatory cattle. *J. Am. Vet. Med. Assoc.* **2007**, *231*, 227–234.
17. Zobil, B.B. Acting Productions Manager, Kumasi Abattoir Company Limited. Kumasi, Ghana. Personal Communication, 17 March 2010.
18. Adzitey, F. MiniReview-Effect of pre-slaughter animal handling on carcass and meat quality. *Int. Food Res. J.* **2011**, *18*, 485–491.
19. Afful, C.R. Kumasi Abattoir Company Limited, Kumasi, Ghana. Personal Communication, 13 July 2009.
20. Obiri-Danso, K.; Hogarh, J.N.; Antwi-Agyei, P. Assessment of contamination of singed hides from cattle and goats by heavy metals in Ghana. *Afr. J. Environ. Sci. Technol.* **2008**, *2*, 217–221.
21. Quilo, S.A.; Pohlman, F.W.; Dias-Morse, P.N. Instrumental colour characteristics of ground beef treated with potassium lactate, sodium metasilicate, peroxyacetic acid or acidified chlorite. *AAES Res. Ser.* **2006**, *545*, 31–33.
22. Okeudo, N.J.; Moss, B.W. Interrelationships amongst carcass and meat quality characteristics of sheep. *Meat Sci.* **2005**, *69*, 1–8.
23. Strappini, A.C.; Metz, J.H.M.; Gallo, C.B.; Kemp, B. Origin and assessment of bruises in beef cattle at slaughter. *Anim. Sci.* **2009**, *3*, 728–736.
24. Miller, M. Dark, Firm and Dry Beef. Beef Facts-Product Enhancements; 2007. Available online: http://www.beefresearch.org/…/BeefResearch/DarkFirmDryBeef.pdf (accessed on 3 May 2010).
25. Immonen, K.; Ruusunen, M.; Puolanne, E. Some effects of residual glycogen concentration on the physical sensory quality of normal pH beef. *Meat Sci.* **2000**, *55*, 33–38.
26. Grandin, T. Livestock-handling quality assurance. *J. Anim. Sci.* **2001**, *79* (E Suppl.), E239–E248.
27. SCAHAW. The Welfare of Animals during Transport. Scientific Report of the Scientific Panel on Animal Health and Welfare on a request from the Commission Related to the Welfare of Animals during Transport, 2004. Available online: http://www.efsa.europa.eu/en/efsajournal/doc/ahaw_report_animaltransportwelfare_en1.pdf?ssbinary=true (accessed on 8 September 2009).
28. Grandin, T. Principles for Low Stress Cattle Handling. AG/Beef/06. 2005. Available online: http://extension.usu.edu/files/publications/beef6stress.pdf (accessed on 22 May 2009).
29. Atkinson, S. The Importance of Animal Handling Technique and Animal Handling Facility Design for the Welfare of Slaughter Animals. NJF Report; 2005. Available online: http://www.njf.nu/filebank/files/20060904$211818$fil$TeQq2b6EMZ55RzFnx4YL.pdf (accessed on 7 April 2010).
30. Maltin, C.; Balcerzak, D.; Tilley, R.; Delday, M. Determinants of meat quality: Tenderness. *Proc. Nutr. Soc.* **2003**, *62*, 337–347.
31. MSA. Australian Beef Carcass Appraisal System. Meat and Livestock Australia. 2006. Available online: http:www.primex.net.au/Primex_2/encoded/MSA%2016pp.pdf (accessed on 25 March 2010).

32. Aradom, S.; Gebresenbet, G.; Bulitta, F.S.; Bobobee, E.Y.; Adam, M. Effect of Transport Times on Welfare of Pigs. *J. Agric. Sci. Technol. A* **2012**, *2*, 544–562.
33. Grandin, T. Handling methods and facilities to reduce stress on cattle. *Vet. Clin. North Am. Food Anim. Pract.* **1998**, *14*, 325–341.
34. Owens, C.M.; Sams, A.R. The influence of transportation on turkey meat quality. *Poult. Sci.* **2000**, *79*, 1204–1207.
35. Mallia, J.G.; Barbut, S.; Vainllancourt, J.P.; Martin, S.W.; McEwen, S.A. A dark, firm dry-like condition in turkeys condemned for cyanosis. *Poult. Sci.* **2000**, *79*, 281–285.
36. Costa, L.N.; Lo Fiego, D.P.; Russo, V. Study on the Relationship between Pre-Slaughter and Carcass Bruising in Calf and Bull Carcasses. NJF Report; 2005. Available online: http://www.njf.nu/filebank/files/20060904$211818$fil$TeQq2b6EMZ55RzFnx4YL.pdf (accessed on 7 April 2010).
37. Grandin, T. Bruising on southwestern feedlot cattle. *J. Anim. Sci.* **1981**, *53* (Suppl. 1), 213.
38. Reynolds, J. Dealing with Downers. *AABP Proc.* **2006**, *39*, 28–31. Available online: http://ansci.colostate.edu/files/dairy_news/v13_4/Downers.pdf (accessed on 26 March 2010).

8

Fatal Canine Leptospirosis on St. Kitts

Amanda Loftis [1,2], Fernanda Castillo-Alcala [1], Lewis Bogdanovic [1,3] and Ashutosh Verma [1,*]

[1] Department of Biomedical Sciences, Ross University School of Veterinary Medicine, P.O. Box 334, Basseterre, St. Kitts, West Indies; E-Mails: adloftis@gmail.com (A.L.); fcastillo@rossvet.edu.kn (F.C.-A.); lewis.bogdanovic@gmail.com (L.B.)

[2] Department of Microbiology & Immunology, Midwestern University, Glendale, AZ 85308, USA

[3] Banfield Pet Hospital, 10520 Trinity Parkway, Stockton, CA 95219, USA

* Author to whom correspondence should be addressed; E-Mails: averma@rossvet.edu.kn; ashutosh.verma@gmail

---

Abstract: Through prospective enrollment of canine patients at the Ross University Veterinary Clinic, on St. Kitts, four cases of acute fatal leptospirosis were diagnosed. Clinical, pathological, and diagnostic findings in these cases are summarized in this case series. Icterus, thrombocytopenia, hyperphosphatemia, pulmonary hemorrhage, and both hepatocellular and renal damage were noted in all four cases. Interestingly, extensive myocardial involvement was also observed in one case. To our knowledge, this is the first documentation of myocarditis in a dog with leptospirosis, and the first report of fatal leptospirosis in any animal species on the Caribbean island of St. Kitts.

Keywords: canine leptospirosis; *Leptospira*; spirochetes

---

1. Introduction

Leptospirosis, a waterborne zoonotic infection that affects dogs and many other mammalian species, is caused by infection with pathogenic *Leptospira*. Leptospires live in the kidneys of reservoir animals and are shed in the urine, contaminating surface water. Susceptible hosts acquire the infection following mucous membrane or percutaneous exposure to infected animal urine or *Leptospira*-contaminated water [1,2].

The incidence of leptospirosis is significantly higher in warmer climates and parts of the world with greater interaction between people and animals. For these reasons, the Caribbean is considered to be one of the major foci of leptospirosis in the world [3]. A recent serosurvey of pregnant women from 10 Caribbean countries reported antibodies against *Leptospira* in every country, including St. Kitts and Nevis [4]. Reports from other Caribbean islands have documented leptospirosis in wildlife and animal reservoirs, but there is limited information on the presence of *Leptospira* in animals on the island of St. Kitts [5–10]. In this case series, we describe the clinical presentation and diagnostic findings in four dogs with acute leptospirosis.

2. Case Descriptions

From 2010 through 2012, a total of 12 cases of suspected leptospirosis were prospectively enrolled at the Ross University Veterinary Clinics, in accordance with an approved Institutional Animal Care and Use Committee protocol. From this group, four confirmed acute cases and one chronic case of leptospirosis were diagnosed. Another four animals in the group were diagnosed with *Ehrlichia canis* infection, and the remaining cases were undiagnosed [11]. The chronic subclinical case of leptospirosis was described previously [10] and the four acute, fatal cases of leptospirosis are described below. *Ehrlichia*- and *Babesia*-specific PCR tests were performed to rule out other etiologies [12]. None of the cases discussed here were found positive for either of these pathogens.

Results of complete blood count (CBC), serum biochemistry testing, and urinalysis are detailed in Table 1. Full necropsies were performed in fatal cases. A complete set of tissue samples were collected from each case, fixed in 10% neutral-buffered formalin, routinely processed and stained with hematoxylin and eosin (HE). Select sections of the kidney and the liver were evaluated using Warthin-Starry stain.

Table 1. Results of complete blood count (CBC), serum biochemistry testing, and urinalysis.

	Case 1	Case 2	Case 3	Case 4
CBC Results				
TNCC (6–17 × 10^9/L)	12.42	32.28	41.8	18.19
Neutrophils, seg (3–11.4 × 10^9/L)	9.3	29.1	ND	16.6
Neutrophils, band (0–0.3 × 10^9/L)	0.2	0	ND	0.2
Lymphocytes (1–4.8 × 10^9/L)	0.1	0.3	ND	0.9
Monocytes (0.15–1.35 × 10^9/L)	7.2	2.9	ND	0.5
Eosinophils (0.1–0.75 × 10^9/L)	0	0	ND	0
Basophils (0 × 10^9/L)	0	0	ND	0
PCV (37%–55%)	30	49	34	30
RBC (5.5–8.5 × 10^{12}/L)	5.04	7.9	5.68	4.73
Hemoglobin (12–18 g/dL)	10.5	16.7	10.5	9.3
Reticulocytes (0–60 × 10^6/L)	0	0	ND	47.3
MCV (60–77 fL)	56	64	60	62
MCH (19.5–24.5 pg)	20.8	21.1	18.5	19.6
MCHC (31.0–34.0 g/dL)	37.6	33	31.1	31.5
Platelets (200–500 × 10^9/L)	19	156	61	3
MPV (3.9–11.1 fL)	7.9	7.8	9.9	8.2

Table 1. *Cont.*

	Case 1	Case 2	Case 3	Case 4
Serum Biochemistry				
Refractometer protein (6–7.5 g/dL)	6.5	8.8	ND	5.4
Total Protein (5.4–8.2 g/dL)	4.4	ICT	ICT	5.3
Albumin (2.5–4.4 g/dL)	2.8	ICT	ICT	2.1
Globulin (2.3–5.2 g/dL)	1.6	ICT	ICT	3.2
Alkaline phosphatase (20–150 U/L)	1697	545	448	596
ALT (10–118 U/L)	147	ICT	62	217
Amylase (200–1200 U/L)	2536	ND	2387	322
Glucose (60–110 mg/dL)	87	84	112	100
Total Bilirubin (0.1–0.6 mg/dL)	11.2	21.8	18	4.7
BUN (25–180 mg/dL)	>180	>180	125	121
Creatinine (0.3–1.4 mg/dL)	ICT	ICT	ICT	2.6
Calcium (8.6–11.8 mg/dL)	9.7	14.7	>16	13.4
Phosphorus (2.9–6.6 mg/dL)	17.5	>20.0	16.1	16.8
Sodium (138–160 mmol/L)	132	149	146	142
Potassium (3.7–5.8 mmol/L)	8.1	ICT	4.7	4.1
Na: K Ratio	16.3	ICT	31.1	34.6
Urinalysis				
Spec. Gravity	1.011	1.027	ND	1.011
pH	6	5	ND	7
Protein (mg/dL)	15–30	100–300	ND	15–30
Glucose (mg/dL)	Negative	100–250	ND	100–250
Ketones (mg/dL)	≥160	Negative	ND	Negative
Bilirubin (mg/dL)	Negative	≥6.0	ND	Negative
Hemoglobin/Blood (Ery/uL)	50–250	80–250, hm	ND	≥250

ND: Not determined; ICT: icterus; hm: hemolysed.

DNA was isolated from whole blood (200 μL), and tissues (10–20 mg) using a DNeasy Blood and Tissue Mini-Kit (Qiagen, Valencia, CA, USA), following the manufacturer's directions. Urine samples (1–1.5 mL) were centrifuged for 5 min at 10,000 g, and pellets were processed using the DNeasy Blood and Tissue Mini-Kit (Qiagen). A *Leptospira*- specific fluorescence resonance energy transfer-polymerase chain reaction (FRET-PCR) was performed on a LightCycler 2.0 real-time PCR platform using thermal protocol and PCR conditions as described elsewhere [10]. *Leptospira* serovars Canicola, Copenhageni (Icterohaemorrhagiae), Grippotyphosa, Hebdomadis, Autmnalis, Australis, Ballum, and Pomona (NVSL, Ames, IA, USA) were maintained at 30 °C in Polysorbate −80 bovine serum albumin medium (NVSL), and used to perform the microscopic agglutination test (MAT), as described previously [13].

2.1. Case 1

A four-month old, intact male mixed-breed puppy (1.6 kg) presented for acute onset of vomiting, diarrhea, anorexia, and lethargy. The owner reported two prior vaccinations with a DHPPC combination, but not *Leptospira*. The patient was hypothermic (T = 96.6 °F), tachycardic (200/min), and hypotensive (systolic blood pressure of 85 mm Hg). CBC with differential revealed lymphopenia with monocytosis, mild microcytic anemia, and severe thrombocytopenia with no visible platelet clumping or giant platelets. Serum biochemistry revealed several abnormalities, most notably elevated liver enzymes, bilirubin, BUN, and phosphorus, and low sodium with high potassium. Urine was dilute with mild hematuria and trace amounts of protein; waxy casts and clumps of transitional epithelial cells were seen in the sediment. The patient was euthanized and submitted for necropsy.

Gross necropsy findings included poor body condition (1.5/5), generalized icterus, and petechial to ecchymotic hemorrhages in the lungs and kidneys. The liver appeared pale and had an enhanced lobular pattern. The main microscopic lesions were confined to the kidneys and the liver (Figure 1). In the kidneys, there was acute tubular degeneration and necrosis, with multifocal mineralization of the tubular basement membrane. In the liver, there was marked dissociation of the hepatocellular cords, multifocal hepatocellular necrosis, central congestion and prominent vacuolation of hepatocytes. Bile stasis was prominent in major biliary ducts.

Figure 1. Case 1. Multifocal areas of acute renal tubular degeneration and necrosis, with multifocal mineralization of the tubular basement membrane (**A**). Marked dissociation of the hepatocellular cords, multifocal hepatocellular necrosis, central congestion and prominent vacuolation of hepatocytes (**B**). H&E stain 40×.

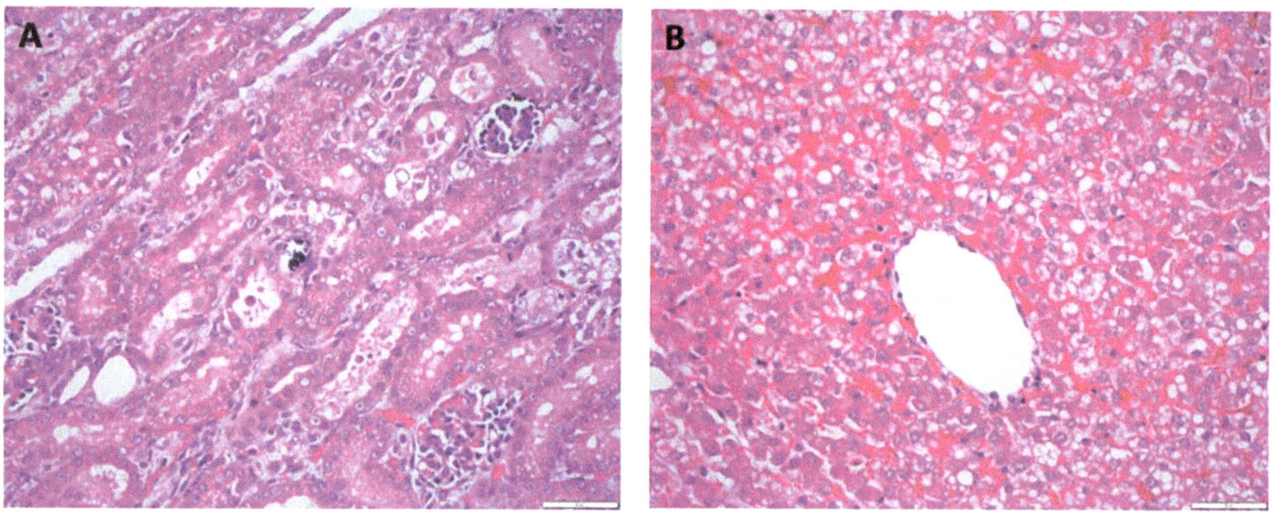

Testing for *Leptospira* using FRET-PCR was performed on blood, liver, and kidney samples. Liver and kidney samples were positive for *Leptospira* DNA, and blood was weakly positive, with detectable DNA on only one of three replicates. No samples were available for serologic testing.

2.2. Case 2

A seven-month-old, intact female mixed-breed dog (9.0 kg) presented for weakness and vomiting. The patient was afebrile (T = 99.7 °F), tachycardic (180/min), hypotensive (blood pressure 90 mm Hg), and icteric on presentation. Neutrophilia, lymphopenia, and monocytosis were noted, along with mild thrombocytopenia and occasional giant platelets. Serum biochemistry was complicated by severe icterus, but liver enzymes, bilirubin, BUN, calcium, and phosphorus were elevated. Urinalysis revealed bilirubinuria and hematuria with granular casts, leukocytes, and bacteria (cocci) seen in sediment. There was no improvement following treatment with intravenous fluids, ampicillin, and famotidine, and the patient was euthanized eight hours after admission.

Gross necropsy findings included only adequate body condition (2.5/5), generalized icterus, petechial to ecchymotic hemorrhages in the subcutaneous tissue, lungs, urinary bladder and kidneys. The liver appeared diffusely congested and there were multifocal, segmental areas of hemorrhage in the gastric and intestinal mucosae. The main microscopic lesions were confined to the kidneys and the liver. In the kidneys, there was acute tubular degeneration and necrosis, with multifocal mineralization of the tubular basement membrane. Multifocal, discrete aggregates of lymphocytes and plasma cells in the renal interstitium were also observed. In the liver, there was marked dissociation of the hepatocellular cords, and multifocal hepatocellular necrosis.

Testing for *Leptospira* DNA using FRET-PCR was performed on blood and urine, and leptospiral DNA was detected in the urine. Serology, using the MAT revealed titers of 1:400 and 1:800 for serovars Icterohaemorrhagiae and Grippotyphosa, respectively.

2.3. Case 3

A four-month old female Bull Mastiff-Rottweiler cross puppy (9.1 kg) was presented for lethargy and anorexia of a few days duration. There was no history of prior vaccination for *Leptospira*; a combination DAPPC vaccine had been given two months prior. The dog was sternally recumbent, afebrile (T = 101.3 °F), severely dehydrated, and tachycardic (250/min). Icterus of the sclera, pinnae, and mucous membranes was noted. The liver was palpably enlarged. CBC was performed but no differential count was included; leukocytosis and thrombocytopenia were detected. Icterus interfered with serum biochemistry testing, but alkaline phosphatase, amylase, bilirubin, BUN, calcium, and phosphorus were all elevated. The patient was euthanized, and necropsy was performed.

Gross necropsy findings included only adequate body condition (2.5/5), generalized icterus, petechial to ecchymotic hemorrhages in the subcutaneous tissue, lungs, and kidneys. The kidneys were slightly enlarged and edematous. The liver was diffusely pale and had an enhanced lobular pattern. There were multifocal areas of hemorrhage in the intestinal mucosa. The main microscopic lesions were confined to the kidneys and the liver. Due to postmortem autolysis, optimal examination of the tissues was prevented. In the kidneys, there was acute tubular degeneration and necrosis, with multifocal mineralization of the tubular basement membrane. There were also multifocal, discrete aggregates of round cells (presumed to be lymphocytes and plasma cells) in the renal interstitium. In the liver, there was marked dissociation of the hepatocellular cords, and multifocal hepatocellular necrosis.

Blood, urine, liver, and kidney samples were tested for *Leptospira* using FRET-PCR, and the urine and liver tested positive for *Leptospira* DNA. No samples were available for serologic testing.

2.4. Case 4

A 7-week-old old male, mixed breed puppy (2.0 kg) presented for acute onset of vomiting, diarrhea, and anorexia. The puppy was afebrile (T = 99.9 °F) and tachycardic (160/min), with generalized lymphadenopathy. Mild neutrophilia and lymphocytopenia, mild anemia, and severe thrombocytopenia were noted on CBC with differential. Liver enzymes, bilirubin, BUN, creatinine, calcium, and phosophorus were all elevated. Abdominal ultrasound revealed hyperechoic kidneys and a hypoechoic, enlarged liver. Upon treatment with intravenous fluids, the patient was noted to be anuric; attempted diuresis with furosemide resulted in only 1 mL of urine; urine was dilute, with significant hematuria, and clumps of transitional epithelial cells were noted in urine sediment. The patient became progressively more icteric, remained anuric, and was euthanized.

Gross necropsy findings included only adequate body condition (2.5/5), generalized icterus and edema (anasarca). There were multifocal petechial to ecchymotic hemorrhages in the lungs, kidneys (Figure 2A,B), urinary bladder, and gastric and intestinal mucosae. The liver appeared pale and had an enhanced lobular pattern. Multifocal small (1–4 mm) areas of pallor were present in the myocardium. The main microscopic lesions were confined to the kidneys, the liver and the heart. In the kidneys, there was acute tubular degeneration and necrosis, with multifocal mineralization of the tubular basement membrane. In the liver, there was marked dissociation of the hepatocellular cords, multifocal hepatocellular degeneration and necrosis. The heart had multifocal to coalescing areas of myocardial degeneration and necrosis, myocarditis and myocardial hemorrhages (Figure 3). Warthin-Starry stain demonstrated spiral organisms in the kidneys and the liver (Figure 2C,D).

Blood, liver, and kidney samples were tested using FRET-PCR, and all three samples were positive for leptospiral DNA. No samples were available for serological testing.

Figure 2. Case 4. Common gross necropsy findings included generalized icterus, petechial to ecchymotic hemorrhages in the lungs (**A**) and kidneys (**B**). In most cases, the liver appeared pale and had an enhanced lobular pattern (**A**). Silver stain showing spiral organisms in the renal interstitium (**C**) and the liver parenchyma (**D**). Warthin Starry Stain 100×.

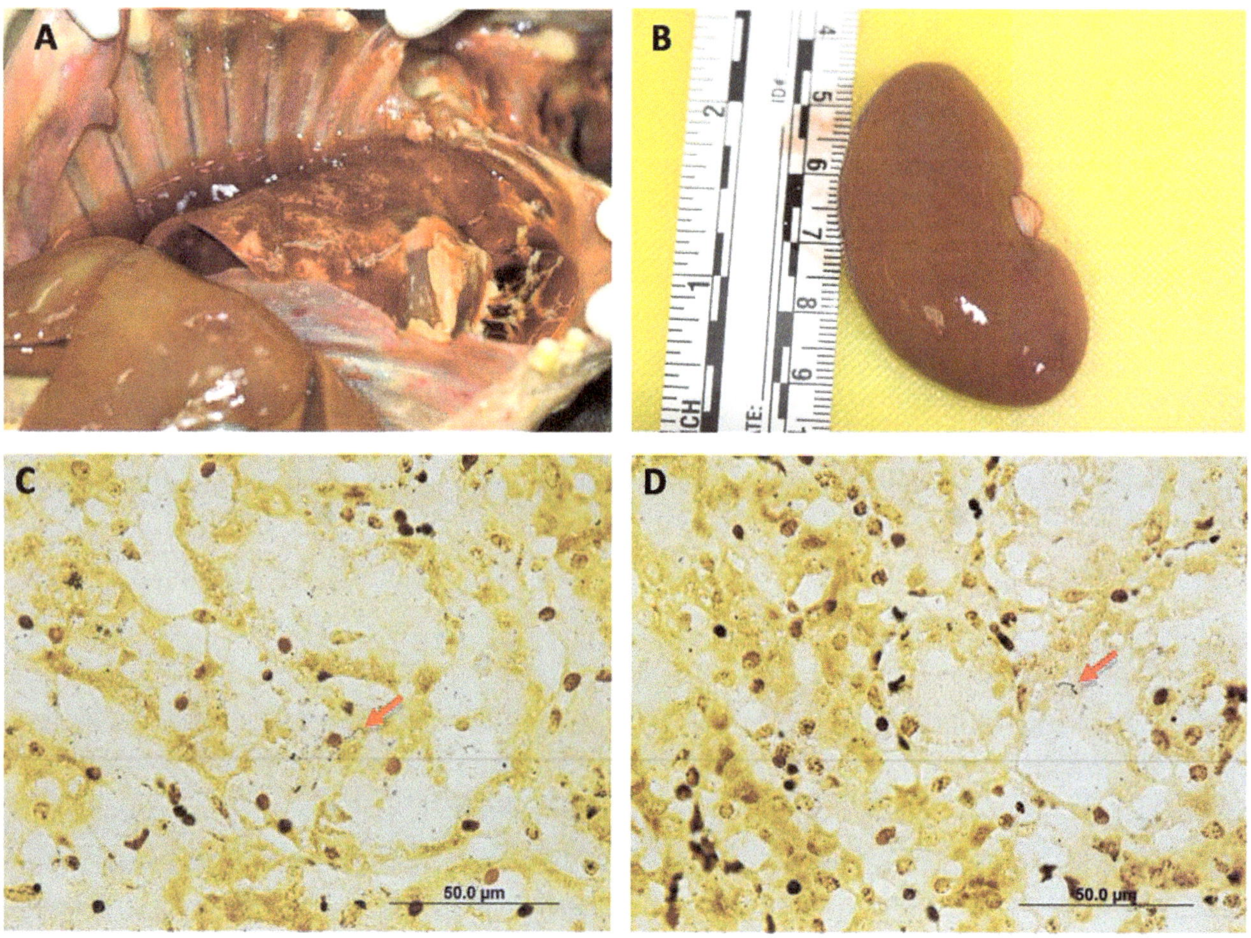

Figure 3. Case 4. Multifocal to coalescing areas of coagulative necrosis within myocardium characterized by the presence of hypereosinophilic and shrunken cardiomyocytes. In addition, there are multifocal hemorrhages that replace and separate the adjacent cardiomyocytes. Also present are aggregates of mixed inflammatory cells, predominantly mononuclear cells, less commonly neutrophils, and occasionally lymphocytes or plasma cells in the interstitium. (**A**). 20×; (**B**). 60×.

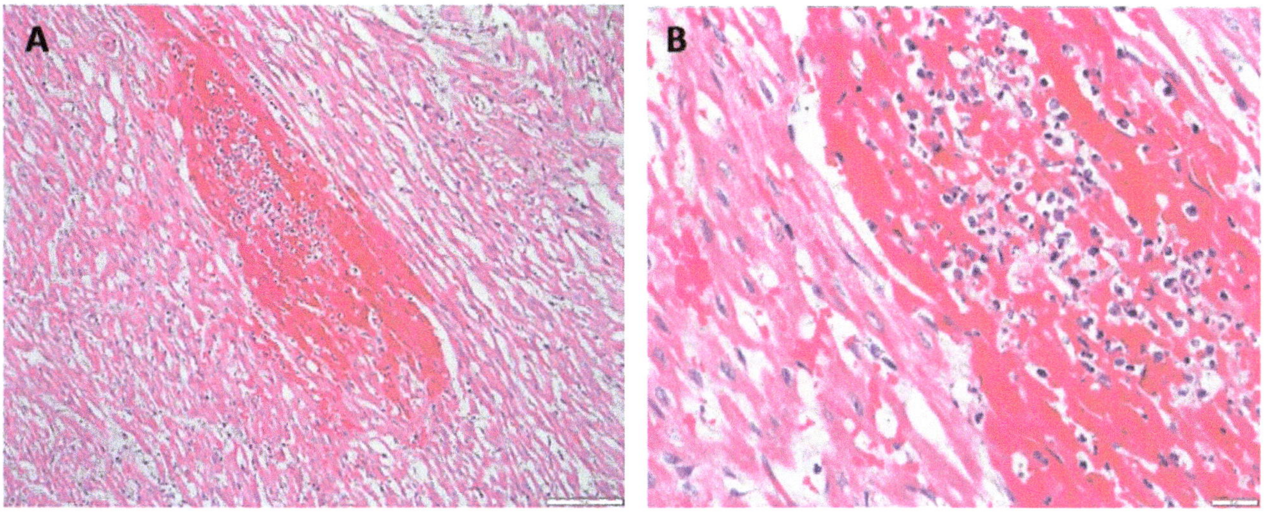

3. Discussion

Initial signs of the leptospiral infection in dogs are protean and include some combination of anorexia, lethargy, depression, fever, and muscle tenderness. The degree of hepatic involvement can vary, as can pulmonary hemorrhage [14,15]. In all four cases described here, hepatic, renal and pulmonary lesions were noted. Generalized icterus, thrombocytopenia, elevated alkaline phosphatase, elevated bilirubin, and hyperphosphatemia were seen in all cases. An inflammatory leukogram, elevated BUN or creatinine, and pancreatic damage were observed in all four patients. In addition to pulmonary hemorrhage, petechial and ecchymotic hemorrhages were commonly present in the kidneys, subcutaneous tissue, gastrointestinal tract and bladder. Commonly, the liver was pale and had an enhanced lobular pattern.

Microscopic lesions were similar in all dogs but varied in extent. Every case exhibited multifocal mineralization of the basement membrane and renal tubular degeneration and necrosis, characterized by swelling and vacuolation of tubular epithelial cells, cytoplasmic hypereosinophilia, and karyorrhexis. Sloughed epithelial cells and cellular debris were present in the lumen of the tubules. Two cases had multifocal, mild lymphocytic and plasmacytic aggregates in the renal interstitium. Lesions present in the liver were characterized by marked dissociation of the hepatocellular cords. Other lesions included hepatocellular necrosis, vacuolation of the cytoplasm of hepatocytes, sinusoidal dilation and congestion and parenchymal hemorrhages.

Interestingly, extensive myocardial damage and myocarditis were observed in one of the cases (case 4). Although abnormal ECG readings in canine leptospirosis and myocarditis in some rare cases of human leptospirosis have previously been documented [14,16], this report describes the first histopathologically confirmed case of canine leptospirosis with myocardial involvement. Other etiologies associated with myocarditis were not investigated in this study.

Taken individually, most of these findings are common in canine leptospirosis [14,15], but the severity and frequency of hemorrhage, thrombocytopenia, and hyperphosphatemia are unusual, possibly reflecting the acute and severe nature of the infections in this case series. The use of qPCR on blood, urine, and tissue samples allowed the accurate diagnosis of *Leptospira* and revealed that tissue samples, followed by urine, are the most appropriate sample for PCR-based diagnosis of acutely fatal cases. Further work is needed to identify the circulating leptospiral strains on St. Kitts, and to determine if the severity of these cases is due to the infecting strain of *Leptospira* or to host-associated factors. Young age of the animals in this case series reflects that of the patient base on the island. In a previous study we found that the average age of "healthy" control-group dogs presented to the Ross University Veterinary Clinics was 1.93 ± 2.17 years [12].

The public health implications of canine leptospirosis depend on various factors, such as geographical location, climate, rainfall, and socioeconomic factors. In a recent study, we showed that one-fifth of tested water sources on St. Kitts were contaminated with leptospiral DNA [17], and 9.1% of serum samples from pregnant women on St. Kitts and Nevis contained antibodies against *Leptospira* [4]. This work documents that *Leptospira* also causes severe, acutely fatal, canine infections on St. Kitts. The presence of stray dogs, feral cats, and several other potential reservoir species, including rats, mongooses, and monkeys, presents a combination of factors that can support enzootic circulation and transmission of the pathogen. This case series is important, as it provides the first evidence of myocarditis in canine leptospirosis, and the presence of fatal cases of canine leptospirosis on this small Caribbean island.

Acknowledgments

We dedicate this work in the memory of Ronald Samuels. This work was supported by the Ross University School of Veterinary Medicine's intramural grant to Amanda Loftis and Ashutosh Verma. We thank Julienne Rawlins, Gillian Carmichael-Branford, Trellor Fraites, and Iona Simmonds for technical assistance and A. Lee Willingham for helpful comments.

Author Contributions

Amanda Loftis and Ashutosh Verma conceived and designed the study. Lewis Bogdanovic, Fernanda Castillo-Alcala, Amanda Loftis and Ashutosh Verma performed the experiments. Amanda Loftis, Ashutosh Verma, Fernanda Castillo-Alcala and Lewis Bogdanovic analyzed the data. Ashutosh Verma, Amanda Loftis and Fernanda Castillo-Alcala wrote the paper.

Conflicts of Interest

The authors declare no conflict of interest.

References

1. Ko, A.I.; Goarant, C.; Picardeau, M. *Leptospira*: The dawn of the molecular genetics era for an emerging zoonotic pathogen. *Nat. Rev. Microbiol.* **2009**, *7*, 736–747.
2. Adler, B.; de la Peña Moctezuma, A. *Leptospira* and leptospirosis. *Vet. Microbiol.* **2010**, *140*, 287–296.

3. Pappas, G.; Papdimitriou, P.; Siozopoulou, V.; Christou, L.; Akritidis, N. The globalization of leptospirosis: Worldwide incidence trends. *Int. J. Infect. Dis.* **2008**, *12*, 351–357.
4. Wood, H.; Drebot, M.A.; Dewailly, E.; Dillon, L.; Dimitrova, K.; Forde, M.; Grolla, A.; Lee, E.; Loftis, A.; Makowski, K.; *et al.* Short report: Seroprevalence of seven zoonotic pathogens in pregnant women from the Caribbean. *Am. J. Trop. Med. Hyg.* **2014**, doi:10.4269/ajtmh.14–0107.
5. Suepaul, S.M.; Carrington, C.V.; Campbell, M.; Borde, G.; Adesiyun, A.A. Serovars of *Leptospira* isolated from dogs and rodents. *Epidemiol. Infect.* **2009**, *8*, 1–12.
6. Matthias, M.A.; Levett, P.N. Leptospiral carriage by mice and mongooses on the island of Barbados. *West Indian Med. J.* **2002**, *51*, 10–13.
7. Weekes, C.C.; Everard, C.O.; Levett, P.N. Seroepidemiology of canine leptospirosis on the island of Barbados. *Vet. Microbiol.* **1997**, *57*, 215–222.
8. Johnachan, P.M.; Smith, G.S.; Grant, G.; Hugh-Jones, M.E. Serological survey for leptospiral antibodies in goats in St Elizabeth Parish, Jamaica, 1985–1986. *Trop. Anim. Health Prod.* **1990**, *22*, 171–177.
9. Everard, C.O.; Cazabon, E.P.; Dreesen, D.W.; Sulzer, C.R. Leptospirosis in dogs and cats on the Island of Trinidad: West Indies. *Int. J. Zoonoses* **1979**, *6*, 33–40.
10. Xu, C.; Loftis, A.; Ahluwalia, S.K.; Gao, D.; Verma, A.; Wang, C.; Kaltenboeck, B. Diagnosis of canine leptospirosis by a highly sensitive FRET-PCR targeting the lig genes. *PLOS ONE* **2014**, *9*, e89507.
11. Loftis, A.D. Ross University School of Veterinary Medicine, Basseterre, Saint Kitts, West Indies. Unpublished data, 2012.
12. Loftis, A.D.; Kelly, P.J.; Freeman, M.D.; Fitzharris, S.; Beeler-Marfisi, J.; Wang, C. Tick-borne pathogens and disease in dogs on St. Kitts, West Indies. *Vet. Parasitol.* **2013**, *196*, 44–49.
13. Cole, J.R.; Sulzer, C.R.; Pursell, A.R. Improved microtechniques for the leptospiral agglutination test. *J. Appl. Microbiol.* **1973**, *25*, 976–980.
14. Sykes, J.E.; Hartmann, K.; Lunn, K.F.; Moore, G.E.; Stoddard, R.A.; Goldstein, R.E. 2010 ACVIM small animal consensus statement on leptospirosis: Diagnosis, epidemiology, treatment, and prevention. *J. Vet. Int. Med.* **2011**, *25*, 1–13.
15. Tangeman, L.E.; Littman, M.P. Clinicopathologic and atypical features of naturally occurring leptospirosis in dogs: 51 Cases (2000–2010). *J. Am. Vet. Med. Assoc.* **2013**, *243*, 1316–1322.
16. Navinan, M.R.; Rajapakse, S. Cardiac involvement in leptospirosis. *Trans. R. Soc. Trop. Med. Hyg.* **2012**, *106*, 515–520.
17. Rawlins, J.; Portanova, A.; Zuckerman, I.; Loftis, A.; Ceccato, P.; Willingham, A.L.; Verma, A. Molecular detection of leptospiral DNA in environmental water on St. Kitts. *Int. J. Environ. Res. Public Health* **2014**, *11*, 7953–7960.

9

A Physician's View of One Health: Challenges and Opportunities

Barbara Natterson-Horowitz

Professor of Medicine, Division of Cardiology, David Geffen School of Medicine at UCLA, Los Angeles, CA 90095, USA; E-Mail: bnatterson@mednet.ucla.edu;

Academic Editors: Duncan C. Ferguson and Margarethe Hoenig

One Health is one of the most important movements and emerging concepts in health today. The convergence of the fields of human and animal medicine has the potential to generate novel scientific hypotheses, create effective new therapies and potentially transform how physicians, veterinarians and their patients understand health and disease. Despite this potential, One Health has not yet gained significant awareness or traction in human medical communities. From its inception, One Health, sometimes also called One Medicine, has been piloted primarily by leaders from the world of veterinary medicine. Although the specific term was coined perhaps 10 years ago, comparative medicine has been quietly evident on university campuses with veterinary and medical schools for decades longer. Although a few physicians have played major leadership roles in One Health, in the United States, despite over ten years of the movement's robust growth, many have still not heard of it. Furthermore, physicians with some awareness of One Health often believe it to be primarily and exclusively about zoonotic infections and global health. The much broader scope and potential of One Health as also including comparative physiology and medicine is not being communicated effectively. Consequently, the human medical community remains largely disengaged. This is problematic because without significant engagement from physicians, nurses and other human health care professionals, the potential of One Health cannot be realized. To advance One Health it is imperative that we first understand the roots of under-engagement of the human medical community. This, in turn, can guide the development of novel and engaging opportunities for physician which demonstrate the power relevance of One Health's comparative, collaborative and cooperative approach.

One of the most fundamental challenges to bringing individual physicians into One Health is to demonstrate that it is relevant to their daily practice of medicine. It is important to remember that the vast majority of physicians are not infectious disease specialists or public health officials. They are internists, pediatricians, obstetrician-gynecologists, cardiologists, dermatologists, and oncologists, among others. There are countless connections between the physiology and pathology of humans and animals in all of these fields. Yet, an informal survey of One Health conferences and journals over the past two years reveals content that is dominated by infectious disease, zoonoses, food safety, and environmentally-related concerns [1,2]. While these issues are tremendously important to human populations, the relative paucity of content from other comparative medical fields is a lost opportunity. Demonstrating the many intersections between animal and human health which are non-infectious is essential to counter physician under-engagement in One Health.

How can the human medical community's awareness and engagement in One Health be strengthened? I faced this question ten years ago as I became increasingly aware and interested in One Health. At the time, I was a faculty cardiologist at the David Geffen School of Medicine at UCLA. I became fascinated by the intersection of human and veterinary medicine. Through my lecturing about One Health to groups of medical students and physicians, I found that while there was mild interest in the topic in general, interest surged when I focused the on comparative studies of the diseases they were dealing with in their human patients. I began tailoring my One Health lectures to their areas of focus and interest. Indeed, when speaking with cardiology fellows, I would discuss hypertrophic cardiomyopathy in cats, mitral regurgitation in Cavalier King Charles spaniels, and ventricular tachycardia in boxers [3–5]. When speaking with psychiatry residents, the discussion would focus on compulsive disorders in Doberman pinchers, feather plucking in parrots and separation anxiety in young dogs [6–8]. I began targeting the content of my lectures to help these physicians-in-training recognize the deep connections between the two medical fields. This tailored, specialty-specific approach led to many requests by students for clinical and research opportunities in One Health.

The increased interest that followed these lectures led to the creation of the Zoobiquity Conferences in 2011 [9]. The conferences are designed to bring together physicians and veterinarians taking care of the similar diseases in different species. The past four U.S.-based conferences cases have included sessions about breast cancer, obsessive-compulsive disorder, heart failure, melanoma, self-injury, infertility and many others. The Zoobiquity Conferences are designed to feature the benefits of the comparative method and to formulate models of interdisciplinary collaboration. For example, a veterinarian presented a case of glioblastoma multiforme in a Rhodesian ridgeback; a physician also presented a case of glioblastoma in a high school principal. They shared with one another imaging, histology, treatment protocols and outcomes through an engaging discussion about similarities in people and non-human animals. The audiences at the conferences comprised of nearly equal distributions of professionals from clinical human and veterinary medicine. The conferences also include a medical field trip in which attendees are led "on rounds" by leading academic and zoological veterinarians at local zoos and on veterinary school facilities.

Developing programs and educational opportunities tailored for physicians is crucial to the development of One Health in the coming years. Helping physicians recognize that the diseases they treat in their patients are often not uniquely human and that animal health experts have important insights to share will advance the One Health concept. Programming which exposes practicing physicians to veterinarians taking care of the same disorders in their patients is one effective way to drive this point home.

These conversations and debates provide a necessary boost to pull One Health from the periphery of the human medicine to the central position where it belongs. There is so much opportunity, yet the gap between the two professions persists. Taking stock of where the barriers are and developing programming to remove them, will do much to promote One Health across the health professions.

References

1. One Health Initiative. "Events". Available online: http://www.onehealthinitiative.com/events.php (accessed on 28 January 2015).
2. One Health Initiative. "Publications". Available online: http://www.onehealthinitiative.com/publications.php (accessed on 28 January 2015).
3. Kittleson, M.D.; Meurs, K.M.; Munro, M.J.; Kittleson, J.A.; Liu, S.; Pion, P.D.; Towbin, J.A. Familial Hypertrophic Cardiomyopathy in Maine Coon Cats: An Animal Model of Human Disease. *Circulation* **1999**, *99*, 3172–3180.
4. Borgarelli, M.; Savarino, P.; Crosara, S.; Santilli, R.A.; Chiavegato, D.; Poggi, M.; Bellino, C.; La Rosa, G.; Zanatta, R.; Haggstrom, J.; Tarducci, A. Survival Characteristics and Prognostic Variables of Dogs with Mitral Regurgitation Attributable to Myxomatous Valve Disease. *J. Vet. Intern. Med.* **2008**, *22*, 120–128.
5. Basso, C.; Fox, P.R.; Meurs, K.M.; Towbin, J.A.; Spier, A.W.; Calabrese, F.; Maron, B.J.; Thiene, G. Arrhythmogenic Right Ventricular Cardiomyopathy Causing Sudden Cardiac Death in Boxer Dogs: A New Animal Model of Human Disease. *Circulation* **2004**, *109*, 1180–1185.
6. Dodman, N.H.; Karlsson, E.K.; Moon-Fanelli, A.; Galdzicka, M.; Perloski, M.; Shuster, L.; Lindblad-Toh, K.; Ginns, E.I. A canine chromosome 7 locus confirms compulsive disorder susceptibility. *Mol. Psychiatry* **2010**, *15*, 8–10.
7. van Zeeland, Y.R.A.; Spruit, B.M.; Rodenburg, T.B.; Riedstra, B.; van Hierden, Y.M.; Buitenhuis, B.; Korte, S.M.; Lumeij, J.T. Feather damaging behaviour in parrots: A review with consideration of comparative aspects. *Appl. Anim. Behav. Sci.* **2009**, *121*, 75–95.
8. Flannigan, G.; Dodman, N.H. Risk factors and behaviors associated with separation anxiety in dogs. *J. Am. Vet. Med. Assoc.* **2001**, *219*, 460–466.
9. Zoobiquity. Conference Overview. Available online: http://zoobiquity.com/conference-research/conference/conference-overview/ (accessed on 28 January 2015).

Prevalence of Presenting Conditions in Grey Seal Pups (*Halichoerus grypus*) Admitted for Rehabilitation

Marc A. C. Silpa [1,*], Susan M. Thornton [2], Tamara Cooper [3] and Joanna Hedley [4]

[1] Royal (Dick) School of Veterinary Studies, University of Edinburgh, Easter Bush Campus, Roslin, EH25 9RG, UK
[2] International Zoo Veterinary Group, Station House, Parkwood Street, Keighley, West Yorkshire, BD21 4NQ, UK; E-Mail: S.Thornton@izvg.co.uk
[3] Cornish Seal Sanctuary, Gweek, Nr. Helston, Cornwall, TR12 6UG, UK; E-Mail: Tamara.Cooper@merlinentertainments.biz
[4] Beaumont Sainsbury Animal Hospital, Royal Veterinary College, Royal College Street, London, NW1 0TU, UK; E-Mail: jhedley@rvc.ac.uk

* Author to whom correspondence should be addressed; E-Mail: M.A.C.Silpa@gmail.com;

Academic Editor: Margarethe Hoenig

Abstract: A retrospective survey was performed on the presenting conditions of 205 live grey seal pups (*Halichoerus grypus*) admitted to the Cornish Seal Sanctuary in Gweek, United Kingdom between May 2005 and March 2011. The purpose of the survey was to examine the prevalence of various presenting signs at the sanctuary. The presenting signs were classified into nine non-mutually exclusive categories: ocular disorders, nasal disorders, oral disorders, respiratory disorders, orthopaedic disorders, puncture wounds, abrasions, netting injuries, and onychia. The sex ratio of seal pups in this study was 1.35 males per female. Of the 205 examined for rehabilitation, 22 (10.73%) did not survive to release. 68.78% of grey seal pups presented with puncture wounds, 47.80% with respiratory disorders, 46.34% with ocular disorders, 42.63% malnourished, 36.59% with abrasions, 25.37% with oral disorders, 23.90% with nasal disorders, 11.71% with orthopaedic disorders, 9.27% with onychia, and 3.41% presented with netting injuries. 52% were normothermic, 42% were hyperthermic, and 5% were hypothermic. Associations between gender, outcome of rehabilitation, hospitalisation time and presenting disorders were examined. In addition, admissions rates were found to display seasonality. The results of this study will aid in future preparation of grey seal rehabilitation facilities.

Keywords: wildlife; pinniped; rehabilitation; epidemiology

1. Introduction

Grey seals (*Halichoerus grypus*) are common among the shores of United Kingdom (UK) and frequently rehabilitated. The most recent estimate for the total grey seal UK population is between 90,600 and 142,900 [1].

Barnett *et al.* [2] first reported presenting conditions of grey seal pups in UK rehabilitation centres, using data dating from 1992 until 1998. Since that time, a major European outbreak of phocine distemper virus has affected the UK seal population [3,4]. Additionally, climate change and other anthropogenic activities have been implicated in changes to disease patterns of marine mammals [5,6] and other wildlife [7]. With continual changes in disease patterns, it is important for the UK to maintain a well-stocked and informed stranding network for seals. To achieve this goal, rehabilitation centres must be kept aware of expected diseases and conditions. The main purpose of this study was to examine the current prevalence of presenting signs in grey seal pups.

2. Methods

2.1. Seals

Records were examined from all juvenile grey seals which were admitted to the Cornish Seal Sanctuary in Gweek, UK from May 2005 until March 2011. Seals were rescued from along the south-west English coast by trained personnel. Some, but not all, seals were given oral rehydration fluids during rescue depending on the assessment and capability of the rescuer. Following a 30 min resting period post-transport, each seal was given a systematic physical examination upon admission to the sanctuary. The examination was performed by a trained animal handler or veterinary surgeon, and the findings were documented. Body condition score (BCS) was subjectively ranked as good, fair or poor.

2.2. Data

Admission records were entered into an Excel® [8] database format. Age estimation was replaced with age classification based on lanugo coat pattern and umbilicus status as described by Barnett *et al.* [2]: neonate (lanugo coat present, umbilicus present), white-Coat (lanugo coat present, umbilicus not present), mid-moult (lanugo coat partially shed), and moulted (lanugo coat completely shed). Based on wild studies of grey seal pups, neonates are assumed to be younger than five days old, white-coats between five and 14 days old, mid-moult from 16 until 21 days, and pups are moulted from 11 days until 10 months old [9,10]. Temperature was classified as marked hypothermic, mildly hypothermic, normal, mildly hyperthermic, and marked hyperthermic based off reported normal values for grey seals [11]. The presenting signs were classified into nine non-mutually exclusive categories: ocular disorders, oral disorders, nasal disorders, respiratory disorders, orthopaedic disorders, puncture wounds, abrasions, netting injuries, and onychia. Trauma was separated into four categories based on type of wound and anatomical involvement: orthopaedic, puncture, abrasion and wounds caused by nets. Due to the inability to perform extensive radiographic investigation, any injuries that grossly included a bone or any obvious fractured bones were classified as an orthopaedic disorder. Superficial dermal wounds were classified as abrasions. Onychia included any inflammation around the nail. A seal was classified as malnourished if it had a poor BCS. Nasal disorders included nasal discharge. A respiratory disorder was indicated if there was marked effort in respiration or production of respiratory noise. Any lesion in the mouth was classified as an oral lesion.

There were two outcomes of rehabilitation. Either the seal was released or the seal did not survive to release. Any deaths that occurred after release were not considered due to the inability to secure accurate survival reports. Any humane euthanasia of seals at the centre was performed by injecting a lethal dose of pentobarbital intravenously. Hospitalisation time was calculated in days starting from day of admission until day of release or death.

To examine if hospitalisation admission displayed seasonality, a cosinor test was performed using R [12] as described by Barnett and Dobson [13]. For all other statistical calculations, Minitab® version 16 [14] was used. Prevalence with 95% confidence intervals was calculated based on a binary examination of the classification disorders. To examine if age or gender were risk factors for the presenting conditions, univariable binary logistic regression analyses were performed. A similar analysis was also performed on outcome with presenting conditions and other variables. Variables with associations of $p < 0.25$ were placed into a multivariable binary logistic regression model, and the least significant variable excluded until a final statistically significant model was obtained.

3. Results

Between May 2005 and March 2011, a total of 205 grey seal pups were admitted for rehabilitation at the Cornish Seal Sanctuary (Table 1). BCS was reported in 190 pups. Only 22 pups did not survive until release. Of those 22, only one was euthanized. The seal pup was euthanized after 4.5 months due to worsening neurological signs and poor prognosis. Due to the low number neonates ($n = 11$), neonates and white-coat were combined for statistical analysis.

Table 1. Counts of grey seal pup age and gender.

	Neonate	White-Coat	Mid-Moult	Moulted	Total
Female	7	17	11	52	87
Male	4	11	19	84	118
Total	11	28	30	136	205

3.1. Prevalence

The prevalence of each presenting disorder with 95% confidence intervals is shown on Figure 1. The most common presenting condition was trauma. 81.95% of seal pups had at least one form of trauma. 68.78% of seal pups had puncture wounds while 36.59% had abrasions. 11.71% had obvious orthopaedic disorders, and 3.41% has netting injuries. After trauma, respiratory disorders were the second most common presenting sign (47.80%). Ocular disorders (46.34%), malnourishment (42.63%), and oral lesions (25.37%) were also significantly present in this population. Onychia (9.27%) and netting injuries were the least common presenting conditions.

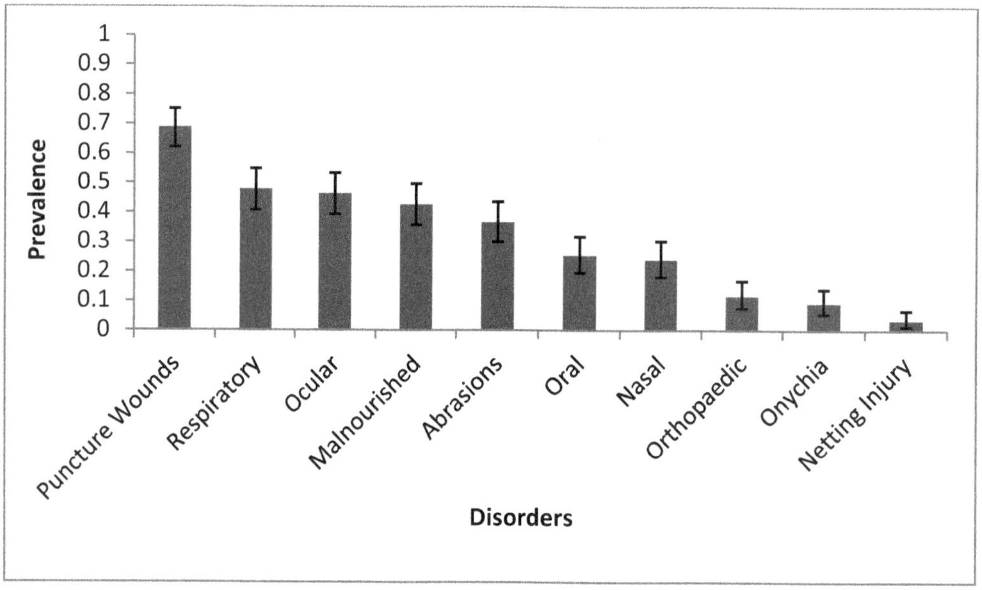

Figure 1. The prevalence and the 95% confidence interval (CI) of each presenting condition observed in rehabilitated grey seal pups. Total for all conditions = 205 pups except malnourishment. Only 190 pups had body condition score (BCS) reported.

3.2. Gender

The significant univariable binary logistic regressions (Table 2) demonstrate that gender is associated with some of the presenting disorders. Females are significantly less likely to have oral disorders and abrasions. In addition, there is a trend of females being half as likely to present with respiratory disorders as males.

3.3. Age

Age was significantly associated with four presenting disorders (Table 2). Younger pups were less likely to have respiratory signs while white-coat pups were significantly less likely to present with nasal disorders, oral disorders and puncture wounds. Seven moulted pups present with netting injuries while no non-moulted pup (neonate, white-coat, and mid-moult) had these injuries. A fisher exact test showed a trend towards an association of age and netting injuries ($p = 0.097$).

3.4. Season

Hospitalisation admissions occurred mainly between October and January (Figure 2). A cosinor test demonstrated that hospital admissions displayed seasonality ($p < 0.001$). The phase of the cosinor test was 11.7, indicating that the peak admissions was during late November. The lowest point of seal admissions occurred in late May.

Table 2. Univariable Binary Logistic Regressions of each presenting disorder observed in rehabilitated grey seal pups.

Disorder	Factor	Variable	*n*	OR (95% CI)	*p*	
Nasal	Age	White-Coat and Neonate	4	0.28 (0.09–0.85)	0.025	**
		Mid-Moult	6	0.62 (0.24–1.64)	0.336	
		Moulted	39	Ref		
Oral	Gender	F	15	0.46 (0.23–0.90)	0.023	**
		M	37	Ref		
	Age	White-Coat and Neonate	4	0.25 (0.08–0.74)	0.012	**
		Mid-Moult	5	0.43 (0.16–1.21)	0.109	
		Moulted	43	Ref		
Respiratory	Gender	F	35	0.59 (0.34–1.03)	0.063	*
		M	63	Ref		
	Age	White-Coat and Neonate	8	0.19 (0.08–0.44)	<0.001	**
		Mid-Moult	11	0.42 (0.18–0.95)	0.036	**
		Moulted	79	Ref		
Puncture Wounds	Age	White-Coat and Neonate	13	0.15 (0.07–0.33)	<0.001	**
		Mid-Moult	24	1.23 (0.46–3.27)	0.677	
		Moulted	104	Ref		
Abrasions	Gender	F	22	0.42 (0.23–0.76)	0.004	**
		M	53	Ref		

F = Female, M = Male, Ref = reference variable; ** = significant at $p < 0.05$, * = significant at $p < 0.10$;
Age: White-Coat and Neonate were combined (Total = 39) due to low neonate count ($n = 11$).

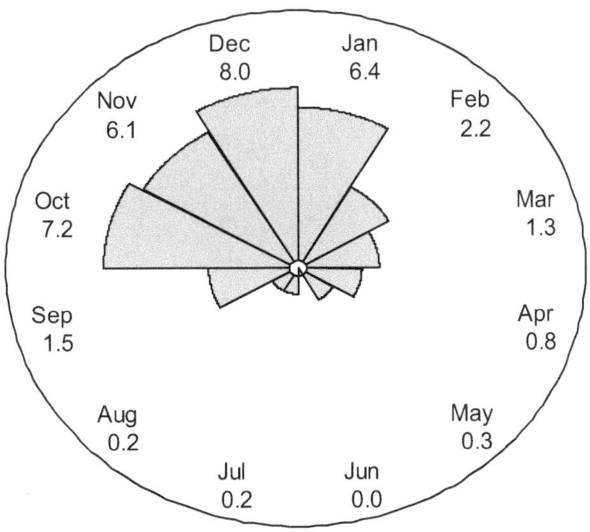

Figure 2. A rose diagram of monthly mean admission rates of grey seal pups from May 2005 through March 2011. Monthly means were adjusted for unequal number of days in each month.

3.5. Temperature

Temperature was recorded on all individuals except three (Table 3). The majority of pups were normothermic. However, almost 42% of pups displayed one form of hyperthermia, while only 5% of pups presented as hypothermic.

Table 3. Recorded temperatures on admissions.

Temperature Classification	Temperature Range (°C)	*n*
Marked Hypothermic	<35	5
Mildly Hypothermic	35–35.9	7
Normal	36–37.9	105
Mildly Hyperthermic	38–38.9	71
Marked Hyperthermic	>39	14
Not Recorded		3

3.6. Outcome

Of the 205 seals admitted for rehabilitation, 22 did not survive to release. Univariate binomial logistic regression of different variables recorded found a significant association with hospitalisation time only. The relative odds for a pup surviving until release increased by 1.06 (95% CI: 1.04–1.09, $p < 0.001$) per day during its stay in rehabilitation. A survival plot (Figure 3) demonstrates that the likelihood of a seal surviving decreased by a significant amount early in rehabilitation. There were no statistically significant associations between presenting condition and whether or not the seal was released.

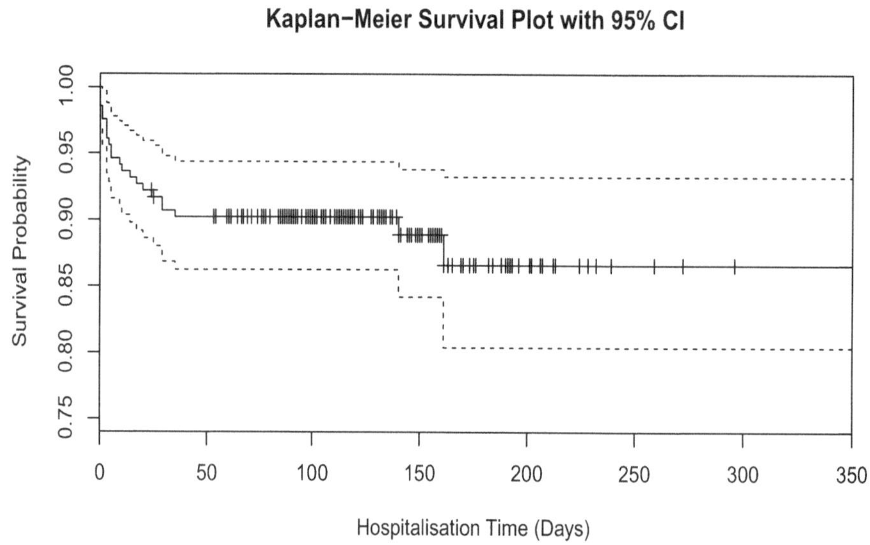

Figure 3. A Kaplan-Meier Survival plot of the seal rehabilitation hospitalisation time with 95% confidence intervals censored for "released". Hatch marks indicate censorship events.

3.7. Multivariable Binary Logistic Regression

Multivariable binary logistic regression analyses could not produce a significant model for any presenting disorder before being reduced to a univariable model. In addition, the multivariable model of outcome did not converge. The low number of seals that did not survive is most likely the cause of the non-convergence. When hospitalisation time was removed, the model did converge insignificantly. Further reductions to the model continued to produce non-significant models until all variables had been removed.

4. Discussion

The main purpose of this study was to examine the presenting signs of grey seal pups found during the initial admission examination. Presenting signs reported in this study, in order of prevalence, are: trauma, respiratory disorders, ocular disorders, malnourishment, oral disorders and onychia.

There was a dramatic difference in the hospitalisation time between seals that were released and those that did not survive. Examination of the survival plot shows that the majority of seals that did not survive died while in the early stages of rehabilitation. This suggests that there could be a critical period during early rehabilitation which could affect the long term outcome of the intervention. This could also indicate that current methods of long term rehabilitation are sufficient to ensure a high survivorship.

Over 80% of the seal pups had one form of trauma. The high level of trauma suggests that rehabilitation centres in the UK need to be prepared to care for wounded seals. With the recent discovery of *Mycobacterium bovis* in a non-healing wound [15] and the high prevalence of puncture wounds (68.78%), rehabilitators should be aware of the potential zoonotic risks and take appropriate protective measures when dealing with infected non-healing wounds.

Grey seal pup admission into the rehabilitation centre was seasonal. The pup production season in south-west England is mid-August through December, with the peak production occurring between August and October [1,16,17]. Admission counts peaked in November. This study found the majority of pups rehabilitated were moulted (Table 1). Pups remain on shore with their mothers until weaned at approximately 3–4 weeks of age. Rescuers are trained not to rescue a seal pup when the mother is present unless the pup has suffered serious trauma or illness [18]. After weaning and moulting, grey seal pups either enter into the water immediately or stay on land for up to a month [1]. Thus shift in the seasonality of seal admissions from pup production would not be unexpected. Non-moulted pups admitted after pup production had ended (e.g., February, March, April, May) may have been pups born post-pup production season. Alternatively, there could be delayed moulting in ill pups. Further investigation into non-moulted pups outside of pup production season is needed.

This study found that 42% of rehabilitated seals presented with hyperthermia. Grey seals spend a majority of their time in the sub-arctic waters of the north Atlantic [1]. Their adapted physiology, used to cope with the cold water, makes them highly susceptible to overheating. Thus, it is expected that a large percentage would present with hyperthermia. Rehabilitation centres should be prepared to treat for hyperthermia.

This study found a significant relationship between age and respiratory conditions. Older seal pups showed increased respiratory signs. A similar relationship with age was found with puncture wounds, oral and nasal disorders. In addition, females were less likely to have abrasions, oral, and respiratory lesions. The reasons behind these relationships are unknown, and suggest further areas of research.

Respiratory disorders increased with age. Unfortunately, this retrospective study was unable identify the cause of the respiratory disorders seen in the pups. However, Baker *et al.* [19] found an increase in pulmonary nematode parasitism in older seals, suggesting a possible cause of the increased odds of respiratory disorders in older pups. Further investigations, including tests for pulmonary nematode infestations in grey seal pups, is required.

Nasal disorders had a similar relationship to respiratory disorders. 50% of white-coat pups that presented with nasal disorders also had a respiratory disorder. This suggests that the nasal discharge observed was most likely caused by a lower respiratory tract lesion. However, this relationship was not observed with moulted pups. Naso-pharyngeal mites (*Halarachne halichoeri*) and symptomatic signs have been found in high prevalence in juvenile grey seals along the Spanish coastline [20]. Thus, it is possible that lower respiratory tract issues are more likely the cause of younger pup nasal discharge, while older pups are more likely to have an upper respiratory tract issue such as Naso-pharyngeal mites.

Puncture wounds were less likely to be found on younger pups. Puncture wounds can be caused by intraspecific interactions, predator/prey interactions, and anthropogenic causes. However, a recent study found 55% free ranging grey seal pups on a breeding beach colony had puncture wounds [21]. This suggests that intraspecific interactions are the most likely cause for puncture wounds; the seal pups had the wounds when anthropogenic and predator causes were unlikely.

Oral lesions found in this data were mostly oral ulcers. *Streptococcus equi* ssp. *zooepidemicus*, has been associated with oral ulcers in the past [19]. It has also been suggested that oral ulcers in the grey seal pup could be due to changes in the gingiva during tooth eruption [2]. Our study found older seal pups were more likely to have oral ulcers, indicating that the effect of tooth eruption could be a valid possibility. No cultures of the oral lesions were performed in this study, and thus the causative agent of the ulcers could not be determined. Further investigations need to be performed to rule out other causative agents (e.g., azotaemic, viral, or autoimmune ulcers).

It should be noted that only moulted pups had netting injuries, though the total number was low. A fishers exact showed a possible significance in this proportion, but a larger sample size is needed for rare events. Grey seal exposure to nets typically occurs in water. Only older, weaned grey seal pups enter into open water by their own choice [10]. Thus, it would be expected that only older pups would have netting injuries. Further research is needed to determine if this association holds to the expectation.

There was a large difference between the prevalence of ocular disorders in this study compared to those of Barnett *et al.* [2]. The ocular lesions noted were similar other lesions observed by Barnett *et al.* [2]. This study found 46.34% of seal pups had an ocular condition (e.g., corneal oedema, corneal ulceration, *etc.*) while in the previous study only 13% had an ocular lesion. Grey seals have large eyes, and these eyes are highly susceptible to trauma [11], which could explain the high prevalence of ocular conditions in pups presented for rehabilitation. The reason behind the difference in the studies is unknown, and should be considered by future research.

Malnourishment was found in 42.63% of seal pups, in comparison to 71% observed by Barnett *et al.* [2]. A study on grey seal mortality found that starvation was the highest probable cause of death in older juveniles [19]. The difference is likely due to different methods used to define malnourishment. This retrospective study relied on the subjective BCS, while Barnett *et al.* [2] used weights and muscle mass cover and Baker *et al.* [19] used post mortem information. The BCS was not standardised before the study, and thus may have caused an under-reporting of malnourished prevalence. Alternatively, the use of weight in sick animals to assess nutritional status may have caused an over-estimation of the malnourished prevalence in Barnett *et al.* [2]. In addition, weight of the pup might reflect the age of the mother instead of the nutritional status of the pup [22]. Further research is needed to determine the true malnourishment prevalence.

There were some limitations to this study due to its retrospective nature. The examination of the seals was not standardised and the examiner on admission was not noted in the record, thus inter-observer reliability could not be assessed. In addition, this study performed multiple comparisons and increased the familywise error rate. However, due to the nature of this exploratory epidemiological survey and the data, no multiplicity adjustment is required [23,24]. Confirmatory studies for this study's findings with appropriate controls should be performed in the future.

5. Conclusions

The rehabilitation of grey seals will continue in the UK in the foreseeable future. The stranding network for seals must maintain a well-equipped and informed system. With climate change, diseases in wild populations are expected to change [5–7]. This study presents an updated prevalence of presenting conditions of seal pups admitted to rehabilitation. Continued assessment of disease prevalence and presenting conditions on admission will allow rescuers to prepare for the continued rehabilitation of grey seals.

Acknowledgments

The authors would like to thank Darren Shaw and Ian Handel for their assistance with the statistical methods and Amanda Stansbury for proofreading the manuscript. This study was performed as part of the Student Selected Component 2 from the Royal (Dick) School of Veterinary Studies' curriculum.

Author Contributions

Marc A. C. Silpa was a veterinary student at the Royal (Dick) School of Veterinary Studies and was involved in project design, data analysis and writing the manuscript. Susan M Thornton and Tamara Cooper were involved in data collection and storage. Joanna Hedley was the project supervisor and was involved in project design and data analysis.

Conflicts of Interest

The authors declare no conflict of interest.

References

1. Sea Mammal Research Unit. *Scientific Advice on Matters Related to the Management of Seal Populations*; Natural Environment Research Council: Swindon, UK, 2013.
2. Barnett, J.E.F.; Woodley, A.J.; Hill, T.J.; Turner, L. Conditions in grey seal pups (*Halichoerus grypus*) presented for rehabilitation. *Vet. Rec.* **2000**, *147*, 98–104.
3. Hammond, J.A.; Pomeroy, P.; Hall, A.; Smith, V.J. Identification and real-time PCR quantification of Phocine distemper virus from two colonies of Scottish grey seals in 2002. *J. Gen. Virol.* **2005**, *86*, 2563–2567.

4. Lonergan, M.; Hall, A.; Thompson, H.; Thompson, P.; Pomeroy, P.; Harwood, J. Comparison of the 1988 and 2002 phocine distemper epizootics in British harbour seal *Phoca vitulina* populations. *Dis. Aquat. Org.* **2010**, *88*, 183–188.
5. Harvell, C.D.; Kim, K.; Burkholder, J.M.; Colwell, R.R.; Epstein, P.R.; Grimes, D.J.; Hofmann, E.E.; Lipp, E.K.; Osterhaus, A.D.; Overstreet, R.M.; *et al.* Emerging marine diseases—Climate links and anthropogenic factors. *Science* **1999**, *285*, 1505–1510.
6. Gulland, F.M.D.; Hall, A. The Role of Infectious Disease in Influencing Status and Trend. In *Marine Mammal Research: Conservation beyond Crisis*; Reynolds, J.E., III, Perrin, W.F., Reeves, R.R., Montgomery, S., Ragen, T.J., Eds.; Johns Hopkins University Press: Baltimore, MD, USA, 2005; pp. 47–62.
7. Harvell, D.; Altizer, S.; Cattadori, I.M.; Harrington, L.; Weil, E. Climate change and wildlife diseases: When does the host matter the most? *Ecology* **2009**, *90*, 912–920.
8. *Microsfot Excel 2010*; Microsoft Corp: Redmond, MA, USA, 2010.
9. King, J.E. *Seals of the World*, 2nd ed.; University of Queensland Press: St. Lucia, Australia, 1983.
10. Westcott, S. *The Grey Seals of the West Country: And Their Neighbours*; Cornwall Wildlife Trust: Truro, England, UK, 1997.
11. Barnett, J. Treatment of sick and injured marine mammals. *Practice* **1998**, *20*, 200–211.
12. R Development Core Team. *R: A Language and Environment for Statistical Computing*; R Foundation for Statistical Computing: Vienna, Austria, 2008.
13. Barnett, A.G.; Dobson, A.J. *Analysing Seasonal Health Data*; *Statistics for Biology and Health*; Springer: Berlin, Heidelberg, Germany, 2010.
14. *Minitab 16 Statistical Software*; Minitab, Inc.: State College, PA, USA, 2009.
15. Barnett, J.E.F.; Booth, P.; Brewer, J.I.; Chanter, J.; Cooper, T.; Crawshaw, T.; Davison, N.J.; Greenwood, A.; Riley, P.; Smith, N.H.; *et al.* Mycobacterium bovis infection in a grey seal pup (*Halichoerus grypus*). *Vet. Rec.* **2013**, *173*, 168–168.
16. Sayer, S.; Hockley, C.; Witt, M.J. *Monitoring Grey Seals (Halichoerus grypus) in the Isles of Scilly during the 2010 Pupping Season*; Natural England Comissioned Reports NECR103; Natural England: Sheffield, UK, 2012.
17. Westcott, S. *Prodcedural Guidelines for Studying Grey Seals in Southwest England*, 2006; Natural England: Sheffield, UK, 2008.
18. Barnett, J.; Knight, A.; Stevens, M. *British Drivers Marine Life Rescue: Marine Mammal Medic Handbook*, 7th ed.; British Divers Marine Life Rescue: Uckfield, UK, 2014.
19. Baker, J.R.; Jepson, P.D.; Simpson, V.R.; Kuiken, T. Causes of mortality and non-fatal conditions among grey seals (*Halichoerus grypus*) found dead on the coasts of England, Wales and the Isle of Man. *Vet. Rec.* **1998**, *142*, 595–601.
20. Alonso-Farré, J.M.; D'Silva, J.I.D.; Gestal, C. Naso-pharyngeal mites Halarachne halichoeri (Allman, 1847) in Grey seals stranded on the NW Spanish Atlantic Coast. *Vet. Parasitol.* **2012**, *183*, 317–322.
21. Baily, J. *The Pathology and Occurrence of Pathogens in Scottish Grey Seals (Halichoerus grypus)*; University of St. Andrews: St. Andrews, UK, 2014.

22. Bowen, W.D.; Iverson, S.J.; Mcmillan, J.I.; Boness, D.J. Reproductive performance in grey seals: Age-related improvement and senescence in a capital breeder. *J. Anim. Ecol.* **2006**, *75*, 1340–1351.
23. Rothman, K. No adjustments are needed for multiple comparisons. *Epidemiology* **1990**, *1*, 43–46.
24. Bender, R.; Lange, S. Adjusting for multiple testing—When and how? *J. Clin. Epidemiol.* **2001**, *54*, 343–349.

11

Feasibility Study of a Standardized Novel Animal Model for Cervical Vertebral Augmentation in Sheep Using a PTH Derivate Bioactive Material

Karina Klein [1,2,*], Jason Schense [3], Peter W. Kronen [1,4,5], Nathalie Fouche [1], Mariano Makara [6], Katharina Kämpf [1], Thomas Steffen [7] and Brigitte von Rechenberg [1,4]

1 Musculoskeletal Research Unit (MSRU), Equine Department, University of Zurich, Winterthurerstrasse 260, CH-8057 Zurich, Switzerland; E-Mails: nathalie.fouche@web.de (N.F.); kkaempf@vetclinics.uzh.ch (K.K.); bvonrechenberg@vetclinics.uzh.ch (B.R.)

2 Graduate School for Cellular and Biomedical Sciences, University of Bern, CH-3012 Bern, Switzerland

3 Kuros Biosurgery AG, Technoparkstrasse 1, CH-8005 Zurich, Switzerland; E-Mail: jason.schense@kuros.ch

4 Center for Applied Biotechnology and Molecular Medicine (CABMM), University of Zurich, Winterthurerstrasse 190, CH-8057 Zurich, Switzerland

5 Veterinary Anaesthesia Services - International (VAS), Zürcherstrasse 39, CH-8400 Winterthur, Switzerland; E-Mail: peter.kronen@vas-int.com

6 Division of Diagnostic Imaging, Vetsuisse Faculty, University of Zurich, Winterthurerstrasse 258c, CH-8057 Zurich, Switzerland; E-Mail: mariano.makara@gmail.com

7 Orthopaedic Research Laboratory, Department of Surgery, McGill University Hospital Center, 687 Pine Avenue West, Montreal, QC H3A 1A1, Canada; E-Mail: tsteffen@orl.mcgill.ca

* Author to whom correspondence should be addressed; E-Mail: kklein@vetclinics.uzh.ch;

Abstract: Prophylactic local treatment involving percutaneous vertebral augmentation using bioactive materials is a new treatment strategy in spine surgery in humans for vertebral bodies at risk. Standardized animal models for this procedure are almost non-existent. The purpose of this study was to: (i) prove the efficacy of PTH derivate bioactive materials for new bone formation; and (ii) create a new, highly standardized cervical vertebral augmentation model in sheep. Three different concentrations of a modified form of parathyroid hormone (PTH) covalently bound to a fibrin matrix containing strontium carbonate were used. The same matrix without PTH and shams were used as controls. The bioactive materials were locally injected. Using a ventral surgical approach, a pre-set amount of material was injected under fluoroscopic guidance into the intertrabecular space of three vertebral bodies. Intravital fluorescent dyes were used to demonstrate new bone formation. After an observation period of four months, the animals were sacrificed, and vertebral bodies were processed for μCT, histomorphometry, histology and sequential fluorescence evaluation. Enhanced localized bone activity and new bone formation in the injected area could be determined for all experimental groups in comparison to the matrix alone and sham with the highest values detected for the group with a medium concentration of PTH.

Keywords: vertebral augmentation; cervical spine; animal model; fibrin matrix; PTH derivate; sheep

---

1. Introduction

Symptomatic compression fractures of vertebral bodies occurring secondary to osteoporosis or neoplasia are a major public health problem in our aging society [1–5]. These fractures may cause persistent, often excruciating pain, spinal instability and kyphotic deformity, all of which potentially impair mobility and reduce the patient's quality of life [5–7]. Nowadays, percutaneous vertebroplasty (VP) is the treatment of choice to mechanically augment the spine. It is a successful, minimally invasive surgical procedure [8–10], which seems to be significantly better than non-surgical treatment in terms of pain relief, reduced hospital stay and recovery period [11]. The VP technique is performed through needle-injection of polymethylmethacrylate (PMMA) bone cement into a collapsed or weakened vertebra, this to stabilize, decompress or avoid further compression fractures (prophylactic VP). Common complications during the surgical procedure are bleeding at the puncture site, local infection and cement leakage into the spinal canal, the paravertebral tissues or the perivertebral venous system [12]. Cement extravasation, as well as bone marrow or fat cells forced out of the vertebra into the systemic circulation may lead to pulmonary embolism (PE), either without clinical signs or with severe cardiac distress symptoms, including death [5].

It is well known that PMMA increases the strength and stiffness of the injected vertebral bodies, but in the absence of osteoinductive properties and the inability to be degraded and replaced by new bone, it will remain just a placeholder. It may also lead to long-term complications, such as damage to neurons, toxicity or fracture of adjacent vertebral bodies [3,13]. Therefore, the search for new, preferably resorbable biomaterials, containing locally-released bioactive agents with osteoinductive properties to strengthen and regenerate weakened vertebral bodies is ongoing. Especially adjacent to the index level that was augmented with PMMA for immediate stability, enhancing local bone formation may in the future avoid in systemically-ill osteoporotic patients a domino effect of adjacent vertebral compression fractures [14].

A truncated form of the human parathyroid hormone ($PTH_{1\text{-}34}$) is already used as a registered pharmaceutical product for osteoporosis treatment. Intermittent systemic injections of $PTH_{1\text{-}34}$ have shown anabolic effects on cancellous bone, resulting in increased bone mineral density [15]. PTH is able to bind directly to a cell surface receptor on osteoblasts, regulating the production of various cytokines (insulin-like growth factor 1, transforming growth factor β1, interleukin 1 (IL-1) and IL-6) and, thus, represents a strong anabolic agent for osteoblast precursors and an indirect anabolic factor for osteoclasts (IL-1 and IL-6) [15–17]. It regulates the balance between osteoblasts and osteoclasts, as well, thereby exerting a direct effect on bone turnover [15], and plays a primary role in calcium homeostasis [18]. In contrast to systemic use, a novel recent strategy is to use an engineered peptide variant of the active fragment of parathyroid hormone (PTH_{1-34}) that is enzymatically incorporated within a fibrin matrix via the coagulation transglutaminase (TG) factor XIIIa to translate the systemically used molecule into a local bone-inducing therapeutic agent [19]. The incorporation of a plasmin substrate sequence linker (pl) enables the cleavage of the peptide by endogenous plasmin. Via cell migration and infiltration, the peptide is activated and released only into the surrounding tissue for the local increase of bone formation. In previous *in vivo* studies using a tibia and femur augmentation model in sheep, various concentrations of this engineered parathyroid hormone ($TGplPTH_{1-34}$), incorporated in different formulations of fibrin matrices, has already shown good results [20]. However, it was unknown whether these results could actually be reproduced in the vertebral bodies, this due to its different anatomical structure, including high vascularity and sinus formations.

Safety aspects concerning the augmentation procedure must be considered, such that good visibility of the material during injection is key to avoid leakage into the spinal canal and damage to the spinal cord. Furthermore, the rheological properties of the material during injection are critical to avoid leakage into the vascular system, possibly causing pulmonary embolism or death. The radiopaque inorganic salt powder strontium carbonate has proven to be a good contrast agent. Strontium is also known to have positive effects on bone formation and for its capability to decrease bone resorption [21,22]. Different studies have shown that strontium could induce the replication of osteoblasts [23] and, concurrently, the apoptosis of osteoclasts [24] using a pathway involving the extracellular calcium-sensing receptor (CaR). An *in vivo* study of Yang *et al.* using a calvarial defect model in rats showed that locally-delivered strontium was able to act as a bone anabolic agent and could activate the Wnt/*β*-catenin signaling pathway, resulting in an accumulation of extracellular matrix, as well as enhanced osteogenesis and bone remodeling [25].

Good animal models for vertebral augmentation are rare. The sheep has been used as an experimental animal model for augmentation in the lumbar spine, although mainly for studying acute cardiovascular changes and embolization with immediate sacrifice on the table after augmentation [26–30]. Due to the different morphology of ovine vertebral bodies with a more trapezoid and slim vertebral body format compared to a round, solid and almost rectangular human vertebral body, a transpedicular approach for vertebral augmentation is highly hazardous and difficult to standardize in the lumbar area in sheep. Therefore, a new, highly standardized augmentation model in the cervical spine of sheep was developed for these experiments, where a ventral approach and customized instrumentation guaranteed the high reproducibility of the augmentation procedure. Apart from the safe deposition of the augmentation material, this model also involved a risk of pulmonary embolism similar to that found with human vertebral augmentation. Therefore, the study results may be better transferable to the human vertebral bone structure.

The aim of this study was to: (i) investigate the scaled effects of PTH derivate bioactive material as an enhancer for new bone formation in sheep; and (ii) create a novel, highly standardized animal model for vertebral augmentation in sheep. To reach aim (i), different concentrations of $TGplPTH_{1-34}$, incorporated in the best performing fibrin matrix formulation from previous studies, were used as bioenhancers. For aim (2), cervical vertebrae in sheep were targeted focusing on the reproducibility and standardization of the model, including the surgical technique and overall evaluation. To the knowledge of the authors, this is the first report for both using the local application of an engineered peptide variant ($TGplPTH_{1-34}$) as a bioactive agent and reporting a standardized animal model in the cervical spine of sheep.

2. Material and Methods

2.1. Study Design and Experimental Animals

Seventeen adult female Swiss alpine sheep with a mean age of 3.2 years (range from 2 to 5 years) and a mean weight of 72.6 kg (54–89 kg) were used for this study, conducted adhering to the Swiss regulations of Animal Welfare (TSchG 455), with a specific permission granted by the federal authorities (Application No. 151/2009).

Using a cervical vertebral augmentation model in sheep, three different concentrations of a modified form of parathyroid hormone ($TGplPTH_{1-34}$) covalently bound to a fibrin matrix containing strontium carbonate, the same matrix without any $TGplPTH_{1-34}$, as well as sham controls were tested and compared. Three vertebrae per sheep were augmented. Each group consisted of three sheep, with the exception of Group 2, where two sheep died during surgery, and therefore, two additional sheep were used (for the group distribution, see Table 1).

Table 1. Group distribution and clinical signs of pulmonary embolism. PTH, parathyroid hormone; PE, pulmonary embolism.

Group	Material	Number of animals	Number of evaluated vertebra	Clinical signs of pulmonary embolism
Matrix alone	FS+SrCO3	3	8	2× mild clinical signs
Low	FS+SrCO3+PTH low conc.	5	9	2× severe clinical signs led to death, 1× mild clinical signs
Medium	FS+SrCO3+PTH low conc.	3	8	1× mild clinical signs
High	FS+SrCO3+PTH low conc.	3	9	1× mild clinical signs
Sham	No materials	3	9	

FS: Fibrin scaffold; SrCO3: Strontium carbonate; PTH low-high: TGplPTH1-34 concentration low-high; Mild clinical signs of PE: intermittend bradycardia, Hypercapnia and mild oxygen desaturation

Using a ventral surgical approach and a customized aiming device, a fixed amount of biomaterial per vertebra (1–1.5 mL) was injected under fluoroscopic guidance in a standardized trajectory and to a standardized depth into the intertrabecular space of three vertebral bodies per sheep (between C2–C6). For the sham controls, the same procedure was performed without material injection. To detect pulmonary emboli, non-invasive airway dead space measurements were performed during surgery, as well as CT angiography of the thorax in all sheep prior to and after surgery [31]. After 16 weeks of follow-up, the sheep were sacrificed, and the harvested vertebral bodies were further processed for macroscopic assessment (signs of inflammation and irritation), μCT analysis and histology, including histomorphometry and evaluation of fluorescent dye incorporation.

2.2. Test Material

Three different concentrations (low, medium, high) of a modified inactivated form of PTH_{1-34} ($TGplPTH_{1-34}$) with a transglutaminase hook (TG-Hook) were evaluated (pending patent application) [19]. Using the TG-hook, the peptide was covalently bound and immobilized onto a fibrin matrix during the coagulation process and later locally released *in vivo* and activated by plasmin-induced proteolytic cleavage (via a plasmin substrate sequence linker (pl)) after cellular infiltration and replacement of the fibrin matrix with a newly secreted extra-cellular matrix. As a contrast agent for better radio-opacity and to improve the rheological properties during the injection procedure, 40% weight volume (w/v) strontium carbonate was added to the formulation. In one of the test groups, only the fibrin matrix including the strontium carbonate was used without PTH_{1-34}.

2.3. Instruments/Equipment

In addition to the routine surgical instruments, a customized aiming device was developed to guarantee the reproducibility of surgical access and to standardize the access point on the bone surface for injection into the trabecular bone of the vertebral body (Figure 1a–c). Using a ventral surgical approach, the aiming device allows an exact drilling and subsequent positioning of the injection needle. This can be achieved via a central drill guide that is positioned on the promontorium of the caudal aspect of the vertebral body (Figure 1a), an aiming targeting tip lined up with the vertebra midline and two sharp long fixation dents (beside the midline) resting on the cranial deeper part of the vertebral body. An oval hole allows monitoring the drill guide tip placed on the promontorium while the drill guide remains positioned (Figure 1b).

Figure 1. This figure shows the aiming device in a correct position using a ventral approach to the vertebral body. (**a**) The lateral view represents the central drill guide in the correct position on the promontorium of the caudal aspect of the vertebral body. (**b**) The craniocaudal view shows the drill guide positioned on the promontorium, with an aiming targeting tip lined up with the vertebra midline and two sharp long dents, arranged symmetrically lateral of the midline, resting on the cranial deeper part of the vertebral body. In (**c**), the aiming device is shown as a whole with the handle, central drill guide and fixation dents.

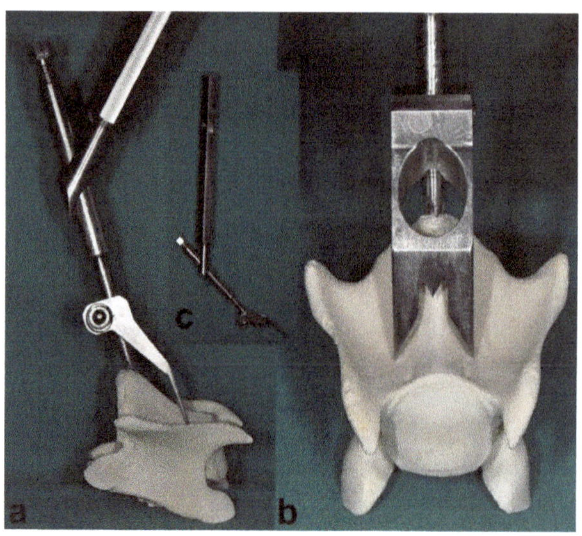

For injection of augmentation material, a 10 G (3.2-mm diameter) 100 mm-long special vertebroplasty needle (1394-1010, Optimed Medizinische Instrumente GmbH, Ettlingen, Germany) (Figure 2b) and an Optimed CementoRE gun (1392-0000, Optimed Medizinische Instrumente GmbH, Ettlingen, Germany) were used (Figure 2c).

Figure 2. The images (**a–e**) show the different steps of the surgical procedure: (**a**) an aiming device was used for repeatable and standardized drilling; (**b**) the vertebroplasty needle was correctly positioned; (**c**) material injection was performed in multiple steps using the Optimed CementoRE gun. Fluoroscopic imaging was used for repeatable and standardized drilling (**d**) and to detect material leakage during injection, as seen in (**e**), where leakage into vertebral vessels was detected at the caudal part of the two injected vertebrae (see the →).

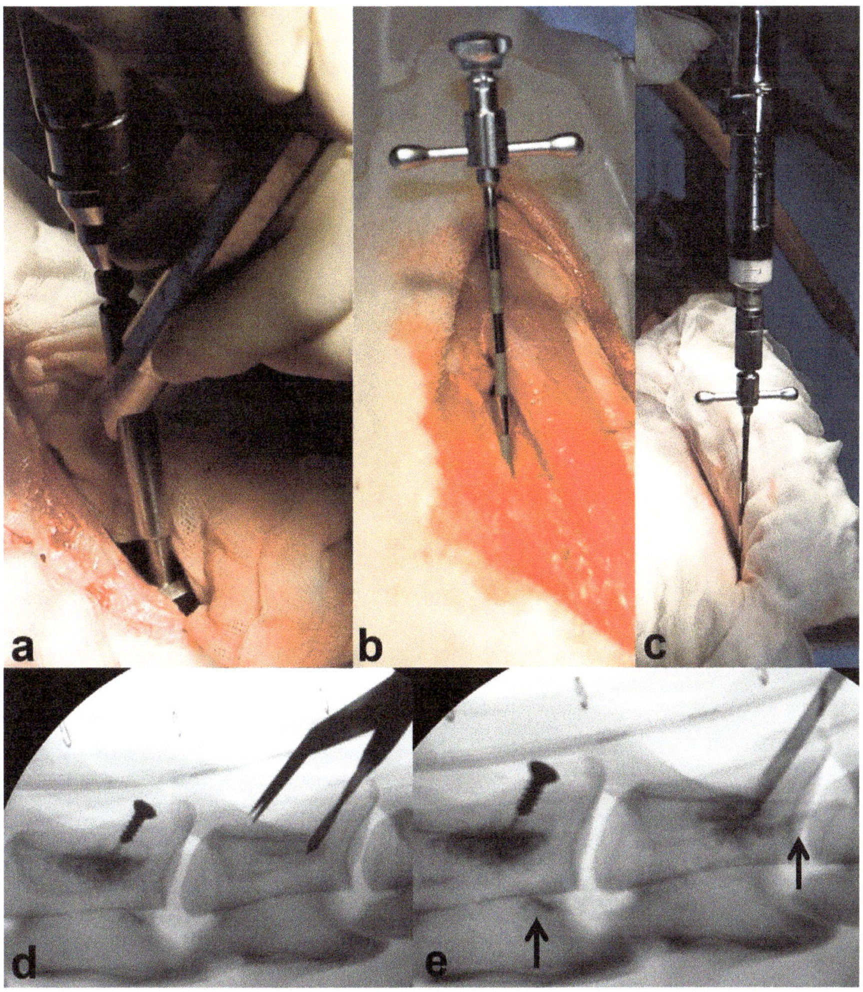

2.4. Anesthesia

A standard anesthetic protocol was used. After 24 hours of fasting and 30 minutes before induction of anesthesia, the animals were premedicated with buprenorphine (Temgesic®, 0.01 mg/kg i.m., Essex Chemie AG, Lucerne, Switzerland) and xylazine (Rompun® 2%, 0.1 mg/kg i.m., Streuli Pharma, Uznach, Switzerland). A catheter was placed into the vena cephalica antebrachii of one of the front legs and prophylactic antibiotics (Penicillin Natrium® 35,000 IU/kg i.v., G. Streuli Pharma, Uznach,

Switzerland; gentamicin, Vetagent®, 4 mg/kg i.v., Veterinaria AG, Zurich, Switzerland), as well as a pre-emptive analgesic drug, carprofen (Rimadyl®, 4 mg/kg i.v., Pfizer SA, Zurich, Switzerland), were given intravenously. A booster for tetanus (Tetanus Serum Intervet, 3,000 IU/sheep s.c., Veterinaria AG Zurich, Switzerland) was administered subcutaneously.

Anesthesia was induced with diazepam (Valium®, 0.1 mg/kg i.v., Roche Pharma AG, Rheinach, Switzerland), ketamine (Narketan 10®, 3 mg/kg i.v., Vetoquinol AG, Belp-Bern, Switzerland) and propofol (Propofol®, 0.4–2 mg/kg i.v., Fresenius Kabi, Stans, Switzerland), the latter administered to effect. After laryngeal desensitization with lidocaine spray (xylocaine spray 10%, 3 pumps of 0.1 mL each, Astra Zeneca AG, Zug, Switzerland), the trachea was intubated and correct placement was confirmed by expired carbon dioxide monitoring ($F_{et}CO_2$). Anesthesia was maintained with a balanced anesthetic protocol employing the administration of isoflurane (1%–2%) in oxygen via an adult F-circuit (circle system, Intersurgical, Berkshire, U.K.), a variable rate infusion of propofol (Propofol®, 0.5–1 mg/kg/h, Fresenius Kabi, Stans, Switzerland), as well as lidocaine given at the beginning of the surgical procedure as bolus (1 mg/kg) and afterwards as constant rate infusion (Lidocaine®, 40 μg/kg/min, Kantonsapotheke, Zurich, Switzerland).

Monitoring parameters included electrocardiogram (ECG), heart rate, pulse rate and invasively measured blood pressures (systolic, mean and diastolic arterial) via an arterial catheter in an auricular artery. Furthermore, inspired and expired concentrations of carbon dioxide, oxygen and isoflurane, as well as esophageal temperature and saturation of arterial blood (SpO_2) were monitored. All parameters were constantly measured and recorded in 10-minute intervals. Intraoperatively, fluids Ringer's lactate solution (Ringer Lactat®, Bichsel, Interlaken, Switzerland) was administered at a rate of 10 mL/kg/h, and heat was applied using a forced-air warming device (Bair Hugger® 505, Augustine Healthcare, Eden Prairie, MN, USA).

Intermittent positive pressure ventilation was applied (if needed) to maintain normocapnia. A Swan-Ganz-catheter was inserted via the jugular vein into the pulmonary artery to allow invasive measurements of pulmonary artery pressure and cardiac output. Physiologic airway dead space measurements were performed with the non-invasive cardiac output monitor, NICO® (Respironics Novametrix, Inc., Wallingford, CT, USA). The results of this comparison between invasive and non-invasive measurements are not included in this paper and will be described elsewhere.

2.5. Surgical Procedure

The anesthetized sheep were placed in dorsal recumbency with the forelimbs retracted caudally and fixed to the surgery table. The neck was bent slightly upwards for an easier approach to the vertebral bodies. The correct position of the sheep was further supported with an inflatable surgery mat, rubber foam rolls and wedges. To prevent bloating and regurgitation, a stomach tube was placed prior to surgery. The tube was maintained throughout the entire surgery until recovery in sternal recumbency. The ventral aspect of the neck was shaved and surgically scrubbed and cleansed. The animals were draped according to routine. A midline skin incision was performed from the pharyngeal region extending caudally to the level of the thoracic inlet. The subcutis and superficial facial planes were bluntly dissected to expose sternohyoid and pharyngeal muscles. A blunt and careful dissection was made in the midline in between the left and right sternohyoid muscles. The jugular vein, carotid artery, vagal nerve, trachea and oesophagus were carefully retracted using a blunt retractor wrapped in gauze. Exposure of the ventral aspect of the vertebral bodies was maintained by securing the retractors in place. The desired vertebra was identified by palpating the transverse processes and the intervertebral spaces. The identification of the area of interest was performed using two anatomical landmarks: the promontorium caudal to the desired vertebral body and the deeper laying cranial aspect of the vertebra. The muscles covering the caudal aspect of the vertebral body were bluntly divided to expose the area of interest. Hemostasis was meticulously kept using electrocautery. The aiming device was placed with the tip of the drill guide at the promontorium in the cranial drill direction (Figure 1a–c).

Under fluoroscopic control, the correct placement of the aiming device and subsequent needle positioning was validated to avoid inaccurate injections. A drill hole with a diameter of 2.8 mm was created in the vertebral body (Figure 2a) followed by placing the special vertebroplasty needle using a Kirschner wire as guide for the correct direction of the needle path. Afterwards, the needle was pushed forward, till its tip was firmly seated and surrounded by bone (Figure 2b).

Material injections were done in multiple steps under fluoroscopic guidance (Figure 2e). Needle filling with augmentation material was done slowly with the aid of the Optimed CementoRE gun (Figure 2c). Subsequently, the gun was removed, and the stylet was used to push the material into the bone, so as to provide exact quantities of injectate. The filling-clearing procedure was repeated one or two times, until a target between 1.5 and 1.8 mL was injected within the intertrabecular space. Using fluoroscopy, the leakage of material into a vessel and thrombus formation was recorded, the injection needle slightly advanced and injection continued. At completion of the procedure, the vertebroplasty needle was removed and the insertion point closed with a 3.5-mm diameter self-tapping screw (8 mm in length, Synthes, Oberdorf, Switzerland) (Figure 2d and 2e). The screw was used to later determine the direction of the needle and insertion point at the time of sacrifice.

Afterwards, the muscles were repositioned, and the closure of the soft tissue was routinely done using resorbable suture material (Vicryl® polyglactin, 2-0, Johnson & Johnson Int., Brussels, Belgium) in a simple continuous fashion, while the skin was closed with a skin stapler (Appose ULV, United States Surgical). The Swan-Ganz catheter was removed, and a normal catheter (Vygonyle S® G14, Vygon GmbH, Aachen, Germany) was placed in the other jugular vein. Intra-operative fluoroscopy images were taken in right lateral view throughout the surgery to document the surgical technique and the injection steps. Immediately after surgery, fluoroscopy images in latero-lateral and ventrodorsal view were taken to document the distribution of the injected material in two projection plans.

2.6. Postoperative Treatment

The animals were supervised during recovery from anesthesia until they could stand on their own, walk around and eat without further complications. They were kept in small groups, and their health status was checked twice daily. Antibiotic and analgesia administrations were continued for 4 days intravenously using the same dosage as perioperatively applied.

Additional analgesia treatment was provided to reduce postoperative pain using intramuscular injections of buprenorphine (Temgesic®, 0.01 mg/kg, Essex Chemie AG, Luzern, Switzerland) every 4 hours for a total of three applications.

2.7. *In Vivo Fluorescence Labeling*

Different fluorescence markers were subcutaneously injected at 6 weeks (calcein green, 5 mg/kg BW s.c., Fluka AG, Buchs, Switzerland), 12 weeks (xylenol orange, 90 mg/kg BW s.c., Fluka AG) and three days prior to sacrifice (oxytetracycline, 20 mg/kg BW s.c., Engemycin® 10%, MSD Animal health GmbH, Lucerne, Switzerland) to dynamically represent new bone formation and remodeling.

2.8. *Sacrifice and Specimen Preparation for Evaluative Procedures*

All animals were sacrificed after a follow up period of 16 weeks, and the three treated cervical vertebrae were harvested for final analysis. Augmentation sites were examined macroscopically, and digital photographs were taken to document tissue reaction at the surgical site (Nikon Digital Camera D5000, 2009 Nikon Corporation©). Radiographs were taken using a Faxitron (Faxitron X-Ray Systems, Hewlett Packard, Mc Minnville Division, OR, USA) to visualize the detailed bone structure and detect remaining augmentation material. Subsequently, each vertebra was cut in a smaller segment containing only the injected vertebral body for evaluative procedures. An additional radiograph was performed to qualitatively assess new bone formation in the vertebral bodies. The bone samples were fixed in 40% ethanol for one week, followed by a series of ethanol dehydration steps (50%–100%) within 6 days. µ-CT analysis of the specimen was performed in 70% ethanol fixation (b-cube AG, Bio-Technopark, Schlieren-Zurich, Switzerland). After complete dehydration, the samples were degreased in xylene and subsequently infiltrated in liquid methymethacrylate (MMA) until polymerization occurred [20]. Using a special band saw (EXAKT® Band System 300/301, EXAKT® Apparatebau GmbH &Co KG, Norderstedt, Germany), cutting of the ground sections (300 µm) and native fluorescence sections (350 µm) were performed. The sections were oriented along the original needle path in the midline of the vertebral body, with the needle path itself, the tip of the needle and the surrounding tissue defined as the region of interest. Before mounting (Cementit® CA 12, Merz + Benteli AG, Niederwangen, Switzerland) the sections on plastic slides (ACROPAL, Maagtechnic, Duebendorf, Switzerland), microradiographs were taken with the Faxitron (27 kV, 11 s; Fuji Photo Film Co Ltd, Tokyo, Japan). Ground sections were polished (Exakt® Mikro- Schleifsystem 400CS, Exakt Apparatebau GmbH, Norderstedt, Germany) and surface stained with toluidine blue. The native sections for fluorescence were mounted on pellucid, acrylic Plexiglas slides (Maagtechnic, Duebendorf, Switzerland) and wrapped in aluminum foil to protect slides from bleaching. For thin section preparation, the remaining bone blocks were cut in smaller segments comprising only the tip of the needle and surrounding tissue. Polymerization was achieved in special customized Teflon forms (D. Nadler, JOSSI AG, Islikon, Switzerland) [20]. Afterwards, the small blocks were mounted on plastic frames and cut using a microtome (Leica® RM 2155, Leica Instruments GmbH). After mounting on glass slides and pressing for two days in the incubator, the sections were stained with either toluidine blue or van Kossa/McNeal.

2.9. Analysis

2.9.1. Micro-Computed Tomography Analysis

Micro-computed tomography (μCT) analysis of the vertebral bodies was performed to qualitatively assess the bone volume density and trabecular thickness, as well as the location and amount of residual augmentation material within the treated levels. The samples were scanned by a micro-computed tomography system (μCT 40, Scanco Medical AG, Brüttisellen, Switzerland). The measured data were filtered and then segmented to separate the bone and the potentially present residual biomaterial from the background using a global thresholding procedure. For samples with identified residual biomaterial, a multi-level segmentation technique was used to segment bone and residual material in two separate phases, whereas for samples without residual material, a simple segmentation procedure was applied to separate bone from background. For all samples, the same thresholds were used. The measurements were performed using semiautomatic masks of nine overlapping hollow sphere shells in different sizes centered at the tip of the needle, used to calculate average bone volume density and trabecular thickness within each sphere shell (Figure 3).

Figure 3. This figure represents one slice through the nine hollow sphere shells used for the analysis. The needle path and the cortical bone areas were excluded from the analysis.

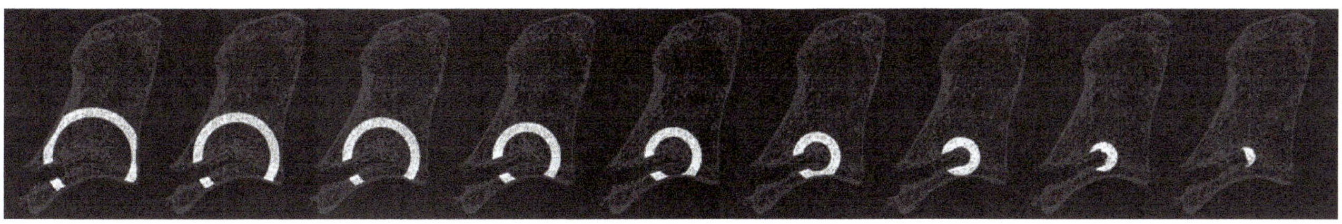

Figure 4. This figure shows the different masks created for density analysis. (**A**) The inner mask to exclude the cortical bone from the analysis. (**B**) The defined cylinder (Ø 3.5 mm) representing the original needle path with two manually determined points "tip" and "base". This cylinder was subtracted from the hollow sphere shells. Furthermore, the part of the sphere shell not lying in the trabecular bone was subtracted from the sphere shell. (**C**) An example of the final sphere shell mask.

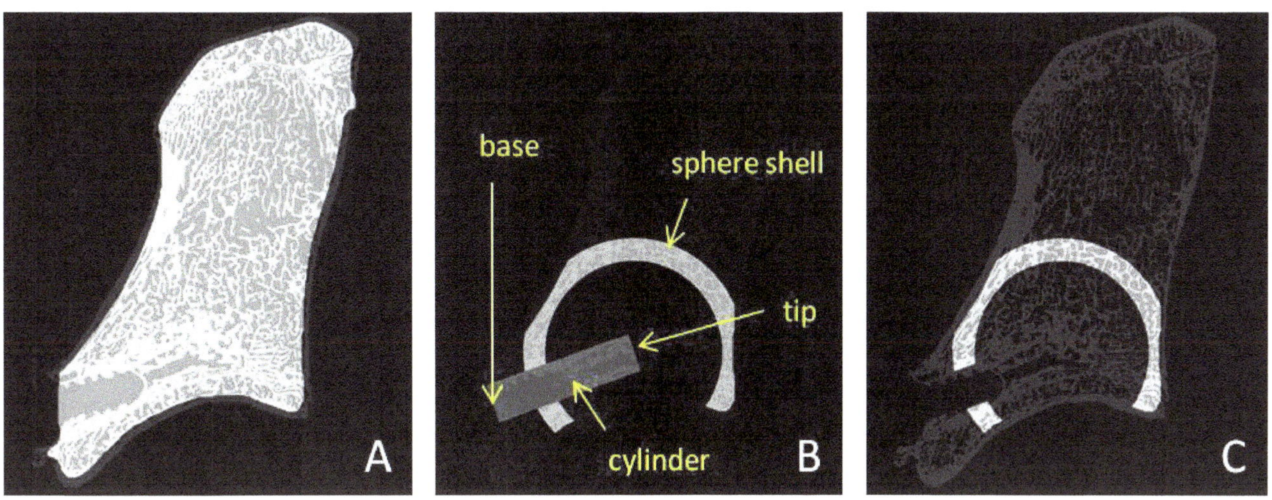

Using these sphere shells, the calculation of average material distribution and bone volume density in correlation to the radial distance from the tip of the needle was possible. To measure only the trabecular bone area, a region correlating to the cylindrical needle path and the cortical bone shell were excluded from the analysis. For the original needle path, a cylinder slightly larger than the original diameter of the needle was chosen, in order to exclude the region of any bone debris produced during the needle insertion procedure (Figure 4).

Integrating the values of the spherical shell data, the bone volume density in full thickness spheres could be computed (Figure 5).

Figure 5. This figure shows one slice with 4 full thickness spheres with 8 mm, 12 mm, 16 mm and 20 mm diameter, respectively.

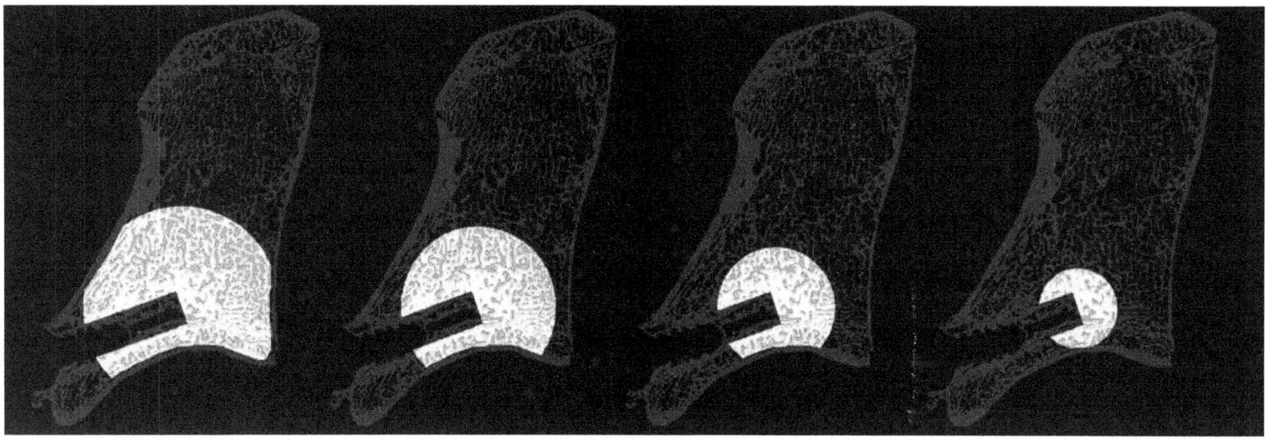

Figure 6. This figure shows a full sphere of 12 mm in diameter and a sphere shell with more than 12 mm in diameter. The inner 'Sphere12' is representative of the injected region of biomaterial, subsequently called 'augmented'. The outer 'Shell12+' is representative of the untreated bone region and used as internal sample reference, subsequently called 'unaugmented'. Needle path and cortical bone regions (grey shaded areas) were excluded from the analysis.

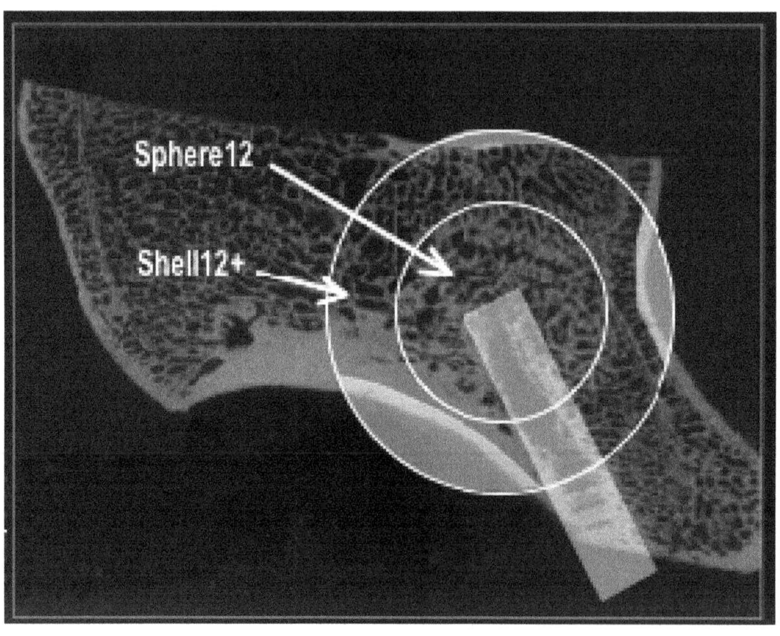

With the injected volume of approximately 1–1.5 mL material, the sum of sphere shells up to 12 mm in diameter were assumed as the injected area (consecutively called the full thickness sphere), whereas the sum of all larger sphere shells were assumed to be non-injected (Figure 6).

2.9.2. Histological Evaluation

Histomorphometry was performed using digitally recorded images of the ground sections (5.6-fold magnification, macroscope Leica Z6 APOA, Leica DFC 420C, Glattbrugg, Switzerland). For standardization of the evaluated area, three circles of 5 mm in diameter were chosen around the tip of the needle (Figure 7). The structures of interest within these circles were manually color-highlighted interactively using Adobe Photoshop Elements 10 (Adobe Systems, San Jose, CA, USA). Old bone was highlighted in blue (R: 0; G: 210; B: 255), newly formed bone in green (R: 34; G: 79; B: 7), granulation tissue in pink (R: 242; G: 40; B: 211) and residual augmentation material in beige (R: 198; G: 156; B: 96) using a standard pixel-detecting tool of Adobe Photoshop. Afterwards, the colored images were analyzed using a special image analysis software (QUIPS/QWIN, Leica standard, V.3.0, 2003, Leica-Microsystems, Heerbrugg, Switzerland), and the colored fractions were automatically detected and measured in pixels using binary segmentation of a standard macro-routine. Afterwards the pixels of each whole circle were set as 100% and the different colored fractions converted into percentages. Circles including the growth plate were excluded from the analysis, to avoid higher rates of new bone present independently of the applied material. Cortical bone in the circles was excluded from the region of interest and the rest of the circle considered as 100%, since disproportional high-density old bone is present in the cortex. The average of all three circles per sample were used for statistical analysis. To reduce any inter-observer variability, only one examiner performed the analysis; certain randomly chosen images were evaluated twice as the control.

Figure 7. Example of a histology ground section for histomorphometric evaluation. Three circles (Ø 5mm) at the tip of the needle were chosen for the evaluation of the percentage of old bone, newly formed bone, total bone and granulation tissue within the area of interest.

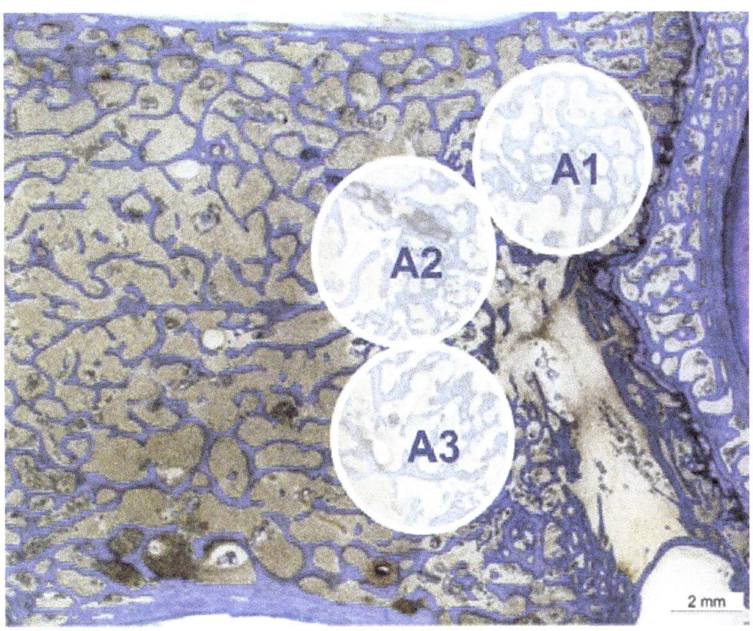

Thin sections were evaluated semi-quantitatively for cellular reactions using a microscope (Leica® DMR, Glattbrugg, Switzerland) in 10- to 20-fold magnification. Scores were given for presence of macrophages, mononuclear cells, osteoclasts, multinucleated foreign body cells, amount of osteoid seam, thickness of osteoid seam and amount of residual material (Table 2). Three power fields per section were assessed with two peripheral and one central in the injected area. The average of all three scoring areas for each augmentation site was statistically evaluated.

Table 2. Indicators for cellular reactions evaluated in the semi-quantitative histology scoring. Low scores indicate low numbers and high scores high numbers of cells, material or osteoid seams.

Indicator	**Observable value** (in the circular scoring area)	**Scoring range** (for each single circular scoring area)
Mononuclear cells	Percentage of mononuclear cells compared to the overall number of cells	0–3
Macrophages	Percentage of macrophages compared to the overall number of cells	0–3
Multinucleated foreign body cells	Absolute number of multinucleated foreign body cells	0–3
Fibroblasts	Percentage of fibroblast compared to the overall number of cells	0–3
Osteoclasts	Absolute number of osteoclasts	0–3
Amount of osteoid seam	Percentage of bone surface covered by osteoid	0–3
Thickness of osteoid seam	Thickness of the osteoid compared to the average size of an osteoblast	0–3
Residual material	Percentage of surface occupied by residual material	0–3

Fluorescent sections were evaluated semi-quantitatively for the differences of dye integration between groups and at different time points (calcein green at 6 weeks, xylenol orange at 12 weeks and oxytetracycline at 16 weeks post-surgery). Digital images of the region of interest at the tip of the needle were recorded. Therefore, 30 single images were taken in a 1.25 magnification and merged together using a special microscope, camera and specific merging software ("Stitching function"; Leica® DM 600B, Leica® DFC 350 FX, Leica® Microsystems CMS GmbH, Mannheim, Germany). Scores were given for the percentage of each fluorescent dye in the region of interest (considered as 100%) with 0% = 0, 1%–25% = 1, 26%–50% = 2, >50% = 3.

2.9.3. Statistical Analysis

Results were analyzed statistically by means of PASWStatistics® software (Base for Mac OS X, Version 21.0, Chicago, IL, USA). Overall differences between groups were assessed using a factorial analysis of variance (ANOVA). Differences between individual groups were calculated with *post hoc* tests according to Scheffe. p-values < 0.05 were considered statistically significant.

3. Results

3.1. Surgery, Postoperative Period and Sacrifice

A total of 17 female adult sheep were treated with the cervical vertebral augmentation model. Out of these 17 animals, two (11.8%) died during surgery after augmentation of the first vertebra. Death was attributed to severe cardiac distress, including a sudden decrease in arterial blood pressure and end-expired CO_2 by approximately 50%, followed by cardiac arrest. The other 15 sheep completed the 16-week follow-up period successfully. Out of these, 5/15 animals (29.4%) developed mild symptoms of pulmonary embolism, but recovered while still in surgery without further complications. No significant difference between treatment groups for the incidence of pulmonary embolism was found. Although only seven animals showed clinical signs of pulmonary embolism, the leakage of biomaterial (0.1–0.5 mL) into the venous circulation was observed in 19/36 (52.7%) material-treated augmentation sites (*i.e.*, sham group excluded) using fluoroscopy during the injection procedure.

In total, 43/45 augmentation sites were treated. Using the aiming device and fluoroscopic imaging for standardized needle placement and material injection, the needle could be positioned successfully during the first attempt in 42/45 augmentation sites (three vertebrae per sheep, 15 remaining sheep). Only in 3/45 augmentation sites (medium and high concentration groups and sham group), needle positioning was unsuccessful in the first attempt. In these cases, the drill guide was repositioned and drilling was repeated due to a misalignment of the first drilling. In one of these injection sites (medium conc. group), no material could be injected in the vertebra, because the first drilling had perforated the opposite cortical bone with a disproportional high risk of leakage outside the vertebral body into the spinal canal. Another unplanned deviation of the surgical procedure occurred in the first sheep of the study, where only two vertebrae were treated due to a very long anesthesia and surgery period. For health and survival reasons, the surgery was stopped after the augmentation into the second vertebra.

Another minor surgical complication at one augmentation site was the breaking of the needle during the extraction procedure from the bone. The small broken part of the needle remained within the bone. However, no further clinical complications resulted from this event, and the augmentation site was evaluated according to the standard protocol.

Under fluoroscopic guidance during surgery, all formulations showed good radio-opacity and a sphere-like shape distribution around the tip of the needle with an injected amount between 1 and 1.5 mL of augmentation material.

The overall surgical procedure for each animal lasted between 45 and 60 minutes. After a short recovery period following anesthesia (approximately 30 minutes), the sheep roamed freely in the stables or on pasture without lameness or other visible discomfort. During the 16-week follow-up, no signs of wound infections or inflammation were noticed in any of the 15 remaining sheep.

The en-bloc harvesting process of the cervical spine, including all treated vertebra, was uneventful, and all samples could be prepared for further evaluation. By setting the screw for needle direction after sacrifice and using the customized aiming device during the surgical procedure, the central area of augmentation within the vertebral bodies could be found in all samples with a longitudinal cut through the original needle path.

3.2. Analysis

3.2.1. Micro-Computed Tomography

Results of μCT are given in Table 3. With the μCT images, the suitability of the surgical method could be confirmed with respect to a consistent, standardized needle placement in the desired and predicted trabecular bone space. For all treatment groups, a higher bone volume density and an increased trabecular thickness was found when compared to the sham group, indicating a bone enhancing effect of all material formulations (Table 3, Figure 8). Trabecular thickness was similar in the treated groups and the matrix alone group. This was combined with a radial distribution for both parameters with higher values central in the augmented area (until sphere 12) and decreasing values to the unaugmented area (sphere >12). Residual augmentation material was only detected in the matrix-only treatment group (no $TGplPTH_{1-34}$, 4/7 samples) and the low concentration group (2/9 samples). No other treatment group had residual material detected.

Table 3. Means and SD of the morphometric μCT measurements for BV/TV (bone volume density) and Tb.Th. (trabecular thickness) for three spheres: 8 mm, 12 mm and 16 mm. Note that the BV/TV in the larger 12 mm sphere is higher for the treated groups, while trabecular thickness is equal to the matrix alone group and only higher compared to the sham.

Group	BV/TV [%] (sphere 8 mm)	BV/TV [%] (sphere 12 mm)	BV/TV [%] (sphere 16 mm)	Tb.Th [mm] (sphere 8 mm)	Tb.Th [mm] (sphere 12 mm)	Tb.Th [mm] (sphere 16 mm)
Matrix alone	52.2 ± 9.0	44.7 ± 11.0	41.0 ± 8.9	0.43 ± 0.07	0.38 ± 0.08	0.34 ± 0.06
Low	52.9 ± 8.6	47.3 ± 6.0	45.6 ± 5.1	0.34 ± 0.07	0.30 ± 0.06	0.31 ± 0.08
Medium	61.5 ± 3.8	55.1 ± 4.8	50.3 ± 4.7	0.40 ± 0.10	0.37 ± 0.08	0.34 ± 0.08
High	50.2 ± 16.6	46.7 ± 15.5	43.8 ± 14.1	0.34 ± 0.11	0.31 ± 0.10	0.28 ± 0.08
Sham	43.6 ± 10.3	45.0 ± 9.1	46.5 ± 8.6	0.27 ± 0.07	0.27 ± 0.07	0.28 ± 0.06

Figure 8. Three representative sagittal sections of the μCT scans: (**a**) a sample of the control group; (**b**) a sample of the group with medium $TGplPTH_{1-34}$ concentration is illustrated; (**c**) a sample of the group with high $TGplPTH_{1-34}$ concentration is shown. A denser bone area in the injected region could be distinguished for the samples in (b) and (c), where the augmentation material was injected. Increased trabecular thickness is visible in the circles of the outlined augmentation area.

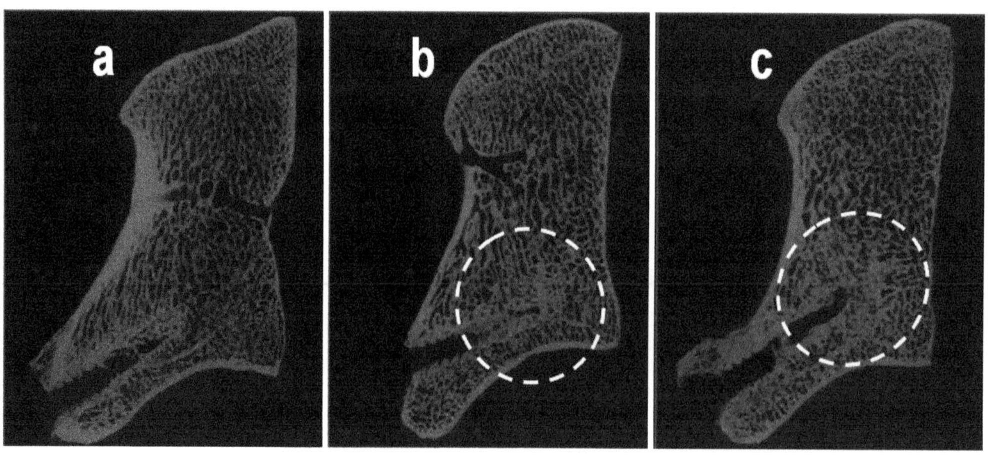

3.2.2. Histomorphometry

Exact percentages of new bone formation, old remaining bone matrix, granulation tissue and total bone are reported in Table 4 and Figure 9.

Table 4. Histomorphometrical measurements of old bone, new bone, total bone and granulation tissue (in percentage of total area measured).

Group	Old bone matrix	New bone matrix	Total bone matrix	Granulation tissue
Matrix alone	22.4 ± 3.4	19.6 ± 8.6	42.0 ± 8.0	58.0 ± 8.0
Low	15.3 ± 2.3	26.3 ± 5.5	41.9 ± 5.2	58.4 ± 5.2
Medium	15.5 ± 3.5	32.0 ± 3.6	47.6 ± 3.6	52.5 ± 3.6
High	9.6 ± 10.5	27.5 ± 9.7	37.1 ± 12.9	62.9 ± 12.9
Sham	34.2 ± 6.9	7.1 ± 8.2	41.4 ± 12.4	58.7 ± 12.4

Figure 9. The bars show the mean and SD values of the histomorphometrical measurements of old bone, new bone and granulation tissue (as a percentage of the total area measured). All treatment groups showed significantly higher percentages of new bone than the control group. In contrast, the sham group had the highest percentage of old bone (significant differences compared to the sham group are highlighted with asterisks; the bracket illustrates the significant difference between the matrix alone group and the group with medium $TGplPTH_{1-34}$).

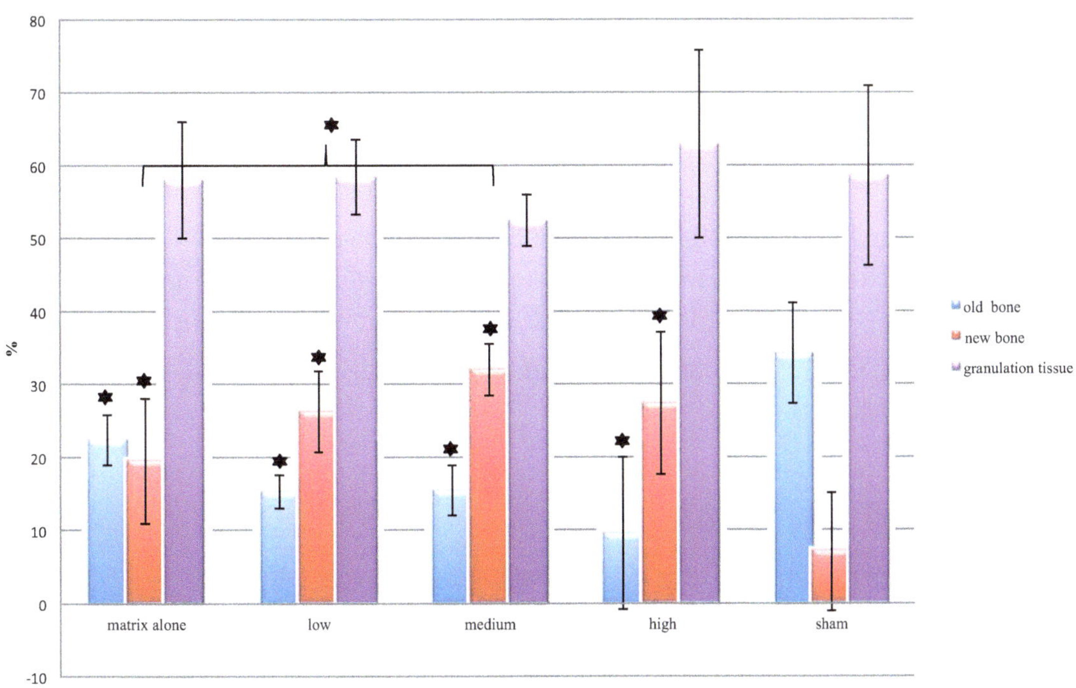

As in the μCTs overall, a high percentage of new bone was found in the augmented region (19.6%–32%) for all treatment groups, whereas in the sham group, new bone was only detected at the border of the needle path (7.1%). In all treatment groups, the area adjacent to the tip of the needle seemed to be mainly filled with new bone, partly due to proliferation and partly to an enhanced remodeling and bone formation process (Figure 10).

Figure 10. Examples of toluidine blue-stained ground sections of all groups; the area at the tip of the needle of all treatment groups showed mainly newly formed bone (indicated by darker blue areas), whereas for the sham group, new bone only was detectable at the border of the needle path. Note the increased trabecular thickness in the augmented area.

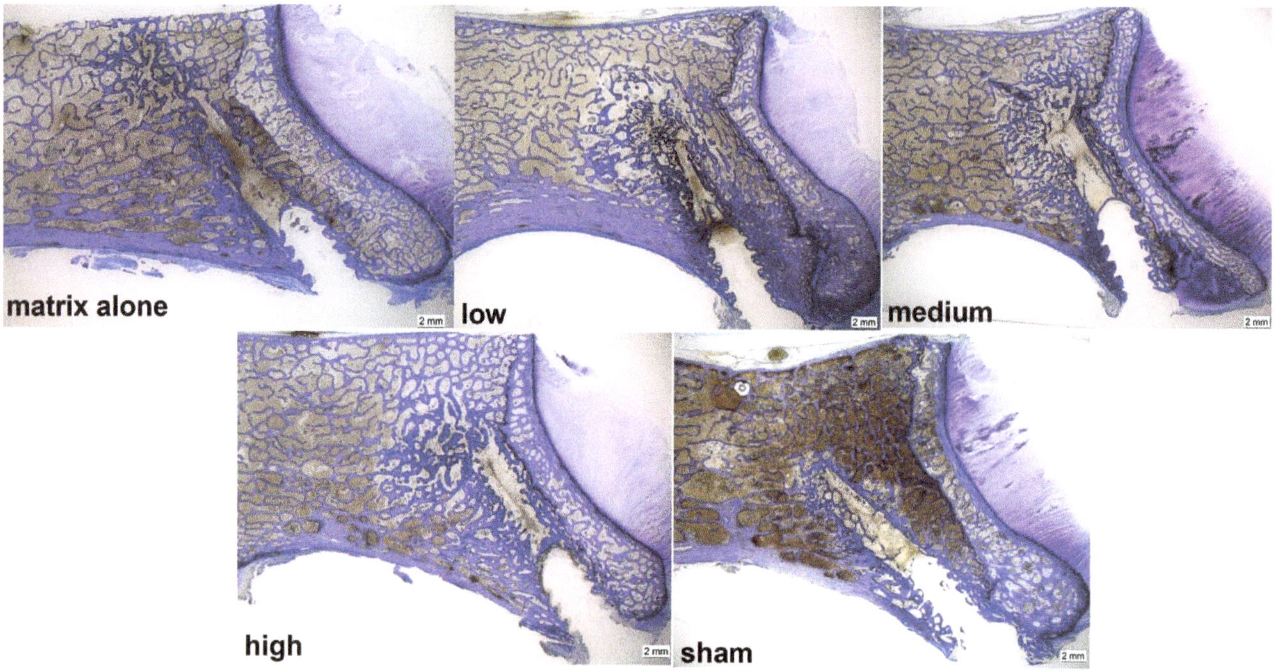

Overall differences between groups in percentage for old and new bone were significant at $p = 0.000$. When compared individually, all treatment groups showed significantly higher percentages of new bone than the sham group (p-value ranging between 0.000 and 0.029). In contrast, the sham group had the highest percentage of old bone compared to all treatment groups (p-value ranging between 0.000 and 0.009). No significant differences between groups were found for the percentages of granulation tissue (52.4%–62.9%) and of total bone (37.1%–47.56%). The bone remodeling process was pronounced in all specimens of the treatment groups, but especially for the groups with higher concentrations of $TGplPTH_{1-34}$. The highest average for new bone (32%) was found for the group with a medium concentration of $TGplPTH_{1-34}$. with statistical significant differences also for the group with matrix alone (19.6%) ($p = 0.042$) (Figure 9).

3.2.3. Fluorescence

Means and SD from semi-quantitatively scoring fluorescence sections are reported in Table 5. No fluorescent dye (tetracycline) was detected at 16 weeks, so that it was left out of the table.

The fluorescence images of all treatment groups demonstrated the sphere-like shape distribution of the biomaterial with a red colored area in the middle and a green area towards the periphery. This pattern indicated a radial progression of new bone formation with enhanced bone activity, and precipitation of the fluorescence markers starting in the periphery and the biomaterial being progressively degraded, starting from the periphery towards the middle of the injected region (Figure 11).

Table 5. Means and SD of the semi-quantitative fluorescence scores for all groups and at different time points show that increased new bone formation occurred mainly at the early time point at six weeks in all PTH derivates compared to controls. At 12 weeks, new bone deposition was lower in all groups, except the matrix alone group.

Group	Calcein green (6w.p.OP)	Xylenol orange (12w.p.OP)
Matrix alone	0.8 ± 0.4	0.9 ± 0.9
Low	1.0 ± 0.0	1.1 ± 0.8
Medium	1.5 ± 0.8	0.8 ± 0.7
High	1.4 ± 0.5	0.9 ± 0.9
Sham	0.7 ± 0.5	0.1 ± 0.3

Figure 11. This figure shows representative fluorescence images of all groups at the three different time points, as well as one image merged, respectively overlaid together. At six weeks, enhanced bone activity in the injected region could be detected especially for the treatment groups with a medium and high concentration. This localized bone activity decreased at 12 weeks and, with the degradation of the material, finally disappeared at 16 weeks. In the sham group, only the area next to the needle track was enhanced. Note that the area of bone deposition is broader in its diameter in the treated groups compared to the matrix alone.

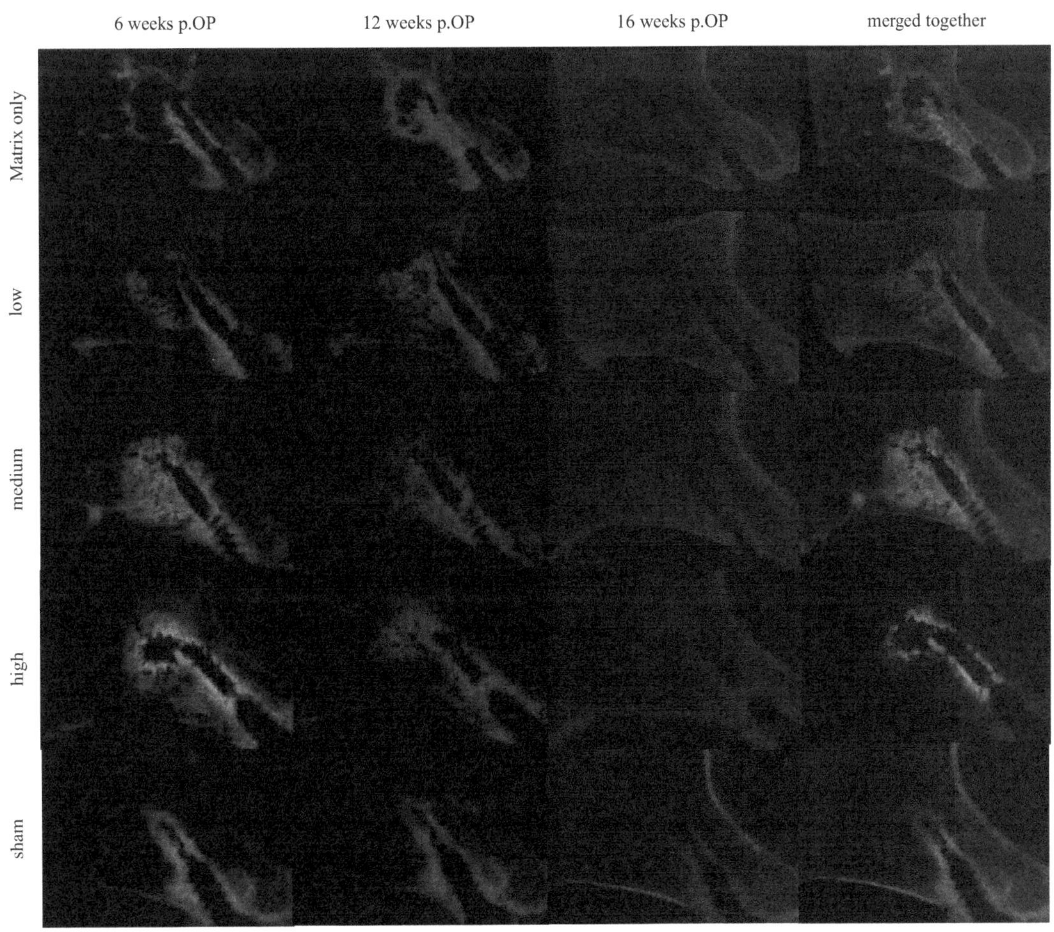

At six weeks, all treatment groups showed enhanced bone activity in the injected area, as indicated by calcein green precipitation. Overall differences between groups in bone activity were significant at $p = 0.003$. Especially in the groups with medium and high TGplPTH$_{1-34}$ concentrations, the bone activity was enhanced with significantly higher values in comparison to the sham group ($p = 0.029$ and $p = 0.040$ for groups with medium and high concentration, respectively). This localized bone activity decreased at 12 weeks (xylenol orange) and finally disappeared at 16 weeks (tetracycline) proportional to the degradation of the material. For the treatment group with matrix only and for the group with a low concentration of TGplPTH$_{1-34}$, higher scores were given at 12 weeks *versus* six weeks, with other treatment groups maintaining stable values during that period. In the sham group, only the area next to the needle track was enhanced for bone activity, which was attributed to the remodeling process of bone debris created by the needle.

3.2.4. Histologic and Cellular Evaluation

Means and SD of the semi-quantitative histology scoring are summarized in Table 6.

Table 6. Means and SD of the semi-quantitative histology scoring are given using the average of the three scoring areas for each augmentation site.

Group	Mononuclear cells	Macro-phages	Multinucleated foreign body cells	Fibro-blasts	Osteo-clasts	Amount of osteoid seam	Thickness of osteoid	Residual material
Matrix alone	1.2 ± 0.4	1.1 ± 0.6	0.0 ± 0.0	0.2 ± 0.3	0.3 ± 0.4	0.7 ± 0.5	0.7 ± 0.5	0.3 ± 0.5
Low	1.3 ± 0.3	1.2 ± 0.5	0.2 ± 0.2	0.0 ± 0.0	0.5 ±0.3	1.2 ± 0.6	1.3 ± 0.6	0.1 ± 0.1
Medium	1.2 ± 0.4	1.0 ± 0.2	0.1 ± 0.2	0.0 ± 0.0	0.5 ± 0.4	1.1± 0.7	1.2 ± 0.7	0.0 ± 0.0
High	1.0 ± 0.2	0.6 ± 0.3	0.0 ± 0.0	0.0 ± 0.0	0.5 ± 0.4	1.2 ± 0.4	1.3 ± 0.3	0.0 ± 0.0
Sham	0.9 ± 0.8	0.2 ± 0.4	0.0 ± 0.0	0.0 ± 0.0	0.5 ± 0.4	0.4 ± 0.3	0.5 ± 0.3	0.0 ± 0.0

The semi-quantitative histology scoring revealed similar values for all groups. Overall differences between groups were only found for scores of macrophages ($p = 0.000$). Due to the degradation process of the biomaterial, the number of macrophages was significantly higher in 3/4 treatment groups compared to the sham group (the p-value was 0.003, 0.001 and 0.009 for groups with matrix only, low and medium concentrations, respectively). However, the low scores of all treatment groups in comparison to the sham group for mononuclear cells and multinucleated foreign body cells indicated an excellent biocompatibility for all formulations. Thick osteoid seams and activated round-shaped osteoblasts evidenced an improved bone activity with higher scores found for all material groups containing TGplPTH$_{1-34}$ (Figure 12). Residual biomaterial was found only for the matrix only and low concentration groups.

Figure 12. This figure shows a thin section with many macrophages (→) and a thick osteoid seam with activated round-shaped osteoblasts (→).

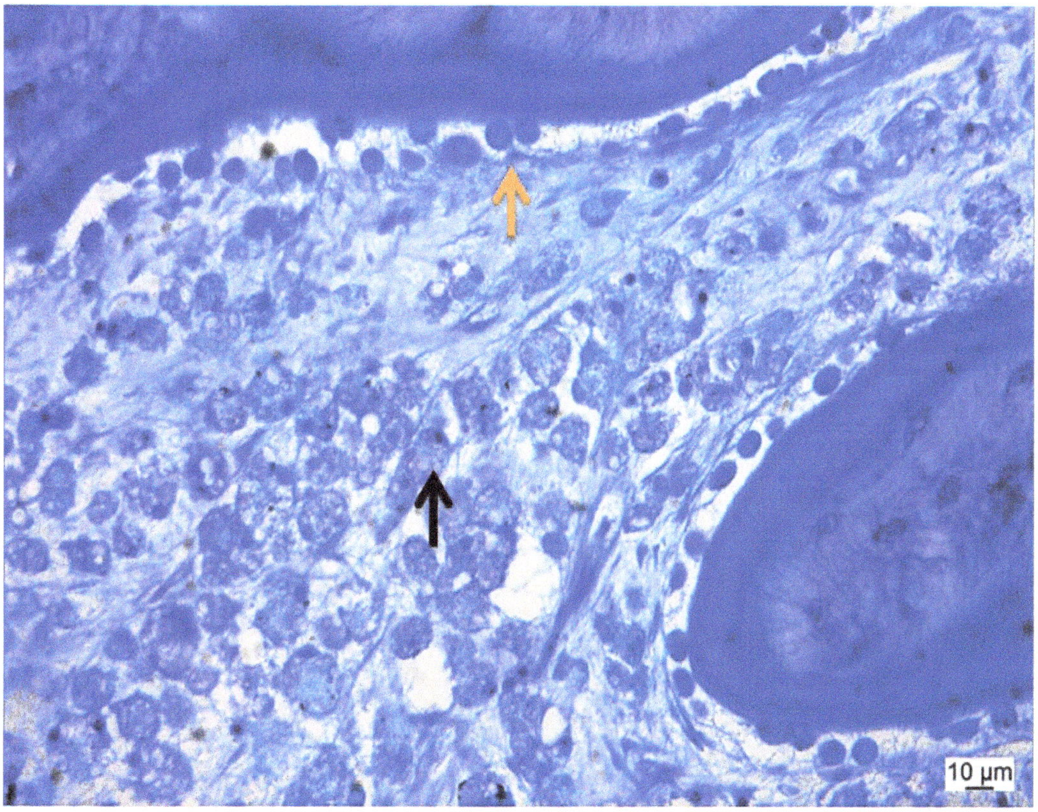

4. Discussion

In this study, a novel animal model in sheep was successfully established by using the cervical vertebrae of 17 sheep for the augmentation of cancellous bone with a biomimetic agent. The surgical and evaluation methods proved to be well standardized and highly reproducible. In addition, the efficacy of locally-delivered $TGplPTH_{1-34}$ incorporated in a fibrin matrix containing strontium carbonate was demonstrated to be a potentially suitable augmentation material for the cervical vertebra.

The surgical method was straightforward and easy to apply, with the aid of the specially developed aiming device. Using fluoroscopic imaging during the surgical procedure, combined with the various analyses, such as µCT, histomorphometry and sequential fluorescence dye staining, we were able to demonstrate that drilling and subsequent needle placement was accurate and reproducible. Consequently, we were able to inject test materials in 43/45 augmentation sites into the intertrabecular spacing of cervical vertebral bodies again with accuracy and reproducibility. However, as already discussed in a previous study concerning the tibia and femur augmentation in sheep [20], the trabecular bone density, as well as the trabecular thickness is much higher in sheep than in humans, such that the needle placement and material injection is more difficult to achieve in comparison to humans. In osteoporotic, brittle human bone, the injection needle can be placed in position using manual pressure only, whereas in sheep, a hole had to be drilled with a burr first in order to be able to push the needle forward into the healthy and dense trabecular bone. However, in contrast to the tibia and femur augmentation study, where a mallet had to be used after drilling to push the needle forward into the bone, this was not required for cervical bone augmentation. Therefore, the frequently observed surgical complications in the previous study, where the rather frail needle broke during the extraction procedure, were significantly less frequent in the current study (1/45). The harvesting method of the treated vertebrae was easy, fast and highly reproducible, with no need for an additional aiming device to define the region of interest as needed in the previous study [20].

Cardiovascular emboli are noticed in human patients after vertebral augmentation, even with a reported mortality rate of 2%. Emboli were also reported in our previously established femoral and tibia augmentation model [20]. Nevertheless, this cervical vertebral model presented more challenges regarding cardiovascular complications in comparison. Although the same material was used in both studies, the cervical augmentation model revealed a relatively high rate of pulmonary emboli, with two animals (11.76%) dying immediately on the table with severe signs of PE and five animals (29.4%) still showing mild signs of PE. In the femoral and tibia augmentation model, a higher leakage of material into the vessels was observed. This may be attributed to the different anatomical location, but probably also to the higher volume of material injected in the femoral and tibia augmentation model (3.5 mL per augmentation site). In human patients, reported emboli are less, but then, they are not routinely followed by lung CT after augmentation and, therefore, may often go unnoticed as long as no life threatening complication jeopardizes the patient's life. The higher mortality rate in sheep compared to humans may be related to the fact that injection of a relatively high material volume was performed in healthy cancellous bone of the vertebral body and that the sheep have denser bone compared to humans. Nevertheless, the cervical augmentation model presented the valuable opportunity to study the development of PE and its consequences, as they also occur in humans during vertebroplasty [32].

Mechanical testing of the vertebral bodies was not performed. Apart from technical problems to develop an adequate testing system with highly standardized cubes, it also was not of high priority in this study. One of the main reasons was that we did not treat osteoporotic sheep, since there is no adequate large animal model for this disease. Although we assumed that new bone formation with highly active osteoblast activity on new osteoid seams would be visible, it was not expected to significantly change trabecular thickness in healthy animals, since the mechanical load on the vertebrae had not changed. Trabecular thickness was only measured in μCT, where only calcified tissue is measured. However, in the histology sections, the increased trabecular thickness due to osteoid deposition is clearly visible in the ground and thin sections.

The three different concentrations (low, medium, high) of $TGplPTH_{1-34}$ proved to be suitable for cervical augmentation in sheep and showed indications of enhanced localized bone activity in all groups, especially during the first six weeks after surgery. Micro CT analysis, histomorphometry, as well as the evaluation of fluorescent incorporation indicated an increased bone formation and remodeling activity spatially limited to the injected area. As in the previous study [20], sequential fluorescent dye images indicated a radial propensity for new bone forming gradually over time from the periphery towards the middle of the injected regions. These findings support the hypothesis of Arrighi *et al.* that cell migration and infiltration into the fibrin matrix activate and release $TGplPTH_{1-34}$ into the surrounding tissue [19]. Our results further confirm those of Yang *et al.* showing that locally applied strontium has inherent osteoinductive properties itself [25]. However, combining strontium with high and probably even better medium concentrations of $TGplPTH_{1-34}$ enhanced the overall proliferative effect that was already previously demonstrated by our group in the femoral and tibia augmentation model [20]. The exact mechanism by which this co-effect is exerted is not fully known. However, we hypothesize that the accumulation of extracellular matrix induced by strontium increases the migration and infiltration of cells into the fibrin matrix and may also reduce osteoclast activity via apoptosis, again enhancing bone formation [25]. PTH, on the other hand, has anabolic activities on osteoblasts, increasing remodeling activity, as clearly shown in our previous study [20]. Taken together, bone forming properties are therefore enhanced by both ways: the increased osteoblastic activity through PTH and the increased population of living cells throughout the extracellular matrix population via strontium. Our evaluation methods did not allow distinguishing between increased remodeling activity and true new bone formation, as would be found in true osteoinduction. However, if in our current study, the different groups are compared to each other, it is obvious that the groups treated with TGplPTH$_{1\text{-}34}$ showed considerable increased bone formation compared to the matrix alone group. If the material alone in combination with trabecular microdamage would be the reason for the new bone formation, the matrix alone and with TGplPTH$_{1\text{-}34}$-treated groups would be equal in their response. However, the differences in new bone deposition are clearly visible in the fluorescent sections. Therefore, it is safe to assume that the new bone formation is in response to both remodeling activity after material injection and new bone formation after local application of TGplPTH$_{1\text{-}34}$.

The broad precipitation of fluorescence markers at six weeks post-surgery for the groups with medium and high concentrations of TGplPTH$_{1\text{-}34}$ indicate an enhanced, early and fast bone formation, which could be confirmed by histomorphometry with the highest percentage of new bone formation (32.0%) found for the medium concentration of TGplPTH$_{1\text{-}34}$, followed by 27.5% new bone formation found for the high concentration of TGplPTH$_{1\text{-}34}$. In comparison, groups with fibrin matrix only or with low concentration of TGplPTH$_{1\text{-}34}$ revealed less overall bone activity and at a later time point (12 weeks). This seems connected to the findings in the μCT analysis, where low quantities of residual material for the groups without or with a low dose of TGplPTH$_{1\text{-}34}$ could be related to higher amounts of remaining material. We assume that the degradation of these formulations is decelerated and therefore reduces the bone enhancing activity due to the delayed release of activated TGplPTH$_{1\text{-}34}$. To prove this theory in a future study, an earlier time point for the first fluorescence injection could be taken into consideration in order to confirm that the enhanced bone activity of medium and high concentrations of TGplPTH$_{1\text{-}34}$ shows a faster degradation of material, in correlation with a stronger enhanced bone activity.

In systemic applications of TGplPTH$_{1\text{-}34}$, a great concern is that high PTH concentrations may increase osteoclast activity [33]. This may be reflected by a lower percentage of newly formed bone, in addition to increased bone resorption zones and higher numbers of osteoclasts. Due to the mechanism of PTH, the influence on osteoclasts must be evaluated, when PTH is applied as a local peptide. In this study, no increase of osteoclasts and no resorption zones were found for any of the PTH concentrations. These findings were attributed to the use of the peptide covalently bound to the fibrin matrix that is only released and activated via local cell invasion and enzymatic cleavage. We therefore suggest that the osteoclast-enhancing effect of PTH shown by others depends not only on the higher dose, but mainly on the route of administration, which could be avoided by delivering the peptide locally and covalently bound to the fibrin matrix.

5. Conclusion

The cervical augmentation model in sheep described in this study proved to be a suitable animal model to evaluate the biocompatibility and new bone formation properties of new biomaterials, intended for vertebral bone augmentation. Although the model revealed to be more challenging, due to cardiovascular complications compared to the femoral and tibia augmentation model, this reflected well the human situation. Nevertheless, the results demonstrated that the TGplPTH$_{1-34}$ was safe to use in sheep, since no signs of inflammation were detected and fast biomaterial degradation took place. All treatment groups were more effective than the sham control. Among these, the medium concentration of TGplPTH$_{1-34}$ induced the best bone enhancing effect. Whether this effect would also be elicited in osteoporotic bone in humans is speculative at this point. Due to the absence of a true osteoporotic large animal model, this could only be verified in a clinical trial study in humans.

Acknowledgments

The authors thank their industrial partners for financing the study.

Author Contributions

K.Kl. was the Ph.D. student and involved in all aspects of the study, including writing the manuscript. J.S. was involved in developing the biomaterial. P.W.K. was the anesthetist and was involved in demonstrating embolization. N.F. was the anesthetist and was involved in demonstrating embolization. K.K. performed histology and was involved in developing bone sampling. M.M. was the radiologist and performed all CT including evaluation. T.S. designed the device and was involved in all aspects of the study. B.R. was the head of the experiment, supervisor of the Ph.D. program and was involved in all aspects of the study.

Disclosure

The study was financed by our industrial partner, Kuros Biosurgery AG, Technoparkstrasse 1, 8005 Zurich, Switzerland.

Conflicts of Interest

The authors declare no conflict of interest.

References and Notes

1. Rapado, A. General management of vertebral fractures. *Bone* **1996**, *18*, 191S–196S.
2. Old, J.L.; Calvert, M. Vertebral compression fractures in the elderly. *Am. Fam. Phys.* **2004**, *69*, 111–116.
3. Lewis, G. Percutaneous vertebroplasty and kyphoplasty for the stand-alone augmentation of osteoporosis-induced vertebral compression fractures: Present status and future directions. *J. Biomed. Mater. Res. B Appl. Biomater.* **2007**, *81*, 371–386.

4. Lavelle, W.; Carl, A.; Lavelle, E.D.; Khaleel, M.A. Vertebroplasty and kyphoplasty. *Anesthesiol. Clin.* **2007**, *25*, 913–928.
5. Hulme, P.A.; Krebs, J.; Ferguson, S.J.; Berlemann, U. Vertebroplasty and kyphoplasty: A systematic review of 69 clinical studies. *Spine (Phila Pa 1976)* **2006**, *31*, 1983–2001.
6. Predey, T.A.; Sewall, L.E.; Smith, S.J. Percutaneous vertebroplasty: New treatment for vertebral compression fractures. *Am. Fam. Phys.* **2002**, *66*, 611–615.
7. Silverman, S.L. The clinical consequences of vertebral compression fracture. *Bone* **1992**, *13* (Suppl 2), S27–S31.
8. Garfin, S.R.; Yuan, H.A.; Reiley, M.A. New technologies in spine: Kyphoplasty and vertebroplasty for the treatment of painful osteoporotic compression fractures. *Spine (Phila Pa 1976)* **2001**, *26*, 1511–1515.
9. Lemke, D.M. Vertebroplasty and kyphoplasty for treatment of painful osteoporotic compression fractures. *J. Am. Acad. Nurse Pract.* **2005**, *17*, 268–276.
10. Phillips, F.M.; Todd Wetzel, F.; Lieberman, I.; Campbell-Hupp, M. An *in vivo* comparison of the potential for extravertebral cement leak after vertebroplasty and kyphoplasty. *Spine (Phila Pa 1976)* **2002**, *27*, 2173–2178; discussion 2178–2179.
11. Jensen, M.E.; Evans, A.J.; Mathis, J.M.; Kallmes, D.F.; Cloft, H.J.; Dion, J.E. Percutaneous polymethylmethacrylate vertebroplasty in the treatment of osteoporotic vertebral body compression fractures: Technical aspects. *AJNR Am. J. Neuroradiol.* **1997**, *18*, 1897–1904.
12. Cotten, A.; Boutry, N.; Cortet, B.; Assaker, R.; Demondion, X.; Leblond, D.; Chastanet, P.; Duquesnoy, B.; Deramond, H. Percutaneous vertebroplasty: State of the art. *Radiographics* **1998**, *18*, 311–320; discussion 320–323.
13. Frankel, B.M.; Monroe, T.; Wang, C. Percutaneous vertebral augmentation: An elevation in adjacent-level fracture risk in kyphoplasty as compared with vertebroplasty. *Spine J.* **2007**, *7*, 575–582.
14. Nardi, A.; Tarantino, U.; Ventura, L.; Armotti, P.; Resmini, G.; Cozzi, L.; Tonini, G.; Ramazzina, E.; Rossini, M. Domino effect: Mechanic factors role. *Clin. Cases Miner. Bone Metab.* **2011**, *8*, 38–42.
15. Poole, K.E.; Reeve, J. Parathyroid hormone—A bone anabolic and catabolic agent. *Curr. Opin. Pharmacol.* **2005**, *5*, 612–617.
16. Carter, P.H.; Schipani, E. The roles of parathyroid hormone and calcitonin in bone remodeling: Prospects for novel therapeutics. *Endocr. Metab. Immune Disord. Drug Targets* **2006**, *6*, 59–76.
17. Pfeilschifter, J.; Laukhuf, F.; Muller-Beckmann, B.; Blum, W.F.; Pfister, T.; Ziegler, R. Parathyroid hormone increases the concentration of insulin-like growth factor-i and transforming growth factor beta 1 in rat bone. *J. Clin. Investig.* **1995**, *96*, 767–774.
18. Whitfield, J.F. Osteoporosis-treating parathyroid hormone peptides: What are they? What do they do? How might they do it? *Curr. Opin. Investig. Drugs* **2006**, *7*, 349–359.
19. Arrighi, I.; Mark, S.; Alvisi, M.; von Rechenberg, B.; Hubbell, J.A.; Schense, J.C. Bone healing induced by local delivery of an engineered parathyroid hormone prodrug. *Biomaterials* **2009**, *30*, 1763–1771.

20. Klein, K.; Zamparo, E.; Kronen, P.W.; Kampf, K.; Makara, M.; Steffen, T.; von Rechenberg, B. Bone augmentation for cancellous bone—Development of a new animal model. *BMC Musculoskelet. Disord.* **2013**, *14*, 200.
21. Ammann, P. Strontium ranelate: A physiological approach for an improved bone quality. *Bone* **2006**, *38*, 15–18.
22. Marie, P.J. Strontium ranelate: A physiological approach for optimizing bone formation and resorption. *Bone* **2006**, *38*, S10–S14.
23. Brown, E.M. Is the calcium receptor a molecular target for the actions of strontium on bone? *Osteoporos. Int.* **2003**, *14* (Suppl 3), S25–S34.
24. Hurtel-Lemaire, A.S.; Mentaverri, R.; Caudrillier, A.; Cournarie, F.; Wattel, A.; Kamel, S.; Terwilliger, E.F.; Brown, E.M.; Brazier, M. The calcium-sensing receptor is involved in strontium ranelate-induced osteoclast apoptosis. New insights into the associated signaling pathways. *J. Biol. Chem.* **2009**, *284*, 575–584.
25. Yang, F.; Yang, D.; Tu, J.; Zheng, Q.; Cai, L.; Wang, L. Strontium enhances osteogenic differentiation of mesenchymal stem cells and *in vivo* bone formation by activating wnt/catenin signaling. *Stem Cells* **2011**, *29*, 981–991.
26. Benneker, L.M.; Gisep, A.; Krebs, J.; Boger, A.; Heini, P.F.; Boner, V. Development of an *in vivo* experimental model for percutaneous vertebroplasty in sheep. *Vet. Comp. Orthop. Traumatol.* **2012**, *25*, 173–177.
27. Krebs, J.; Ferguson, S.J.; Hoerstrup, S.P.; Goss, B.G.; Haeberli, A.; Aebli, N. Influence of bone marrow fat embolism on coagulation activation in an ovine model of vertebroplasty. *J. Bone Joint Surg. Am.* **2008**, *90*, 349–356.
28. Krebs, J.; Ferguson, S.J.; Nuss, K.; Leskosek, B.; Hoerstrup, S.P.; Goss, B.G.; Shaw, S.; Aebli, N. Plasma levels of endothelin-1 after a pulmonary embolism of bone marrow fat. *Acta Anaesthesiol. Scand.* **2007**, *51*, 1107–1114.
29. Aebli, N.; Krebs, J.; Schwenke, D.; Davis, G.; Theis, J.C. Cardiovascular changes during multiple vertebroplasty with and without vent-hole: An experimental study in sheep. *Spine (Phila Pa 1976)* **2003**, *28*, 1504–1511; discussion 1511–1512.
30. Boger, A.; Benneker, L.M.; Krebs, J.; Boner, V.; Heini, P.F.; Gisep, A. The effect of pulsed jet lavage in vertebroplasty on injection forces of pmma bone cement: An animal study. *Eur. Spine J.* **2009**, *18*, 1957–1962.
31. Measurements are not in the content of this paper and will be published elsewhere.
32. Data not shown here.
33. Robling, A.G.; Kedlaya, R.; Ellis, S.N.; Childress, P.J.; Bidwell, J.P.; Bellido, T.; Turner, C.H. Anabolic and catabolic regimens of human parathyroid hormone 1-34 elicit bone- and envelope-specific attenuation of skeletal effects in sost-deficient mice. *Endocrinology* **2011**, *152*, 2963–2975.

12

Optimizing the Measurement of Colostrum Antibody Concentrations for Identifying BVDV Persistently Infected Calves

Caitlin J. Jenvey *, Michael P. Reichel, Sasha R. Lanyon and Peter D. Cockcroft

School of Animal and Veterinary Sciences, The University of Adelaide, Roseworthy Campus, Roseworthy, SA 5371, Australia; E-Mails: michael.reichel@adeliade.edu.au (M.P.R.); sasha.lanyon@adelaide.edu.au (S.R.L.); peter.cockcroft@adelaide.edu.au (P.D.C.)

* Author to whom correspondence should be addressed; E-Mail: caitlin.jenvey@adelaide.edu.au;

Academic Editors: Duncan C. Ferguson and Margarethe Hoenig

Abstract: Colostrum contains substantially higher concentrations of immunoglobulins compared to serum, which may help to improve the utility of diagnostic tests. The aim of this study was to determine the diagnostic value of colostrum antibody concentrations in identifying Bovine Viral Diarrhoea Virus (BVDV) PI (persistently infected) calf carrying beef heifers following an experimental infection. Colostrum was collected within 12 hours of parturition and tested in undiluted, 1:5, 1:10, 1:100, 1:200, and 1:500 dilutions using an enzyme-linked immunosorbent assay (ELISA) for BVDV antibody. Cows were determined to be carrying a PI calf based on positive quantitative Real Time-Polymerase Chain Reaction and antigen ELISA result on pre-colostral serum and ear notch samples collected from their calf. The median ELISA sample-to-positive (S/P) ratio for colostrum collected from heifers that carried a PI calf were significantly higher than the median ELISA S/P ratio for colostrum collected from heifers that did not carry a PI calf at dilutions of 1:100, 1:200, and 1:500. This study provides further evidence for increased antigenic stimulation *in utero* by the BVDV viraemic PI calf, which can also be identified with 100% diagnostic sensitivity when using 1:500 dilution colostrum.

Keywords: BVDV; colostrum; ELISA; PI calves

---

1. Introduction

Colostrum contains high concentrations of maternal antibodies that are selectively transferred into the mammary gland from the serum of the dam prior to calving. Concentrations of antibodies in bovine colostrum can be up to five [1] to 10 times [2] greater when compared to serum. Due to these high antibody concentrations, colostrum could improve the utility of diagnostic tests by increasing the magnitude of detectable differences between cohorts of individual animals, including, but not limited to, cows infected with Bovine Viral Diarrhoea Virus (BVDV). Dams that are infected with BVDV between 40 and 120 days of gestation may produce persistently infected (PI) offspring that test negative for BVDV-specific antibodies [3]. These PI animals are important reservoirs of infection due to their high persistent levels of viral excretion and infectivity for susceptible cattle [4]. There is evidence to suggest that the BVDV antibody concentration of dams carrying PI calves are elevated during late gestation when compared to previously infected dams carrying non-PI calves [5–7], but this difference has not been convincing enough to be utilised in practice (early detection of PI calves). These studies found that, on average, the antibody levels of cows carrying PI calves and cows not carrying PI calves tended to overlap, and although samples should be collected in the last few months of gestation, there is larger variation in antibody levels between these two groups at parturition compared with early pregnancy [5–7]. There is little research into whether this increase in BVD specific antibody concentrations may also be found in colostrum collected from dams carrying PI calves. It is possible that concentrations found in colostrum may be quantitatively greater compared to serum, thus also allowing identification of the PI-carrying dam using colostrum. The aim of this study was to determine the diagnostic value of colostrum BVDV antibody concentrations in identifying PI calves following an experimental infection of a group of beef heifers.

2. Methods

2.1. Heifers

Twelve beef heifers were experimentally infected with BVDV-type 1c by co-mingling with a PI dairy cow from day 90, post artificial insemination [8]. All cows seroconverted within 28 days of exposure (antibody enzyme-linked immunosorbent assay), at which time the PI cow was removed from further direct or indirect contact with the heifers. Heifers were determined to have been carrying a PI calf based on positive quantitative real-time polymerase chain reaction and antigen ELISA result on serum and ear notch samples collected from their calf prior to colostrum ingestion.

2.2. Antibody ELISA

Colostrum was collected within 12 hours of calving and stored at −80 °C until testing could be performed. The colostrum samples were tested as undiluted samples, as well as at dilutions of 1:5, 1:10, 1:100, 1:200, and 1:500. Samples were diluted using the diluent supplied with the ELISA kit and tested in triplicate using the IDEXX BVDV Total Ab Test. Results were expressed as sample-to-positive (S/P) ratios.

2.3. Statistical Analysis

A Mann-Whitney U test was performed to identify significant differences between colostrum from heifers carrying PI calves and heifers that did not carry PI calves at each dilution, with a p-value < 0.01 considered significant. A two-graph receiver operating characteristic analysis (TG-ROC) was performed to determine DSe, DSp, and 95% confidence interval (CI) of the antibody ELISA for the detection of a PI calf for each dilution, or no dilution. The diagnostic sensitivity (DSe) and diagnostic specificity (DSp) were calculated using the following equations:

$$\text{DSe} = \frac{\text{Number of heifers carrying PI calves that tested ELISA positive}}{\text{Number of heifers carrying PI calves}} \times 100 \quad (1)$$

$$\text{DSp} = \frac{\text{Number of heifers carying non-PI calves that tested ELISA negative}}{\text{Number of heifers carrying non-PI calves}} \times 100 \quad (2)$$

3. Results

Of the twelve beef heifers that were experimentally infected, the calves of three heifers tested virus positive by RT-PCR and antigen positive by ELISA in their serum prior to colostrum ingestion. The calves from the remaining eight heifers tested virus negative and antigen negative and one heifer aborted her fetus 253 days post-AI. The median ELISA S/P ratio for colostrum collected from heifers carrying a PI calf were significantly higher compared to colostrum collected from heifers that were not carrying a PI calf for dilutions of 1:100 ($p < 0.05$), 1:200 ($p < 0.01$), and 1:500 ($p < 0.01$) (Table 1). For undiluted and 1:5 diluted colostrum, the median ELISA S/P ratio for colostrum samples collected from heifers carrying and not carrying PI calves did not differ significantly (Table 1).

Table 1. Median (Range) optical density value for colostrum collected from cows carrying and not carrying PI calves for dilutions of 0, 1:5, 1:100, 1:200, and 1:500.

Dilution	Heifers carrying PI calf	Heifers not carrying PI calf
0	2.08 (1.56–2.13) [a]	2.22 (1.63–2.52) [a]
1:5	2.55 (2.58–2.51) [b]	2.55 (2.38–2.66) [b]
1:100	2.21 (2.31–2.15) [c]	1.81 (1.14–2.19) [d]
1:200	1.98 (2.07–1.89) [e]	1.50 (0.85–1.85) [f]
1:500	1.81 (1.83–1.67) [g]	1.00 (0.37–1.60) [h]

[a] Different superscript letters in the same row are statistically different (Mann-Whitney U Test).

The TG-ROC for DSe and DSp for each dilution are shown in Figure 1. The value of the DSe and DSp at the intercept increased with the dilution of the sample, reaching 100% at a colostrum dilution of 1:500. The DSe, DSp, and S/P threshold at the intercept for each dilution were: 33% at an S/P ratio threshold of 2.10 for undiluted colostrum (Figure 1a), 56% at a 1:5 dilution colostrum at an S/P ratio threshold of 2.60 (Figure 1b), 93.9% at a 1:100 dilution colostrum at an S/P ratio threshold of 2.20 (Figure 1c), 93.9% at a 1:200 dilution colostrum at an S/P ratio threshold of 1.90 (Figure 1d), and 100% at a 1:500 dilution colostrum at an S/P ratio threshold of 1.65 (Figure 1e).

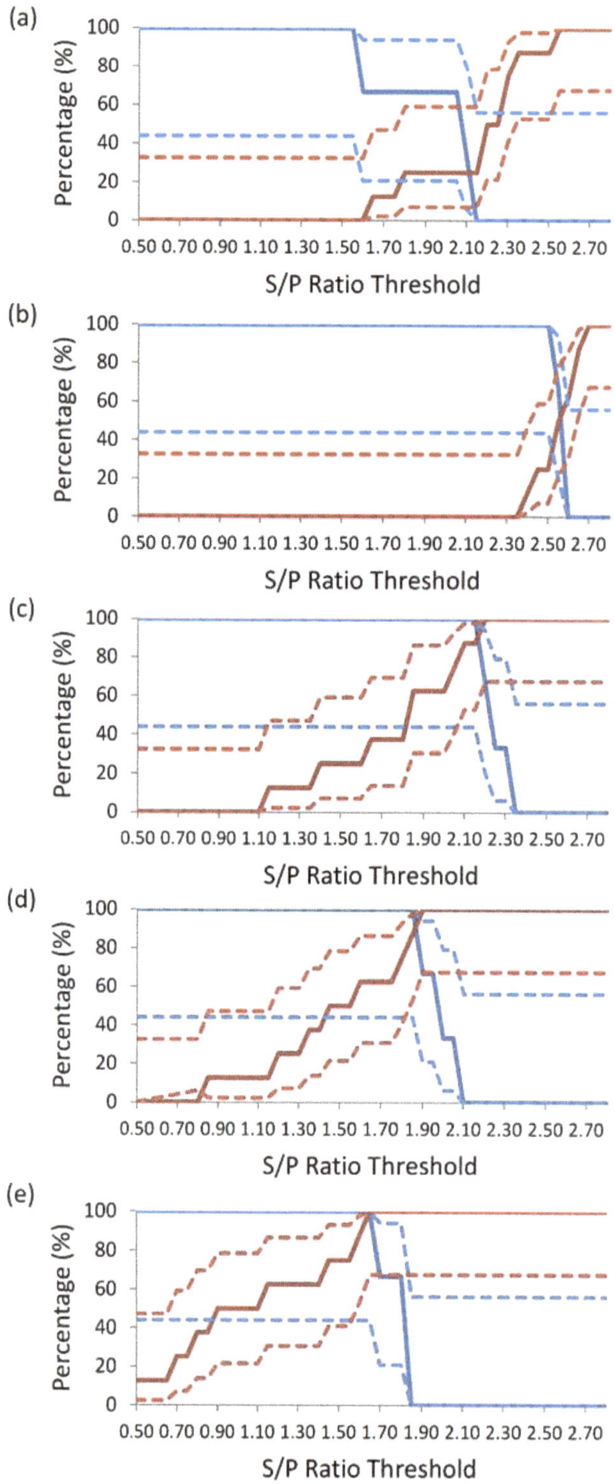

Figure 1. Two-graph receiver operating characteristic analysis of (**a**) undiluted colostrum, (**b**) 1:5 dilution colostrum, (**c**) 1:100 dilution colostrum, (**d**) 1:200 dilution colostrum, and (**e**) 1:500 dilution colostrum, using a commercial enzyme-linked immunosorbent assay for the detection of antibodies specific to BVDV. Diagnostic sensitivity (solid blue line) ± 95 percent confidence interval (dotted blue line) was calculated using sample-to-positive (S/P) ratio results for colostrum collected from heifers carrying PI calves (n = 3) and diagnostic specificity (red line) ± 95 per cent confidence interval (dotted red line) was calculated using S/P ratio results for colostrum collected from heifers carrying non-PI calves (n = 8).

4. Discussion

The purpose of this study was to determine the diagnostic value of colostrum BVDV antibody concentrations in identifying PI calves following an experimental infection of beef heifers. Previous studies [5–7] have demonstrated higher BVDV antibody concentrations in serum collected from seropositive cows carrying PI calves when compared to cows that do not carry a PI calf. However, there is little research into whether this same claim can be made with regards to colostrum samples. These previous studies also demonstrated some overlapping of antibody levels from cows that carried a PI calf and cows that did not carry a PI calf [5–7]. This result was also demonstrated in this study as no significant differences were observed in the median ELISA S/P ratios for heifers that carried a PI calf and heifers that did not carry a PI calf when colostrum was tested undiluted or diluted 1:5. However, the median ELISA S/P ratio for colostrum collected from heifers that carried a PI calf were significantly higher compared to the median ELISA S/P ratio for colostrum collected from heifers that did not carry a PI calf for dilutions of 1:100, 1:200 and 1:500. In addition, DSe and DSp of the ELISA was 100% when using colostrum diluted at 1:500. The results of this study indicate that colostrum, when diluted at 1:500, could be used to identify PI calves immediately following calving. It is possible that further dilution of the serum collected in these previous studies (1:10 [6] and 1:100 [6,7]) may have further increased the differences in antibody levels observed between cows that carried a PI calf and cows that did not carry a PI calf, thus, reducing the overlapping of antibody levels observed between the two groups.

This study provides further evidence for increased antigenic stimulation *in utero* by the BVDV viraemic PI calf. This study does not make any recommendations regarding the replacement of other PI detection methods with colostrum antibody testing, but rather, this study highlights the fact that colostrum can be used for PI calf detection and may be used in conjunction with other methods of detection.

5. Conclusions

The improvement in DSe observed in this study when colostrum was diluted, highlights the ability to improve the diagnostic utility of a test when disease-specific antibody concentrations (*i.e.*, BVDV antibody concentrations) supersede the ability of the ELISA to measure beyond the maximal S/P threshold. Additionally, colostrum may also benefit tests that demonstrate poor test characteristics, such as the poor diagnostic sensitivity experienced when testing for Johne's disease. This approach, while tested here in beef heifers, could most readily be applied in dairy cows, where colostrum is routinely and easily collected by the producer.

Acknowledgements

The author's would like to thank the Roseworthy Campus farm staff and Brenden Johansson for their assistance, as well as Rosemary Santangelo of IDEXX Laboratories for the supply of the ELISA kits used in this study.

Author Contributions

Caitlin J. Jenvey is a PhD candidate from the University of Adelaide and was involved in sample collection, data analysis and writing the manuscript. Michael P. Reichel and Sasha R. Lanyon designed the experimental plan and assisted with data analysis and manuscript editing. Peter D. Cockcroft was the primary supervisor and assisted with data analysis and manuscript editing.

Conflicts of Interest

The authors declare no conflict of interest.

References

1. Beer, A.; Billingham, R.; Head, J. The immunologic significance of the mammary gland. *J. Investig. Dermatol.* **1974**, *63*, 65–74.
2. Baurucker, C.; Burkett, A.; Magliaro-Macrina, A.; Dechow, C. Colostrogenesis: Mass transfer of immunoglobulin G1 into colostrum. *J. Dairy Sci.* **2010**, *93*, 3031–3038.
3. Grooms, D. Reproductive consequences of infection with bovine viral diarrhoea virus. *Vet. Clin. North Am. Food Anim. Pract.* **2004**, *20*, 5–19.
4. Lindberg, A.; Alenius, S. Principles for eradication of bovine viral diarrhoea virus (BVDV) infections in cattle populations. *Vet. Microbiol.* **1999**, *64*, 197–222.
5. Brownlie, J.; Hooper, L.; Thompson, I.; Collins, M. Maternal recognition of foeatl infection with bovine virus diarrhoea virus (BVDV)—The bovine pestivirus. *Clin. Diagn. Virol.* **1998**, *10*, 141–150.
6. Lindberg, A.; Niskanen, R.; Gustafsson, H.; Bengtsson, B.; Baule, C.; Belak, S.; Alenius, S. Prenatal diagnosis of persistent Bovine Viral Diarrhoea Virus (BVDV) infection by detection of viral RNA in fetal fluids. *Vet. J.* **2001**, *164*, 151–155.
7. Stokstad, M.; Niskanen, R.; Lindberg, A.; Thoren, P.; Belak, S.; Alenius, S.; Loken, T. Experimental infection of cows with Bovine Viral Diarrhoea Virus in early pregnancy—Findings in serum and foetal fluids. *J. Vet. Med. Series B* **2003**, *50*, 424–429.
8. Lanyon, S.; Sims, S.; Cockcroft, P.; Reichel, M. Comparison of serum, ear notches, and nasal and salival swabs for Bovine Viral Diarrhoea Virus antigen detection in colostrum-fed persistently infected (PI) calves and non-PI calves. *J. Vet. Diagn. Investig.* **2014**, *26*, 783–787.

13

Governance and One Health: Exploring the Impact of Federalism and Bureaucracy on Zoonotic Disease Detection and Reporting

Heather A. Allen

Center for Food Security and Public Health, College of Veterinary Medicine, Iowa State University, Ames, IA 50011, USA; E-Mail: hallen@iastate.edu;

Academic Editors: Duncan C. Ferguson and Margarethe Hoenig

Abstract: The merits of One Health have been thoroughly described in the literature, but how One Health operates in the United States federal system of government is rarely discussed or analyzed. Through a comparative case-study approach, this research explores how federalism, bureaucratic behavior, and institutional design in the United States may influence zoonotic disease outbreak detection and reporting, a key One Health activity. Using theoretical and empirical literature, as well as a survey/interview instrument for individuals directly involved in a past zoonotic disease outbreak, the impacts of governance are discussed. As predicted in the theoretical literature, empirical findings suggest that federalism, institutional design, and bureaucracy may play a role in facilitating or impeding zoonotic disease outbreak detection and reporting. Regulatory differences across states as well as compartmentalization of information within agencies may impede disease detection. However, the impact may not always be negative: bureaucracies can also be adaptive; federalism allows states important opportunities for innovation. While acknowledging there are many other factors that also matter in zoonotic disease detection and reporting, this research is one of the first attempts to raise awareness in the literature and stimulate discussion on the intersection of governance and One Health.

Keywords: federalism; One Health; public health; animal health; disease reporting; disease detection; zoonoses; institutions; governance

---

1. Introduction

Beginning with Calvin Schwabe, the merits of a One Health approach have been thoroughly described for over three decades [1,2]. In the United States, the government has the duty, obligation, and authority to protect environmental health, public health, as well as animal health [3,4]. However, little has been written on how the U.S. system of governance impacts One Health. This research uses zoonotic disease detection and reporting in the United States to examine to what extent federalism, bureaucratic behavior, and design of U.S. institutions may impact this key set of One Health activities.

Zoonotic disease detection and reporting is critical to One Health; over half of all pathogens known to infect humans are zoonotic and an estimated 75 percent of emerging infectious diseases are zoonotic [5]. Yet, animal and human disease surveillance, detection, and reporting activities in the United States are fragmented, both practically and politically. There are disconnects between the animal health and public health sectors, as well as a myriad of state and federal surveillance systems [6]. The National Strategy for Countering Biological Threats specifically called for improving "coordination between human, plant, and veterinary disease reporting systems" [7] (p. 6) and "fostering information sharing" [7] (p. 12) between different government sectors. A delay in the detection and reporting of a zoonotic disease outbreak can have significant implications for public health and animal health [8]. While quantitative research has been conducted to analyze timeliness in disease detection and reporting [9,10], this research uses a qualitative approach to frame One Health in the context of the U.S. system of governance, exploring the complexities of zoonotic disease detection in the United States.

To start, it is necessary to describe the U.S. system of governance, including theories of bureaucratic behavior and federalism, focusing on potential impacts to zoonotic disease detection. Next, a comparative case study provides further information based on data collected from publicly available literature and a survey/interview instrument. Four zoonotic disease outbreaks from 2000–2006 are selected for further analysis, based on the speed in which they were detected. Then, the factors impeding or facilitating detection are carefully reviewed to describe how or to what extent federalism, institutional design, and bureaucratic behavior may facilitate or impede rapid zoonotic disease detection and reporting. Ultimately, this research (1) provides information to raise awareness regarding the complexity of disease detection and reporting in a federal system and (2) stimulates further discussion and future research on the significant gap in the literature at the intersection of One Health and public policy and administration.

2. U.S. System of Governance & One Health

Many theories regarding both federalism and bureaucracy have been written; this section merely summarizes key points with direct application to zoonotic disease detection and reporting and ultimately One Health.

2.1. Definitions

For the purpose of this paper, zoonotic disease detection and reporting are discussed together, acknowledging they are independent terms/activities, both distinctly important to disease surveillance and response. Detection typically refers to the initial recognition of the disease or a disease outbreak [11]; reporting refers to an individual—regardless of position—reporting this case or outbreak to a regulatory authority at the local, state, or federal level. In theory, if a disease is detected it should be reported (per applicable state and federal regulation), though this is not always the case [12]. Indeed, the detector of the disease and the reporter may be the same entity: for example, both public health and animal health laboratories may detect an outbreak and message these results to a government agency. These two connected but separate activities are discussed in tandem here, as response to an outbreak relies on both detection and reporting.

2.2. Federalism

Federalism is the division or separation of powers between the U.S. federal government and state governments. It is specifically granted in the 10th Amendment to the U.S. Constitution: "The powers not delegated to the United States by the Constitution, nor prohibited by it to the States, are reserved to the States respectively, or to the people" [13]. Federalism was a critical reaction by the framers of the U.S. Constitution to the strong central power in England [14].

On the federal side, "federal public health powers flow from the U.S. constitution" [3] (p. 79). Both the Animal Health Protection Act (7 U.S.C. 8301 *et seq.*) and Public Health Services Act (42 U.S.C. 201) broadly define the authority for the federal government to act on matters of disease and disease transmission in animals and people, respectively. However, these powers are also limited by the 10th Amendment. While there are definitely federal actions related to zoonotic disease detection and reporting, historically the authority over these activities falls to the states.

In particular, states are reserved what are known as police powers [3]. It is these police powers which enable state governments to legally conduct public health infectious disease surveillance within a population of individuals [15]. It is also through these powers that states can and do mandate disease reporting within the state from laboratories, physicians, and sometimes other entities or individuals [3,16]. Typically, disease reporting in states occurs in two executive agency pipelines—one for animal diseases to animal health/agriculture departments, and one for human diseases to public health/human services departments. While state to federal disease reporting is generally voluntary (from a purely regulatory perspective), federally accredited veterinarians and others do have the obligation to report specific animal diseases to the federal government [16].

While discussing the merits of different political science theories could fill a book, it is useful to note several positions. Some argue we are in an era of competitive federalism, where states and the federal government compete over various domestic policy areas [17]. In general, the enumerated powers of the federal government have been widely interpreted by the Supreme Court [3]. Moreover, it is possible that federal authority could be much more expansive on issues of disease surveillance and reporting if there was the desire (or perhaps necessity) to act [18]. However, the federal government has historically been the provider of mere performance standards to encourage consistency across state disease surveillance and reporting activities.

2.3. Bureaucratic Behavior & Institutional Design

Similarly, there is extensive literature on the role of institutional design in policy-making and intergovernmental relations, for example [19,20]. Because zoonotic disease detection and reporting is largely an executive-branch activity, the most important aspect is the behavior of these executive agencies. At both the state and the federal level, policy responsibilities are dispersed amongst executive agencies, sometimes with functions that broadly overlap. For example, different agencies may each have infectious disease surveillance systems for various populations or diseases. Human health and animal health issues are delegated to separate agencies. Often, wildlife disease issues are in yet another agency/entity. At the federal level in the United States, just to provide an example of the many agencies involved in zoonotic disease detection, the U.S. Department of Health and Human Services, U.S. Department of Agriculture, U.S. Department of Homeland Security, U.S. Department of Defense, and U.S. Department of the Interior all play some role in the surveillance and detection of zoonotic diseases (and this list is certainly not all inclusive) [21].

However, executive agencies are not designed—nor do they function—equally: some receive significantly more support (financial and/or political) than others, based on their area of authority and jurisdiction. Indeed, human health agencies at the state and federal level are typically significantly better funded than agencies devoted to the policy areas of agriculture or wildlife [22,23]. Additionally, some executive agencies are significantly more influenced by the stakeholders they serve than are others. A popular hypothesis of bureaucratic behavior is that agencies constantly seek greater autonomy and authority *vis-à-vis* other agencies [24,25]. This type of behavior can lead to a lack of cooperation, or at the least, little enthusiasm for shared tasks between agencies, even with regard for a common goal. Practically, this may result in a critical lack of information sharing or communication between executive agencies, at both a state and a federal level. However, there are also theories which suggest that this battle for power is not fully explanatory: agencies act in specific ways for many different reasons, including the organizational culture, resources at hand, leadership, and reputation. Regardless of which theory one might subscribe to, it is clear that bureaucratic behavior that results from the design of our institutions may foster impediments to effective coordination and communication.

2.4. Potential Implications of Federalism, Bureaucratic Behavior, and Institutional Design for One Health

With regard to federalism, there are two primary issues which arise as concerns for the practice of zoonotic disease detection and reporting. First, because these powers are reserved for the states, the federal government does not have direct power—or has not typically exercised direct power—over how they are exercised. Second, when powers are reserved for the states, each state can, and does, choose to exercise these powers in various manners. Indeed, these issues are plainly observed by the widely varying requirements and capabilities for zoonotic disease detection and reporting in each state [12,16].

Bureaucracy and institutional design also may have important implications for One Health, specifically zoonotic disease detection and reporting. In particular, executive agencies are designed to often have overlapping responsibilities. Furthermore, they are often poor coordinators and cooperators. Due to the competing nature of executive agencies, for funding, influence, or authority, knowledge about specific disease cases can be compartmentalized, rather than shared between practitioners or officials at various levels; state or federal executive agencies may not cooperate or coordinate effectively on detection and reporting efforts [26].

Now that the stage has been set regarding how federalism and bureaucratic behavior may influence zoonotic disease detection and reporting, the research that follows works to unravel whether these potential implications are supported by empirical evidence.

3. Methods

A qualitative case study approach is employed, using a comparative case study as described in [27]. This research was accepted as exempt by The George Washington University Institutional Review Board, #0011107. A case study approach is not appropriate to examine "the prevalence of phenomena"; it is intended to provide a detailed description of how and why [27] (p. 10). This method uses a set of individual outbreaks to explore any impact of the U.S. system of governance on zoonotic disease detection and reporting.

3.1. Cases

The unit of analysis—or case—is a zoonotic disease outbreak. From prior research [28], the most rapidly detected outbreaks and the least rapidly detected outbreaks are identified. More than one type of each case is preferred [27], so two cases are identified from each group. In addition to being an outlier, each case also required existing, published literature regarding its detection, reporting, and/or response. With these criteria, the slowest outliers (least rapidly detected) are two salmonella outbreaks, one in 2006–2007 and one in 2003–2004. The two fastest outliers (most rapidly detected) are a case of rabies in 2006, and a case of anthrax in 2000. For simplicity, these are sometimes referred to as "slow" and "fast" outbreaks or cases, with the clear acknowledgment this is time to detection not speed of disease spread.

3.2. Data Sources

There are three key sources of information for this case study: publicly available literature specifically on the cases, the survey instrument/interviews, and theories of governance (discussed above). For each case, an open-source literature review was conducted, followed by a structured interview/survey for additional information. The information and evidence from these data sources were integrated, subsequently embedding qualitative results in a theoretical context.

3.3. Interview/Survey

Subjects were contacted by email and provided details on the research and an informed consent form. The subjects were identified from published articles and professional references (with express permission of the individual being contacted), and included practitioners, state officials, diagnostic laboratory personnel, and federal officials. Both animal health and public health subjects participated. Initially all potential respondents were involved in the fast and slow outlier cases. However, to improve sample size, the population was expanded to those who had specific experience responding to one of the zoonotic disease outbreaks identified in [28]. These participants were referred by other respondents.

Both structured interviews and a survey instrument were employed. The questions were the same whether the interview was conducted orally or the respondent replied to an online survey. This option was provided to offer individuals flexibility and improve the response rate. Respondents were asked about the factors they thought improved or impeded zoonotic disease outbreak detection and reporting in the specific zoonotic disease outbreak (case). They were also asked about the interaction between the animal health and human health sector and explicitly about whether federalism and institutional design impacted zoonotic disease detection and reporting. All questions were open-ended.

All responses were analyzed using frequency counts; thematic analysis was also conducted to identify key concepts. Survey responses were anonymous; interviews were not recorded. Most subjects offered information that would be considered identifying to others in the field. As such, all data was de-identified and aggregated, removing references to specific events or locations.

3.4. Limitations

There are limitations to the external validity and generalizability of case study results [5], particularly with regard to the small sample size of survey/interview respondents. Any inferences drawn from differences between the groups of respondents (outbreaks detected quickly, slowly, and other) should be considered with caution, given small sample sizes. Indeed, these case studies may not be generalizable to all zoonotic disease outbreaks: each outbreak is unique. Additionally, due to confidentiality concerns, detailed information cannot be provided on specific aspects of each outbreak. Finally, this analysis may not be generalizable to other systems of governance—particularly those that are not federalized.

4. Results and Discussion

4.1. Literature Review of Cases

In terms of the two slow cases, the first outbreak affected only humans; both humans and domestic pets (such as hamsters and mice) were affected during the second outbreak. The literature highlighted that both were foodborne infectious that were ultimately identified through PulseNet, a system operated by the Centers for Disease Control and Prevention which uses DNA information to detect outbreaks [29]. The pulsed-field gel electrophoresis (PFGE) subtyping allowed astute epidemiologists to identify an increase in specific strains of Salmonella in PulseNet. However, there was a significant lag between the first symptoms and PulseNet analysis to detect the outbreak. In large part, this is due to the fact that cases—initially not thought to be related—were later linked to the outbreak through retrospective analysis of PFGE patterns in PulseNet.

Both slow cases involved many states—as many as 21 in one outbreak [30]. States were geographically dispersed, such as cases in both Minnesota and South Carolina [31]. The literature indicates the detection of the outbreak was impeded by the extent to which the cases were "dispersed temporally and geographically" [32]. Additionally, Salmonellosis typically has low fatality rates in humans, though many rodents died in one of the two cases [31]. This may have contributed to the delay in detection. Ultimately, without the PFGE suptyping that was aggregated in PulseNet for further analysis, it is unlikely that either of these outbreaks would have been characterized or successfully investigated to a source.

In terms of the fast cases, the rapid onset of severe rabies symptoms probably aided in detection; additionally, the astute clinician rapidly identified confounding risk-factors for the disease [33]. Even though rabies is not frequently observed in the United States, unlike many tropical diseases, clinicians are frequently aware of clinical signs that may indicate rabies infection. The second fast case—like the second slow case—affected both humans and animals, in this case, livestock. This outbreak affected areas historically unaffected by anthrax, and resulted in a significant increase in anthrax cases in cattle [34]. Given the large outbreak and the patient's direct contact with dead cattle, the clinician rapidly gave a presumptive diagnosis of anthrax which was later confirmed in the laboratory. This was the first case of cutaneous anthrax in the United States for eight years [34], and preceded the 2001 attacks with *Bacillus anthracis.*

The literature provides important information which aids in describing the detection of these four cases. It is clear that consistent and multi-state use and access to PulseNet is critical for detection, and that the frontline providers are often key in making rapid detections. However, the literature does not provide much insight into whether federalism, bureaucratic behavior, or institutional design that may have impacted detection. As such, we turn now to the interview and survey which specifically explored these intersections.

4.2. Interview and Survey Results

Thirty individuals, with a direct role in detecting zoonotic disease outbreaks, were asked to participate in the research, with a response rate of 60 percent (n = 18). Of these respondents, eight were from the fastest cases to detection (44%), six from the slowest cases (33%), and four from other outbreaks (22%). Additionally, three individuals were not willing to participate in the research due to confidentiality concerns, or because they did not feel as if they could recall the events correctly. This response rate is typical of survey instruments [35]. Of these respondents, 50 percent completed the survey and 50 percent were interviewed by phone. While there is no doubt this is a small sample size, there are a limited number of individuals that have been directly involved in the detection of a zoonotic disease outbreak, and this sample represents a key number of those individuals.

Table 1 provides a breakdown of respondents by level of government and sector. Table 2 indicates role of respondent. Further disaggregation of these results is not possible due to confidentiality concerns.

Table 1. Response Information for Survey/Interview by Level of Government and Sector.

Sector/Level	Local	State	Federal	Total
Human Health	2	7	2	11
Animal Health	0	5	2	7
Total	2	12	4	18

Table 2. Role of Respondent.

Role	Total
Laboratory	3
Official/ Practitioner	15
Total	18

4.2.1. Impediments to and Facilitators of Detection

Respondents were specifically asked to identify impediments and facilitators to detecting zoonotic disease outbreaks, in order to ascertain whether issues of governance arose naturally. They were requested to answer with a specific outbreak in mind—either one of the slow or fast cases identified previously, or another outbreak as identified in their response. Table 3 lists the top three impediments identified; Table 4 lists the top three facilitators for each group of respondents (outbreaks detected slowly, outbreaks detected rapidly, and other outbreaks).

Table 3. Top Three Impediments for Zoonotic Disease Outbreak Detection and Reporting.

Impediment	Response Percentage (*n* = 18)	For Outbreaks Detected Rapidly (*n* = 8)	For Outbreaks Detected Slowly (*n* = 6)	For Other Outbreaks (*n* = 4)
Knowledge/obligation to report	44%	38%	17%	100%
Diagnostics	33%	50%	17%	25%
(tie) Astute, Aware, Educated Providers	22%	25%	33%	0%
(tie) Funding	22%	13%	33%	25%

Table 4. Top Three Facilitators for Zoonotic Disease Outbreak Detection and Reporting.

Facilitator	Response Percentage (*n* = 18)	For Outbreaks Detected Rapidly (*n* = 8)	For Outbreaks Detected Slowly (*n* = 6)	For Other Outbreaks (*n* = 4)
Diagnostics	44%	63%	50%	0%
Communication and Collaboration between Agencies and Practitioners/Laboratories	39%	50%	50%	0%
Astute, Aware, and Educated Providers	33%	25%	33%	50%

For impediments, respondents specifically mentioned the lack of knowledge regarding both federal and state reporting requirements and how to report diseases. Specific impediments included the lack of awareness amongst providers and practitioners about reporting requirements and law, resource or time burdens of reporting, and the pressure from clients (both on the veterinary and human side) not to report. For diagnostics, respondents primarily mentioned the need for and lack of rapid, cost-effective, sensitive, and specific diagnostic tests, particularly for diseases less commonly observed in the United States. A lack of electronic reporting was also noted as a gap. Respondents also cited the gap of awareness, education, and training amongst providers and practitioners regarding zoonotic disease threats, and the understaffed and under-resourced nature of many local and state departments which work to detect zoonotic disease outbreaks.

It is possible to note some differences between the groups of respondents. Those involved in "fast" outbreaks more frequently cited that a lack of knowledge regarding reporting requirements and diagnostics impeded rapid outbreak detection more than those who responded from "slow" outbreaks. Those involved in "slow" outbreaks spoke more often about a lack of astute and trained providers and funding issues. Given the criticality of diagnostics and electronic reporting in detecting the "slow" outbreaks, it is not surprising that this group of respondents did not cite this as a significant impediment to detection. Interestingly, all of the respondents involved in the "other" disease outbreaks cited that a lack of knowledge about disease reporting requirements impeded outbreak detection.

Diagnostics emerged at the top of the list for facilitators. Rapid, sensitive, and specific diagnostic testing was cited by both groups of respondents ("slow" and "fast" cases) as a key factor that facilitated outbreak detection and reporting. Interestingly, those responding from the "other" group did not mention diagnostics. Respondents from both the rapidly and slowly detected outbreaks frequently mentioned that communication and cross-agency cooperation, as well as collaboration between practitioners and laboratories facilitated detection. Just "picking up the phone to discuss" was often mentioned as a way to facilitate detection. Finally, astute and trained providers can be critically important to rapidly detecting and reporting outbreaks with the appropriate training and keen knowledge particularly on asking the right questions to capture suspected zoonotic disease exposures. However, it is interesting that the respondents for the rapidly detected outbreaks did not mention this more frequently, given the importance of this factor in the detection and reporting of those rapidly detected outbreaks.

4.2.2. Collaboration between Sectors

Next, respondents were specifically asked about the collaboration and coordination between animal health and human health agencies/entities in detecting the specific outbreak. This question resulted in some of the most diverse responses characterizing the relationship, from "miserable" to "contentious" to "we worked great together" and "there were and are no issues". Interestingly, nearly all respondents (89%) volunteered that they felt as if this issue varied dramatically by state.

The majority of respondents from both the human health side (63%) and animal health side (57%) reported that their working relationship between the two sectors was positive. Many provided concrete observations of bilateral press releases, publications, and outreach to ensure a consistent public message. Of those reporting a problem (n = 6), most were linked to outbreaks that were detected slowly (67%). Interestingly, the individuals noting problems between the two sectors focused on response to zoonotic disease incidents rather than detection to the incidents. Additionally, respondents stated problems with not working towards a common goal successfully and problems or barriers to effective information sharing.

4.2.3. Federalism

When explicitly asked about the role of federalism in zoonotic disease detection and reporting, only a single respondent suggested that federalism played a role. Interestingly, this respondent also noted that federal reporting requirements for specific diseases did impact detection and reporting. However, an additional three respondents noted that federalism was not important in detection or reporting, but was critically important in response; collaboration between state and federal agencies during the response phase was problematic. Though respondents did not recognize federalism as playing a role when questioned explicitly, four individuals did offer that individuals at the local level are not provided enough deference by state and federal officials, who must conduct their own investigations into the disease outbreak. Responses were equally distributed across the fast, slow, and other cases.

4.2.4. Institutional Design and Bureaucratic Behavior

In comparison to federalism, many more respondents (50 percent or $n = 9$) suggested that institutional design and bureaucratic behavior play a role in zoonotic disease detection and reporting. These nine respondents included respondents from the slow ($n = 3$), fast ($n = 4$), and other ($n = 2$) cases; or 50% of the respondents from each of these groups. Of these nine respondents, 44 percent ($n = 4$) noted that they felt that institutional design and bureaucracy was actually a positive factor; three others suggested it was negative, and two thought it was both positive and negative. In all, six of the nine respondents stated that institutional design and bureaucratic behavior could or did play a positive role; in their remarks, respondents cited their own state system as a "model" of a bureaucracy that was effective for practice. Regarding the potential negative influence of bureaucratic behavior on zoonotic disease detection, comments specifically focused on behavior and lack of coordination or communication amongst executive agencies, resulting in "siloes" and "misguided budget priorities".

4.2.5. Other Factors

Finally, respondents were asked if there were other factors, not yet discussed, that could improve U.S. zoonotic disease detection and reporting, based on their experience in the field. These responses were not broken out between the groups as respondents replied "in general" rather than with reference to a specific outbreak. Interestingly, 10 of the 18 respondents specifically cited interpersonal relationships: knowing the person on the other end of the phone, in a different sector, that they could speak to both officially and informally. Table 5 lists the other responses to this question.

Table 5. Top Three Improvements Suggested for Zoonotic Disease Detection and Reporting.

Improvement	Response Percentage ($n = 18$)
Interpersonal Relationships/Communication	67%
Education (Practitioner and Public)	22%
Resources	16%

Resources and education/training (which requires resources) are commonly discussed factors for improving zoonotic disease detection and reporting for example, [36]. While outside the scope of this research, it is unclear to what extent the outcome—faster disease detection, reporting, and ultimately response—is linked back to specific inputs. Given an era of fiscal uncertainty and tight budgets—particularly at the state and local level—it is important that resources be used as effectively as possible. However, while the argument can most definitely be made that zoonotic disease detection requires more resources [7,8], determining the most appropriate allocation of these resources remains difficult.

4.3. Discussion

Theoretical literature suggests that federalism, institutional design, and bureaucratic behavior could play a significant—and by most accounts—detrimental role in zoonotic disease detection. Indeed, there are pieces of empirical evidence that suggest the same. However, there is also information which suggests that these factors could play a role in facilitating rapid zoonotic disease detection. This section connects the gathered empirical evidence on outbreak detection—in particular, the responses to the interview/survey instrument—with the theoretical literature on federalism, bureaucratic behavior, and institutional design.

The factors listed in Tables 3 and 4 are well in line with those involved in zoonotic disease detection and reporting. Indeed, the literature review on these outbreaks also indicated the importance of diagnostics (including electronic reporting, as indicated in the outbreaks that were detected slowly) and astuteness of providers in disease detection. However, the more important question is: are these factors influenced by federalism, bureaucratic behavior, or institutional design? Certainly, three of the factors can be connected back to issues of governance.

First, and perhaps most importantly, is the knowledge or willingness to report notifiable diseases (Table 3). This factor was listed by respondents as the number one impediment to rapid detection. As a direct result of a federalized system where powers are reserved to the states, each state has varying requirements for reporting (e.g., how fast and who has to report); reporting of many notifiable diseases is often voluntary from the state level to the federal level. This regulatory framework may be detrimental to rapid zoonotic disease detection, particularly in multi-state outbreaks where these inconsistencies across states can easily delay recognition and/or response. It has been suggested that a more consistent regulatory approach and additional state to federal reporting requirements (and penalties for failure to report) would "encourage" and facilitate detection and reporting.

Second, respondents cited communication and collaboration across agencies and roles as an important facilitator in detecting and reporting past outbreaks. Interestingly, many theories of bureaucratic behavior indicate that executive agencies may choose to compete or compartmentalize information rather than cooperate. Indeed, this was reflected in the responses to the question regarding collaboration between the sectors (animal and human): one respondent suggested that absolutely no interaction occurred between the two sectors (animal health and human health) in the zoonotic disease outbreak which hampered detection and response; a concerning matter which has also been identified in past research [37]. However, respondents also suggested that effective cooperation between agencies occurs regularly in certain states, leading to positive outcomes for human and animal health.

Third, funding was reported as an impediment by respondents as well as a top three need to improve zoonotic disease detection and reporting. Resources were also mentioned in the outbreak literature review and predicted by theories of institutional design and behavior: some agencies have significantly more resources and/or influence, based on their design and behavior interacting with stakeholders. Moreover, in a federal system, each state operates with different capabilities and funding allocations based on the interests of the state. As noted by respondents and literature on zoonotic disease, deficient levels of funding can result in a lack of personnel, old IT systems, insufficient diagnostic equipment, or an absence of zoonotic disease education in either the animal or human health sectors—all of which could potentially delay zoonotic disease detection.

Despite the fact that implicitly some of the respondents' remarks regarding factors that facilitate or impede zoonotic disease detection can be identified as a consequence of federalism, respondents did not explicitly state that federalism played an important role in facilitating or impeding zoonotic disease detection. This is particularly interesting given the number of comments about state-specific success in zoonotic disease detection—a result of a federal system where states are independent actors with delegated and reserved powers. Some states may develop highly effective ways to facilitate interaction and collaboration facilitating disease detection. However, these comments are consistent with other research, where states have emerged as innovators [38] in both disease detection and reporting practices. Federalism—with the ability for states to create their own infrastructure, processes, regulations, and organizations—can facilitate detection. Electronic reporting, formal pathways between animal health and human health agencies, close relationships with producers and farm veterinarians, as well as informal training and workshops were all mentioned as specific mechanisms to facilitate zoonotic disease detection within a state.

Respondents did both implicitly suggest and explicitly state that bureaucratic behavior and institutional design affected the detection and reporting of the zoonotic disease outbreak: half of the respondents believed there was an impact. However, six of these nine respondents suggested that their experiences with bureaucratic behavior were not negative. This empirical evidence reinforces results found in an examination of the 1999 West Nile Virus outbreak in New York State [39], where initially the author notes questions of jurisdiction and authority (both between levels of government and across sectors of government) but finds that intergovernmental operations were also flexible, adapting and acting effectively across jurisdictions and sectors. While this is a divergence from what is commonly suggested in the theoretical literature—that executive agencies tend to compartmentalize information and fail to coordinate effectively—it is important to note that there were also respondents who clearly indicated that coordination problems and information siloes remain. It appears that certain states have better communication and collaboration processes in place across executive agencies, and as such, the behavior of bureaucracies and institutions and experience of officials and practitioners varies by state. Flexibility and adaptability of regulatory processes and ease of communication in matters of disease detection and reporting appears critical to rapid detection.

In sum, it is clear that federalism may impact the timeliness of zoonotic disease detection and reporting: while respondents did not explicitly cite federalism, implicitly they relayed multiple remarks demonstrating that regulatory differences across states and between states and the federal government is problematic, as also indicated in the outbreak and theoretical literature review. However, the ability of states to form and shape their own institutions and processes can also facilitate rapid detection through efficient collaboration. A federal system of governance therefore has multiple consequences for zoonotic disease detection with opposite effects. The evidence collected here on the impact of bureaucratic behavior and institutional design also remains mixed, though ultimately the impact of these factors appears to vary by state and outbreak circumstances. It seems likely that effective behavior and well-designed institutions and processes can facilitate detection, while compartmentalization of information, funding issues, and poor cooperation between executive agencies (between the animal and human sectors) can all impede detection of zoonotic disease outbreaks.

5. Conclusions

While researchers and policy analysts yearn for clear conclusions, the extent to which the U.S. system of governance impacts zoonotic disease detection and reporting deserves significantly more attention. Characteristics of the U.S. system of governance do matter in the success or failure of One Health approaches to key problems in policy and practice. This is the first attempt in the literature to describe the area of intersection between public policy and administration and One Health.

While empirical evidence suggests compartmentalization of knowledge within the animal health and human health sectors, as well as within different levels of government, innovative local and state systems can facilitate efficiency and flexibility. Bureaucracies can be flexible and adaptable, while also being prone to funding issues and overlapping regulations. After action reviews and reports of lessons learned for disease outbreaks must not only capture the technical side of outbreak detection—including the effectiveness of surveillance systems, epidemiological investigations, and disease control—but also the public policy and administration aspect to fully comprehend the facilitators and impediments to rapid detection and reporting. Moreover, other factors matter beyond those of governance, including technical advances and interpersonal relationships.

Further research on the topic is crucial, particularly from those federal, state, and local personnel responding to zoonotic disease outbreaks in the United States. This research can help to inform improvements in zoonotic disease detection, reporting, and response at the local, state, and federal levels by raising awareness of these complex issues. Systematic analysis of this intersection is critical to better understanding how to successfully execute One Health activities in a complex U.S. federal system of governance.

Acknowledgments

This research was conducted when the author was a PhD candidate at The George Washington University. The author would like to thank Professors Taylor Burke, Rebecca Katz, and Kathryn Newcomer at The George Washington University for aiding and improving this research with their expertise in law, public health, and case studies respectively. Comments from two anonymous reviewers greatly improved this manuscript.

Conflicts of Interest

The author declares no conflict of interest.

References and Notes

1. Schwabe, C.W. *Veterinary Medicine and Human Health*; Williams & Wilkins: Baltimore, MA, USA, 1984.
2. Kahn, L.H. Confronting zoonoses, linking human and veterinary medicine. *Emerg. Infect. Dis.* **2006**, *12*, 556–561.
3. Gostin, L.O. *Public Health Law: Power, Duty, Restraint*; University of California Press: Berkley, CA, USA, 2008.
4. United States Department of Agriculture Animal and Plant Health Inspection Service: About APHIS. Available online: http://www.aphis.usda.gov/wps/portal/banner/aboutaphis (accessed on 6 February 2015).
5. Taylor, L.H.; Latham, S.M.; Woolhouse, M.E. Risk factors for human disease emergence. *Phil. Trans. R. Soc. B* **2001**, *356*, 983–989.
6. Dato, V.; Wagner, M.M.; Fapohunda, A. How outbreaks of infectious disease are detected: A review of surveillance systems and outbreaks. *Public Health Rep.* **2004**, *119*, 464–471.

7. National Security Council. National Strategy on Countering Biological Threats. November 2009. Available online: http://www.whitehouse.gov/sites/default/files/National_Strategy_for_Countering_BioThreats.pdf (accessed on 10 February 2015).
8. Halliday, J.; Daborn, C.; Auty, H.; Mtema, Z.; Lembo, T.; Bronsvoort, B.M.; Handel, I.; Knobel, D.; Hampson, K.; Cleaveland, S. Bringing together emerging and endemic zoonoses and surveillance: shared challenges and a common solution. *Phil. Trans. R. Soc. B* **2012**, *367*, 2872–2880.
9. Chan, E.H.; Brewer, T.F.; Madoff, L.C.; Pollack, M.P.; Sonricker, A.L.; Keller, M.; Freifeld, C.C.; Blench, M.; Mawudeku, A.; Brownstein, J.S. Global capacity for emerging infectious disease detection. *Proc. Natl. Acad. Sci. USA* **2010**, *107*, 21701–21706.
10. Jajosky, R.A.; Groseclose, S.L. Evaluation of reporting timeliness of public health surveillance systems for infectious diseases. *BMC Public Health* **2004**, doi:10.1186/1471-2458-4-29.
11. Ashford, D.A.; Kaiser, R.M.; Bales, M.E.; Shutt, K.; Patrawalla, A.; McShan, A.; Tappero, J.W.; Perkins, B.A.; Dannenberg, A.L. Planning against biological terrorism: Lessons from outbreak investigations. *Emerg. Infect. Dis.* **2003**, *9*, 515–519.
12. Doyle, T.J.; Glynn, M.K.; Groseclose, S.L. Completeness of notifiable infectious disease reporting in the United States: An analytical literature review. *Am. J. Epidemiol.* **2002**, *155*, 866–874.
13. U.S. Const. amend. X. Print.
14. Hamilton, A. Federalist Paper: No. 70. The Executive Department Further Considered, 1788. Available online: http://avalon.law.yale.edu/18th_century/fed70.asp (accessed on 11 May 2015).
15. Lee, L.M.; Heilig, C.M.; White, A. Ethical justification for conducting public health surveillance without patient consent. *Am. J. Public Health* **2012**, *102*, 38–44.
16. Allen, H.A. Reportable animal diseases in the United States. *Zoonoses Public Health* **2012**, *59*, 44–51.
17. Rivlin, A.M. *Reviving the American Dream*; The Brookings Institution: Washington, DC, USA, 1992.
18. Katz, R.; Rosenbaum, S. Challenging custom: Rethinking national population surveillance policy in a global public health age. *J. Health Politics Policy Law* **2010**, *35*, 1027–1055.
19. Anderson, J.E. *Public Policymaking*, 6th ed.; Houghton Mifflin Company: Boston, MA, USA, 2006.
20. Wright, D.S. Federalism, intergovernmental relations, and intergovernmental management: historical reflections and conceptual comparisons. *Public Adm. Rev.* **1990,** *50,* 168–178.
21. Dudley, J.P. Global zoonotic disease surveillance: An emerging public health and biosecurity imperative. *Bioscience* **2004**, *54*, 982–983.
22. Campbell, C. The Complex Organization of the Executive Branch: The Legacies of Competing Approaches to Administration. In *The Executive Branch*; Aberbach, J.D., Person, M.A., Eds.; Oxford University Press: Oxford, UK, 2005; pp. 243–282.
23. Riley, D.D.; Brophy-Baermann, B.E. *Bureaucracy and the Policy Process*; Rowman and Littlefield Publishers, Inc.: Oxford, UK, 2006.
24. Rourke, F.E. *Bureaucracy, Politics, and Public Policy*; Little, Brown, and Company: Boston, MA, USA, 1968.
25. Wilson, J.Q. *Bureaucracy: What Government Agencies Do and Why They Do It*; Basic Books, Inc.: New York, NY, USA, 1989.
26. Stone, A.B.; Hautala, J.A. Meeting Report: Panel on the potential utility and strategies for design and implementation of a national companion animal infectious disease surveillance system. *Zoonoses Public Health* **2008**, *55*, 378–384.

27. Yin, R.K. *Case Study Research: Design and methods*; 3rd ed.; SAGE Publications: Los Angeles, CA, USA, 2003.
28. Allen, H.A. Characterizing zoonotic disease detection in the United States: Who detects zoonotic disease outbreaks & how fast are they detected. *J. Infect. Public Health* **2014**, doi:10.1016/j.jiph.2014.09.009.
29. Centers for Disease Control and Prevention: About PulseNet. Available online: http://www.cdc.gov/pulsenet/about/index.html (accessed on 16 February 2015).
30. Behravesh, C.B.; Ferraro, A.; Deasy, M.; Dato, V.; Moll, M.; Sandt, C.; Rea, N.K.; Rickert, R.; Marriott, C.; Warren, K.; *et al.* Human *Salmonella* infections linked to contaminated dry dog and cat food, 2006–2008. *Pediatrics* **2010**, *126*, 477–483.
31. Centers for Disease Control and Prevention. Outbreak of multidrug-resistant *Salmonella typhimurium* associated with rodents purchased at retail pet stores—United States, December 2003—October 2004. *MMWR Morb. Mortal. Wkly. Rep.* **2005**, *54*, 429–433.
32. Centers for Disease Control and Prevention. Multistate outbreak of human *Salmonella* infections caused by contaminated dry dog food—United States, 2006–2007. *MMWR Morb. Mortal. Wkly. Rep.* **2008**, *57*, 521–524.
33. Centers for Disease Control and Prevention. Human rabies—Indiana and California, 2006. *MMWR Morb. Mortal. Wkly. Rep.* **2007**, *56*, 361–365.
34. Centers for Disease Control and Prevention. Human anthrax associated with an epizootic among livestock—North Dakota, 2000. *MMWR Morb. Mortal. Wkly. Rep.* **2001**, *50*, 677–680.
35. Newcomer, K.E.; Triplett, T. Using Surveys. In *Handbook of Practical Program Evaluation*, 2nd, ed.; Wholey, J.S., Hatry, H.P., Newcomer, K.E., Eds.; Jossey-Bass: San Francisco, CA, USA, 2010.
36. Chomel, B.B.; Belotto, A.; Francios-Xavier, M. Wildlife, exotic pets, and emerging zoonoses. *Emerg. Infect. Dis.* **2007**, *13*, 6–11.
37. Lipton, B.A.; Hopkins, S.G.; Koehler, J.E.; DiGiacomo, R.F. A survey of veterinarian involvement in zoonotic disease prevention practices. *J. Am. Veterinary Med. Assoc.* **2008**, *233*, 1242–1249.
38. Holahan, J.; Weil, A.; Wiener, J.M. Federalism and Health Policy: An Overview. In *Federalism and Health Policy*; Holahan, J., Weil, A., Wiener, J.M., Eds.; The Urban Institute Press: Washington, DC, USA, 2003; pp. 1–24.
39. Bidjerano, M. The Metaphors of Federalism Revisited: The Web And Intergovernmental Relations. In Proceedings of the Thirty-Sixth Annual Meeting of the Northeastern Political Science Association and the International Studies Association, Boston, MA, USA, 11–13 November 2004.

14

Development and Evaluation of a Novel Taqman Real-Time PCR Assay for Rapid Detection of *Mycoplasma bovis*: Comparison of Assay Performance with a Conventional PCR Assay and Another Taqman Real-Time PCR Assay [‡]

Hemant Naikare [†,*], Daniela Bruno [†], Debabrata Mahapatra, Alesia Reinisch, Russell Raleigh and Robert Sprowls

Texas A&M Veterinary Medical Diagnostic Laboratory, 6610 Amarillo Blvd West, Amarillo, TX 79106, USA; E-Mails: danirbruno@gmail.com (D.B.); debabrata77@gmail.com (D.M.); areinisch@tvmdl.tamu.edu (A.R.); r-raleigh@tvmdl.tamu.edu (R.R); r-sprowls@tvmdl.tamu.edu (R.S.)

† These authors contributed equally to this work.

‡ Some of the data included in this manuscript was presented at the 55th American Association of Veterinary Laboratory Diagnosticians (AAVLD) Annual Meeting, Greensboro, NC, USA, 18–24 October 2012.

* Author to whom correspondence should be addressed; E-Mail: hnaikare@tvmdl.tamu.edu;

Academic Editors: Duncan C. Ferguson and Margarethe Hoenig

Abstract: The objective of this study was to develop and validate a Taqman real-time PCR assay for the detection of *Mycoplasma bovis* (*M. bovis*). Unique primers targeting the highly conserved house-keeping gene (*uvrC*) were designed and the probe sequence was derived from a previously published microarray study. There was 100% agreement in the outcome between our assay and the other two published assays for *M. bovis* detection. The analytical limit of detection of our assay is 83 copies of the *uvrC* gene. This assay was validated on a total of 214 bovine clinical specimens that were submitted to the Texas A&M Veterinary Medical Diagnostic Laboratory (TVMDL), Texas, USA. The specificity of the assay was assessed to be 100% since no cross-reactivity occurred with 22 other bacterial and other *Mycoplasma* species. We conclude that the *uvrC* gene serves as a good and reliable diagnostic marker for the accurate and rapid detection of *M. bovis* from a wider variety of specimen matrices.

Keywords: *Mycoplasma bovis*; cattle; *Taqman* real-time PCR; *uvrC* gene

1. Introduction

Mycoplasma bovis (*M. bovis*) continues to be a significant economic burden to the beef and dairy cattle industries. It is a major bovine mycoplasma pathogen associated with pneumonia, mastitis, arthritis, and abortion. It has been reported that *M. bovis* accounts for monetary losses of about 150 million euros across Europe and more than $100 million/year in the US due to mastitis and respiratory disease [1].

M. bovis, which belongs to the family *Mycoplasmataceae* in the class Mollicutes, is characterized by its small genome size (580–1380 kb), devoid of cell wall, and require complex growth media [2]. *M. bovis* is widespread within the bovine population in enzootically infected areas. Infection is usually introduced into *M. bovis*-free herds by asymptomatic calves or adult carrier cattle that are actively shedding the organism. Organisms can be shed via the respiratory tract for many months or even years, and such animals act as a reservoir of infection. Contact animals become infected via the respiratory tract, the teat canal, genital tract or artificial insemination with infected semen [1].

Infections caused by *M. bovis* are difficult to treat by antibiotic therapy. Their lack of cell wall makes them resistant to antimicrobials that target the cell wall such as beta-lactams [1,3]. Control methods rely mainly on culling infected animals and testing newly purchased animals before addition to the herd and maintaining extensive hygiene within the premises [4]. Hence, rapid and reliable diagnostic tools are in constant demand to detect infected animals and control the disease caused by *M. bovis*.

In comparison to the other bacterial pathogens that affect cattle, *M. bovis* are slow growers, and their fastidious growth requires the addition of sterols. It may take 3 to 10 days to grow at 37 °C in presence of 5%–10% CO_2. They produce "centered" colonies that give a "fried-egg" like appearance [5]. Although scientific literature cites culture as the gold standard method for detection of *M. bovis*, culture offers limited sensitivity and specificity due to multiple factors [1,6,7]. Serological tests determine previous exposure to *M. bovis* and are considered to be more sensitive than culture in diagnosing chronic infections. Different types of ELISA tests with whole cell or treated antigen have been described to detect antibodies in milk and serum and are also commercially available. Antibodies to *M. bovis* can be detected with various immunological methods including counter current electrophoresis, ELISA, immunoblotting, immunobinding and immunohistochemistry methods [8]. Although serology can help in identifying mycoplasma negative herds, the presence of high sero-prevalance in many populations limits the utility of serological tests [7].

The complete genome sequence of the international reference strain of *M. bovis* PG45 (ATCC 25523) has been reported [9]. Several PCR based molecular tests have been published which allow *M. bovis* identification using conventional, SYBR, Taqman real-time PCR or loop-mediated isothermal amplification (LAMP) platforms with varying sensitivity and specificity indices [10–15]. The known diagnostic targets for *M. bovis* detection primarily include 16S *rRNA* and *uvrC* genes. The *uvrC* gene is a highly conserved housekeeping gene that encodes for a DNA repair enzyme "deoxyribodipyrimidine photolyase" [10]. Subramaniam and colleagues have demonstrated that although the *uvrC* gene is well conserved in *M. bovis* and in another small ruminant pathogen *Mycoplasma agalactiae*, this gene differs significantly between the two phylogenetically closely related *Mycoplasma* species [10]. Thomas and colleagues [16] have demonstrated the *uvrC* gene to be a conserved target suitable for PCR based diagnostics by PCR amplification and sequencing from ninety-two and twenty *M. bovis* strains respectively. Interestingly, Marenda and colleagues [17] have demonstrated the limitation of *uvrC* target's universality for *M. bovis* detection since the *uvrC* gene sequences are only slightly divergent making it difficult to differentiate *M. bovis* and *M. agalactiae*. Based on their suppression subtractive hybridization study, Marenda and colleagues have further proposed that the *polC* target based PCR should be included as a complement to the *uvrC* target based detection of *M. bovis* [17]. Other diagnostic markers that have been reported for PCR based identification of *M. bovis* include an ATP binding protein *oppD*/*F* and membrane protein 81 [7].

Our objective was to develop and evaluate a rapid and accurate *uvrC* gene-based Taqman real-time PCR assay for the detection of *M. bovis* in a wide variety of clinical specimen matrices that can be utilized for routine diagnostic testing, molecular surveillance, and export testing.

2. Experimental Section

2.1. Clinical Specimens

A total of 214 specimens comprising milk samples: individual animals and bulk tanks (78); fresh lungs (45); joint fluids (5); semen (8); and nasal swabs (78) submitted to the TVMDL laboratory for culture and/or *M. bovis* PCR were included in this study. These specimens originated from dairy farms, beef feed lots, and from bison farms across Texas and other states in the US.

2.2. DNA Extraction

The clinical specimens were prepared for nucleic acid purification as follows: (i) milk: ~25 to 50 mL of milk sample was pelleted by centrifuging at 3000–4000 g for 15–20 min. The supernatant fat and excess liquid were removed, and the pellet was washed twice with sterile phosphate buffered saline (PBS). The washed pellet was re-suspended in 200 µL of sterile PBS and then used for nucleic acid purification; (ii) Lung tissues: ~1–2 grams of tissue was aliquoted and mixed with 10–20 mL of sterile PBS and homogenized using a stomacher (10% w/v) (Stomacher® Lab Blender Model 8.0 Seward Medical Limited, London-UK 10/94). Following disruption, 200µL of the tissue supernatant was used for nucleic acid purification; (iii) Nasal swab samples were directly re-suspended in ~ 400 to 500 µL of sterile PBS and 200 µL of it was used for nucleic acid extraction; (iv) semen and joint fluid specimens: 200 µL of specimen was directly used for nucleic acid extraction; (v) *Mycoplasma* sp. isolates/colonies: ~1–4 colonies were transferred into 200 µL of sterile PBS using sterile disposable loop, and subjected to nucleic acid purification.

The nucleic acid purification from 200 µL of processed clinical specimens was performed using QIAamp DNA mini kit (Qiagen #51306) as per the manufacturer's instructions. DNA was eluted in 100 µL of sterile water and stored at −20 °C until the PCR amplification could be performed.

2.3. TaqMan Real-Time PCR Assay

The *M. bovis uvrC* gene sequence was retrieved from the Genbank accession # AF003959.1. *M. bovis* species specific primers were designed using Primer3 software (http://frodo.wi.mit.edu/). The probe sequence was derived from a previously published microarray study [18]. The primers and probe were synthesized from IDT-DNA and Life Technologies respectively, and the sequence information is listed in Table 1.

Table 1. Sequences of primers and probes used in this study.

Gene Target	Oligo	Sequence (5'→3')	Reference	Product Size
uvrC	Forward Primer	GAG AAT GCT TCA GTA TTT TGA CGG	This study	170 bp
	Reverse Primer	CAA AAG CAA AAT GTT AAA TTC AGG	This study	
	Probe	(6 FAM) CAT ATA TAA GTG AGA CTA ACT TAT T(MGB)	[18]	
uvrC	F2024	TCT AAT TTT TTC ATC ATC GCT AAT GC	[12]	112 bp
	R2135	TCA GGC CTT TGC TAC AAT GAA C		
	M.bov	(FAM) AAC TGC ATC ATA TCA CAT ACT (MGB)		
16S rRNA	Forward Primer	CCT TTT AGA TTG GGA TAG CGG ATG	[19]	360 bp
	Reverse Primer	CCG TCA AGG TAG CAT CAT TTC CTA T		

Taqman real-time PCR was carried out in Applied Biosystems 7300 or 7500 Fast thermal cycler instruments (Applied Biosystems, Foster City, CA, USA) in a standard mode. The PCR was performed in a 20 μL final reaction volume. The 3 μL of template DNA was added to 17 μL master mix prepared with TaqPCR core kit (Qiagen #201225) containing 2.0 μL 10X PCR buffer, 0.4 μL dNTP (10 mM each), 2.4 μL·$MgCl_2$ (25 mM), 0.8 μL each of forward and reverse primers (25 μM), 0.8 μL of probe (7.5 μM), 0.25 μL Taq DNA Polymerase (5 units/μL) and 9.55 μL of water. The PCR assay was performed using 96-well plates that were sealed with optical sealing tape (Applied Biosystems, Foster City, CA, USA). Reaction mixtures containing water substituted for DNA templates were used as negative controls. The thermocycling conditions were set as per the following parameters: 95 °C for 8 min, 40 cycles of 95 °C for 20 s, and 60 °C for 1 min. Fluorescence was read at the end of each round of the annealing step. Specimens that produced an increase in the fluorescence signal of the reporter dye over the threshold value (set at 10% of the maximum fluorescence of the positive amplification control), auto baseline, and produced a characteristic sigmoidal curve were considered to be positive for *M. bovis*. The DNA extracts from all the specimens were also tested for *M. bovis* by conventional PCR, and its sensitivity and specificity was compared to our Taqman assay. Conventional PCR was carried out in a T3 Thermocycler (Biometra- Göttingen, Germany), and the conditions used were as described by Gonzalez *et al.* [19]. Similarly, our Taqman assay was compared to the Taqman assay of Clothier *et al.* using their recipe and thermocycling conditions [12]. Table 1 provides sequence information of primers and probe used for conventional PCR as per Gonzalez *et.al.* [19] and Taqman PCR as per Clothier *et.al.* [12].

2.4. Culture

Culture was carried out directly from the clinical specimens in accordance with the protocol described previously by Goll and colleagues [2]. The specimens were processed as follows: (i) lung tissues: an incision was made on the tissue surface with a sterile scalpel blade. A sterile cotton tipped applicator was penetrated into the incised tissue to obtain the inoculum, which was then cultured on Hayflick's mycoplasma agar plates; (ii) milk samples, joint fluids, and semen samples: a sterile cotton tipped applicator was dipped into the clinical specimen, and the inoculum was cultured on Hayflick's mycoplasma agar plates; (iii) nasal swabs: they were directly plated onto Hayflick's mycoplasma agar plates. The inoculated plates were incubated at 37 °C with 5% CO_2 for one week and were examined under a dissecting microscope for mycoplasma growth every other day during the incubation. The characteristic "fried egg" like "centered" colony appearance was interpreted as positive culture for *M. bovis* [2].

2.5. Sensitivity and Specificity Analyses

The specificity of the *M. bovis* Taqman assay was assessed using genomic DNA from 22 different bacterial and *Mycoplasma* species that could potentially be encountered with mastitis, arthritis and pulmonary infections in ruminants (Table 2). A subset of clinical specimens ($n = 71$) were also subjected to culture-based detection of *M. bovis*. The limit of detection and analytical sensitivity of the real-time assay was determined using 10-fold serial dilutions of a culture of *M. bovis* strain ATCC 25523 in triplicate. The number of copies of *M. bovis* template DNA was calculated using the online resource "dsDNA copy number calculator" from URI Genomics and sequencing center (http://www.uri.edu/research/gsc/resources/cndna.html).

Table 2. *Mycoplasma* sp. and other bacterial species tested for specificity of the real-time PCR assay.

Number	Species	Strain	Real-Time PCR
1	*Mycoplasma bovis*	ATCC 25523	Positive
2	*Mycoplasma bovis*	ATCC 27369	Positive
3	*Mycoplasma bovis*	Field isolate	Positive
4	*Mycoplasma alkalescens*	ATCC 29103	Negative
5	*Mycoplasma canadense*	ATCC 29418	Negative
6	*Mycoplasma arginini*	ATCC 23838	Negative
7	*Mycoplasma bovigenitalium*	ATCC 27748	Negative
8	*Staphylococcus aureus*	Field isolate	Negative
9	*Streptococcus agalactiae*	Field isolate	Negative
10	*Escherichia coli*	Field isolate	Negative
11	*Corynebacterium pseudotuberculosis*	Field isolate	Negative
12	*Streptococcus uberis*	Field isolate	Negative
13	*Coagulase Negative Staphylococcus*	Field isolate	Negative
14	*Pseudomonas aeruginosa*	Field isolate	Negative
15	*Klebsiella pneumonia*	Field isolate	Negative
16	*Proteus mirabilis*	Field isolate	Negative
17	*Serratia marcescens*	Field isolate	Negative
18	*Entereococcus faecalis*	Field isolate	Negative
19	*Arcanobacterium pyogenes*	Field isolate	Negative
20	*Candida spp*	Field isolate	Negative
21	*Histophilus somnus*	Field isolate	Negative
22	*Salmonella spp*	Field isolate	Negative
23	*Bacillus cereus*	Field isolate	Negative
24	*Pasteurella multocida*	Field isolate	Negative
25	*Mannheimia haemolytica*	Field isolate	Negative

3. Results and Discussion

3.1. Limit of Detection

Using 10-fold serial dilutions of genomic DNA extracted from pure culture of the international reference strain of *M. bovis* ATCC 25523 isolate, we determined the limit of detection for the *uvrC* gene-based Taqman assay similar to the method employed for *Bacillus anthracis* PCR by Moser *et al.* [20]. The extracted DNA was quantified and checked for purity using NanoDrop® ND-1000 Spectrophotometer (Nanodrop Technologies, Inc. Wilmington, DE, USA). The DNA was tested in triplicate to determine the lowest detectable concentration, and the results indicated that the *Taqman assay* was able to detect 900 femtograms of total extracted DNA from all replicates (Figure 1). The genome length of *M. bovis* ATCC 25,523 was recently reported to be 1,003,404 bp [9]. Based on the observed Ct values and the standard curve, the assay demonstrated high sensitivity and was estimated to have a detection limit of ~83 copies of *uvrC* gene (Figure 1) and approximately 4×10^2 cfu/mL. The limit of detection of our Taqman assay is comparable to the limit of detection reported by Clothier *et al.* [12].

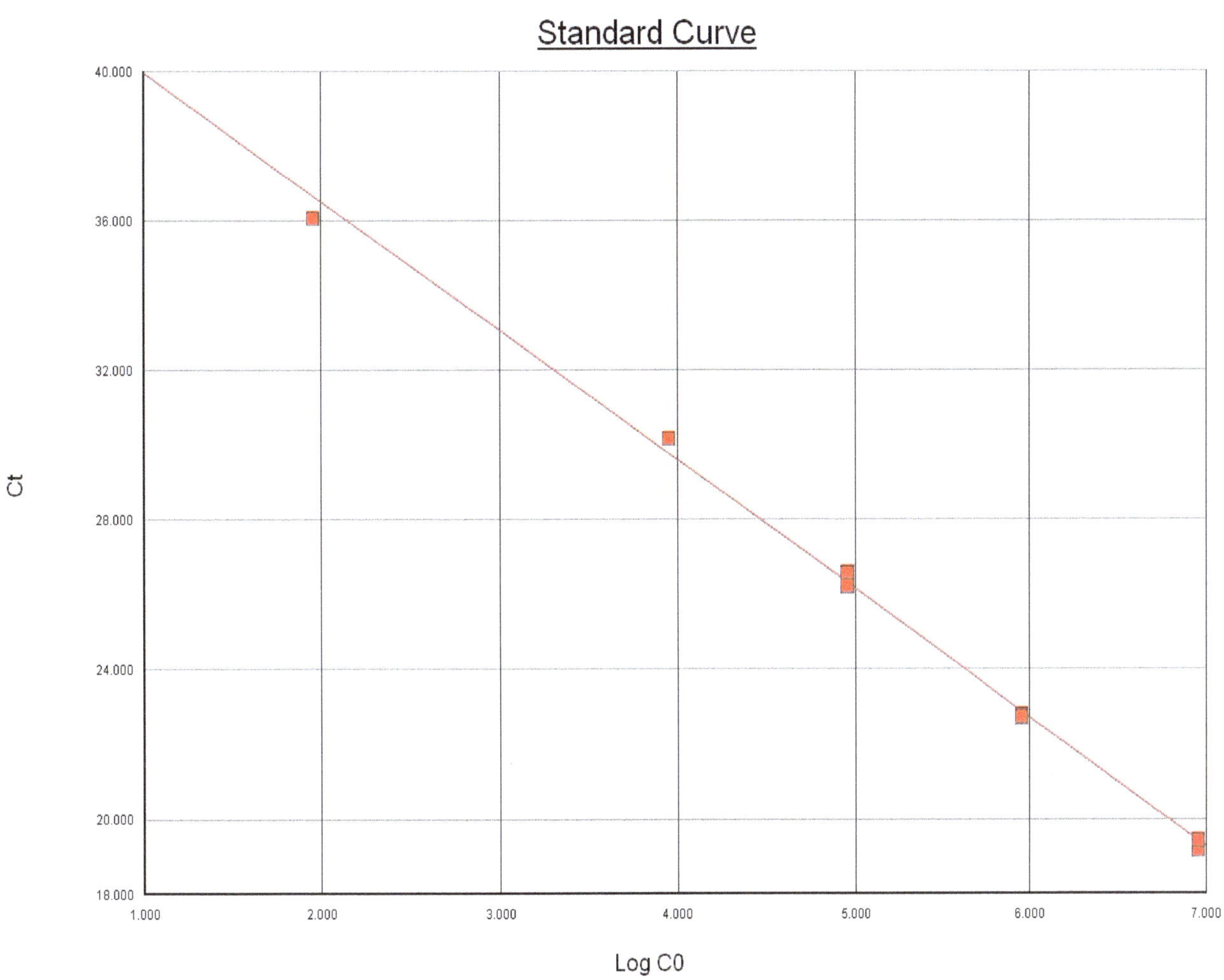

Figure 1. Relationship between the amount of template DNA copies (Log CO) in the Taqman assay and the mean threshold cycle (Ct). Slope: −3.448840; intercept: 43.393936; $R^2 = 0.996695$.

3.2. *Assay Specificity*

The specificity of our Taqman assay was evaluated with genomic DNA from 22 bacterial and *Mycoplasma* species which could likely be present in infections from where *M. bovis* could be detected (Table 2). Both *M. bovis* ATCC isolates and a known clinical isolate of *M. bovis* were detected by the Taqman assay. No cross-reactivity was observed with other DNA targets, suggesting 100% specificity of the Taqman assay. The *uvrC* gene in *M. bovis* has been shown to be stable and resistant to normal mutation process reinforcing its efficacy as a target for PCR assays [16]. Thomas *et al.* [16] have demonstrated the *uvrC* gene to be a conserved target suitable for PCR based diagnostics by PCR amplification and sequencing from 92 and 20 *M. bovis* strains respectively. The specificity of our Taqman assay is similar to the specificity reported for another Taqman assay with *uvrC* target for *M. bovis* detection [12].

3.3. *Assay Performance with Clinical Specimens*

Analysis of the specimens from our study revealed *M. bovis* by Taqman PCR in 82 out of the 214 specimens (Table 3). Out of these 82 positives, the break-up was as follows: 93.3% of lung samples were positive (42 of 45), 19.2% of milk samples were positive (15 out of 78), 28.2% of nasal swabs were positive (22 of 78), 40% of joint fluid samples were positive (2 of 5), and 12.5% of semen specimens were positive (1 of 8). Although transmission of *M. bovis* through infected semen has been cited as a route of infection [1], to our knowledge, this is the first report of a PCR confirmed positive for *M. bovis* from semen.

The performance of our Taqman assay matched 100% (Table 3) with two previously published PCR methods: conventional PCR targeting the 16S rRNA [19] and Taqman real-time PCR targeting *uvrC* gene [12]. This study demonstrates our Taqman assay to have at least equivalent sensitivity and specificity as the other two PCR assays and that either of the two *uvrC* targeting Taqman assays could be utilized for the rapid and accurate detection of *M. bovis*.

Table 3. Comparison between our Taqman PCR assay, conventional PCR and Clothier *et al.* Taqman assay.

Specimen	Our Taqman PCR Assay		Conventional PCR		Clothier *et al.* Taqman PCR Assay	
	Positive	Negative	Positive	Negative	Positive	Negative
Lung (n = 45)	42	3	42	3	42	3
Milk (n = 78)	15	63	15	63	15	63
Nasal swab (n = 78)	22	56	22	56	22	56
Joint fluid (n = 5)	2	3	2	3	2	3
Semen (n = 8)	1	7	1	7	1	7
Total (n = 214)	82	132	82	132	82	132

n = number of specimen of each kind of specimen matrix tested.

3.4. *Performance Comparison of Culture and Taqman PCR Assay*

Gonzalez *et al.* has demonstrated that pre-enrichment does not significantly increase the isolation of *Mycoplasma* sp. but increases the cost of diagnosis based on their comparative study of over 4000 milk samples which were tested for *Mycoplasma* sp. by both: direct inoculation of milk on Hayflick agar plates and pre-enrichment in Hayflick broth before culturing on Hayflick agar plates [21]. Therefore, we directly cultured the clinical specimens without pre-enrichment in the Hayflick mycoplasma broth.

Out of the 214 clinical specimens, a subset (n = 71) was evaluated for the presence of *M. bovis* by culture examination which is cited in the literature as the gold standard test for *M. bovis* detection (Table 4). Interestingly, only 35.21% (n = 25) of these 71 specimens were positive for *M. bovis* by culture method, whereas 70.42% (n = 50) were positive by our Taqman assay. Notably 27 out of the remaining 46 culture-negative specimens were positive by Taqman assay, while two specimens were positive by culture but negative by Taqman assay. Bell *et al.* recently reported similar findings and found PCR to detect 45.28% more of the positive *M. bovis* cases which were negative by the *M. bovis* culture test [22]. It is noteworthy that in addition to *M. bovis,* other bacterial and viral respiratory pathogens were also detected in some of the clinical specimens. However, in this study we did not investigate the concomitant *M. bovis* infections in presence or absence of these respiratory pathogens. The detection of *M. bovis* in clinical specimens may not always correlate with presence of an infectious underlying disease as *M. bovis* has been detected from both, clinically healthy animals and sick animals [23].

Table 4. Comparison between culture and our Taqman PCR assay.

Specimen	Culture		Our Taqman PCR Assay	
	Positive	Negative	Positive	Negative
Lung (n = 40)	17	23	39	1
Milk(n = 18)	4	14	4	14
Swabs(n = 10)	4	6	6	4
Joint Fluid (n = 3)	0	3	1	2
Total (n = 71)	25	46	50	21

Discrepancy between the outcome of culture results and Taqman assay results can be attributed to various factors. Due to the fastidious nature and fragility of *Mycoplasma* sp., suspected clinical specimens need to be promptly received within 24 h of sample collection in chilled condition to prevent loss of viability [7]. Whereas, PCR can detect *M. bovis* DNA from non-viable organisms and provides enhanced sensitivity compared to culture based examination [24]. Interestingly, Castillo-Alcala and colleagues have observed a large number of samples to be culture-positive for *M. bovis*, but were negative for *M. bovis* by hybridization probes based real-time PCR assay on a LightCycler platform [23]. Sensitivity of the PCR assays for *M. bovis* detection thus varies amongst different platforms of PCR. Isolation of *M. bovis* is significantly impaired from antibiotic treated animals and especially from lungs of chronically affected animals. Also co-infection, bacterial overgrowth, and contamination with other bacteria hinders with *M. bovis* isolation. Culture allows growth of all kinds of *Mycoplasma* species, and it is not specific for *M. bovis* detection as is the case with Taqman assay. Species level identification of *M. bovis* is not solely possible based on culture morphology, but requires further testing for confirmation by ELISA, PCR or immuno-histochemistry [7]. Inclusion of an internal extraction/ amplification control is recommended as it will assist in identifying any false negative results. As the internal control co-amplifies with the *uvrC* target gene, it serves in detecting any possible PCR inhibitors derived from the specimen DNA [25].

4. Conclusions

The *uvrC* gene-based Taqman real-time PCR assay described in this study is much faster than conventional PCR and culture based identification of *M. bovis*. The Taqman assay results can be obtained within 2.5 h with greater sensitivity and specificity in identifying *M. bovis* DNA from clinical specimens. We have validated our *uvrC* gene based Taqman real-time PCR assay to serve as a rapid and accurate test for the detection of *M. bovis* from a variety of clinical specimens.

Acknowledgments

We thank Ashlie McCarthy, Carlos Santisteban and Abhijit Gurjar of Quality Milk Production Services, Cornell University, Ithaca, New York for providing some of the reference isolates of *Mycoplasma* species that were used in our assay validation.

Author Contributions

Hemant Naikare contributed to the overall study design and analyses of the data, supervised the laboratory work and wrote the manuscript with Daniela Bruno. Daniela Bruno equally contributed towards study design, data compilation, and assisted in writing the manuscript. Debabrata Mahapatra and Alesia Reinisch extracted nucleic acids and performed P.C.R. experiments. Russell Raleigh performed isolation and identification of *Mycoplasma* sp. Debabrata Mahapatra, Alesia Reinisch and Russell Raleigh also assisted in preparing the manuscript. Robert Sprowls provided assistance with the study design and was involved in drafting the manuscript. All authors read and approved the final version of the manuscript.

Conflicts of Interest

The authors declare no conflict of interest.

References

1. Nicholas, R.A.; Ayling, R.D. *Mycoplasma bovis*: Disease, diagnosis and control. *Res. Vet. Sci.* **2003**, *74*, 105–112.
2. Goll, F., Jr. Identification of mycoplasmas isolated from domestic animals. In *Mycoplasmosis in Animals: Laboratory Diagnosis*; Whitford, H.W., Rosenbusch, R.F., Lauerman, L.H., Eds.; Iowa State University Press: Ames, IA, USA, 1994; pp. 15–27.
3. Rosenbusch, R.F. Biology and Taxonomy of Mycoplasmas. In *Mycoplasmosis in Animals: Laboratory Diagnosis*; Whitford, H.W., Rosenbusch, R.F., Lauerman, L.H., Eds.; Iowa State University Press: Ames, IA, USA, 1994; pp. 3–11.
4. Pfutzner, H.; Sachse, K. *Mycoplasma bovis* as an agent of mastitis, pneumonia, arthritis and genital disorders. *Revue Sci. Tech.* **1994**, *15*, 1477–1494.
5. Nicholas, R.A.J.; Baker, S.E. Recovery of Mycoplasmas from Animals. In *Mycoplasma Protocols*; Miles, R.J., Nicholas, R.A.J., Eds.; Humana Press: Totowa, NJ, USA, 1998; pp. 37–44.
6. Jasper, D.E. Bovine Mycoplasma mastitis. *Adv. Vet. Sci. Comp. Med.* **1981**, *25*, 121–159.

7. Caswell, J.L.; Archambault, M. *Mycoplasma bovis* pneumonia in cattle. *Anim. Health Res. Rev.* **2007**, *8*, 161–186.
8. Kumar, A.; Verma, A.K.; Rahal, A. *Mycoplasma bovis*, A Multi Disease Producing Pathogen: An Overview. *Asian J. Anim. Vet. Adv.* **2011**, *6*, 537–546.
9. Wise, K.S.; Calcutt, M.J.; Foecking, M.F.; Röske, K.; Madupu, R.; Methé, B.A. Complete genome sequence of *Mycoplasma bovis* type strain PG45 (ATCC 25523). *Infect. Immun.* **2011**, *79*, 982–983.
10. Subramaniam, S.; Bergonier, D.; Poumarat, F.; Capaul, S.; Schlatter, Y.; Nicolet, J.; Frey, J. Species identification of *Mycoplasma bovis* and *Mycoplasma agalactiae* based on the *uvr*C genes by PCR. *Mol. Cell. Probes* **1998**, *12*, 161–169.
11. Bashiruddin, J.B.; Frey, J.; Königsson, M.H.; Johansson, K.E.; Hotzel, H.; Diller, R.; deSantis, P.; Botelho, A.; Ayling, R.D.; Nicholas, R.A.; *et al.* Evaluation of PCR systems for the identification and differentiation of *Mycoplasma agalactiae* and *Mycoplasma bovis*: A collaborative trial. *Vet. J.* **2005**, *169*, 268–275.
12. Clothier, K.A.; Jordan, D.M.; Thompson, C.J.; Kinyon, J.M.; Frana, T.S.; Strait, E.L. *Mycoplasma bovis* real-time polymerase chain reaction assay validation and diagnostic performance. *J. Vet. Diagn. Invest.* **2010**, *22*, 956–960.
13. Cai, H.Y.; Bell-Rogers, P.; Parker, L.; Prescott, J.F. Development of a real-time PCR for detection of *Mycoplasma bovis* in bovine milk and lung samples. *J. Vet. Diagn. Invest.* **2005**, *17*, 537–545.
14. McAuliffe, L.; Ellis, R.J.; Lawes, J.R.; Ayling, R.D.; Nicholas, R.A. 16S rDNA PCR and denaturing gradient gel electrophoresis; a single generic test for detecting and differentiating Mycoplasma species. *J. Med. Microbiol.* **2005**, *54*, 731–739.
15. Bai, Z.; Shi, L.; Hu, C.; Chen, X.; Qi, J.; Ba, X.; Peng, Q.; Chen, Y.; Chen, H.; Guo, A. Development of a loop-mediated isothermal amplification assay for sensitive and rapid detection of *Mycoplasma bovis*. *Afr. J. Biotechnol.* **2011**, *10*, 12333–12338.
16. Thomas, A.; Dizier, I.; Linden, A.; Mainil, J.; Frey, J.; Vilei, E.M. Conservation of the *uvr*C gene sequence in *Mycoplasma bovis* and its use in routine PCR diagnosis. *Vet. J.* **2004**, *168*, 100–102.
17. Marenda, M.S.; Sagne, E.; Poumarat, F.; Citti, C. Suppression subtractive hybridization as a basis to assess *Mycoplasma agalactiae* and *Mycoplasma bovis* genomic diversity and species-specific sequences. *Microbiology* **2005**, *151*, 475–489.
18. Lee, K.H.; Lee, J.W.; Wang, S.W.; Liu, L.Y.; Lee, M.F.; Chuang, S.T.; Shy, Y.M.; Chang, C.L.; Wu, M.C.; Chi, C.H. Development of a novel biochip for rapid multiplex detection of seven mastitis causing pathogens in bovine milk samples. *J. Vet. Diagn. Investig.* **2008**, *20*, 463–471.
19. Gonzalez, Y.R.C.; Baccunana, C.R.; Bolske, G.; Mattsson, J.G.; Molina, C.F.; Johansson, K.E. *In vitro* amplification of the 16S rRNA genes from *Mycoplasma bovis* and *Mycoplasma agalactiae* by PCR. *Vet. Microbiol.* **1995**, *47*, 183–190.
20. Moser, M.J.; Christensen, D.R.; Norwood, D.; Prudent, J.R. Multiplexed detection of anthrax-related toxin genes. *J. Mol. Diagn.* **2006**, *8*, 89–96.
21. González, R.N.; Sears, P.M.; Wilson, D.J. Diagnosis of Intramammary Infections Due to *Mycoplasma bovis* in Dairy Cattle. In Proceedings of the 3rd IDF International Mastitis Seminar, 1995; Volume S-2, pp. 23–27.

22. Bell, C.J.; Blackurn, P.; Elliott, M.; Patterson, T.I.; Ellison, S.; Lahuerta-Marin, A.; Ball, H.J. Investigation of polymerase chain reaction assays to improve detection of bacterial involvement in bovine respiratory disease. *J. Vet. Diagn. Investig.* **2014**, *26*, 631–634.
23. Castillo-Alcala, F.; Bateman, K.G.; Cai, H.Y.; Schott, C.R.; Parker, L.; Clark, M.E.; McRaild, P.; McDowall, R.M.; Foster, R.A.; Archambault, M.; *et al*. Prevalence and genotype of *Mycoplasma bovis* in beef cattle after arrival at a feedlot. *Am. J. Vet. Res.* **2012**, *73*, 1932–1943.
24. Justice-Allen, A.; Trujillo, J.; Goodell, G.; Wilson, D. Detection of multiple *Mycoplasma* species in bulk tank milk samples using real-time PCR and conventional culture and comparison of test sensitivities. *J. Dairy Sci.* **2011**, *94*, 3411–3419.
25. Hoorfar, J.; Malorny, B.; Abdulmawjood, A.; Cook, N.; Wagner, M.; Fach, P. Practical considerations in design of internal amplification controls for diagnostic PCR assays. *J. Clin. Microbiol.* **2004**, *42*, 1863–1868.

15

Alkylation and Carbamylation Effects of Lomustine and Its Major Metabolites and MGMT Expression in Canine Cells

Thushara Chakkath [1], Sidonie Lavergne [1], Timothy M. Fan [2], David Bunick [1] and Levent Dirikolu [1,*]

[1] Department of Comparative Biosciences, College of Veterinary Medicine, University of Illinois, Urbana, IL 61802, USA; E-Mails: chakkat1@illinois.edu (T.C.); slavergn@illinois.edu (S.L.); dbunick@illinois.edu (D.B.)

[2] Department of Veterinary Clinical Medicine, College of Veterinary Medicine, University of Illinois, Urbana, IL 61802, USA; E-Mail: T-fan@illinois.edu

* Author to whom correspondence should be addressed; E-Mail: dirikolu@illinois.edu;

Academic Editor: Anthony Blikslager

Abstract: DNA Alkylation is thought to be the reason for the efficacy of lomustine while carbamylation has been implicated as the cause for the side effects seen with lomustine treatment such as hepatotoxicity. In the alkylation study we show that lomustine and its metabolites form similar levels of the DNA adducts N^7 hydroxyethylguanine and O^6 hydroxyethyldeoxyguanosine. In terms of carbamylation, lomustine showed greater extent of carbamylation in the canine hepatocytes and lymphoma cell lines. The DNA repair enzyme O^6 methylguanine DNA methyltransferase (MGMT) causes resistance of tumor cells to bifunctional nitrosourea, like lomustine. There is no data available regarding MGMT expression/activity in canine cells or tissues. Our study shows that there is low MGMT activity in the canine lymphoid cell line 17–71 while the GL-1 cells did not show any detectable enzyme activity or mRNA expression. The MGMT enzyme activity measured in canine hepatocytes is about 250–350 fmol/mg protein as compared to about 90 fmol/mg protein in 17–71 cells. We also show that MGMT mRNA expression in 17–71 cells and canine hepatocytes positively correlates with its enzyme activity in these cells.

Keywords: lomustine; trans-4-hydroxylomustine; cis-4-hydroxylomustine; lymphoma; MGMT

---

1. Introduction

It is known that alkylating agents such as nitrosoureas decompose at physiological conditions to yield alkylating and carbamylating intermediates [1], however the relative contribution of these events to the toxicity and therapeutic effects are unclear [2]. These compounds are electrophilic in nature and attack the nucleophilic sites on the DNA to form alkylated products [3]. The N^7 position of guanine is the most reactive site [3,4] with all alkylating agents and hence about 70%–90% of the adducts are formed at this position [5,6]. However the relative mutagenicity and carcinogenicity of alkylating agents correlate with the reagents ability to bind to the oxygen sites [7,8]. Chloroethylating compounds like lomustine form adducts at the O^6 position of guanine [5]. If not repaired, these adducts form DNA interstrand cross links [3] which may lead to double strand breaks and ultimately, apoptosis of the cell [9].

Decomposition of lomustine in aqueous medium produces chloroethyl carbonium ions which is an alkylating intermediate and also cyclohexyl isocyanate which is a carbamylating agent [10–12]. It is believed that the dominant role of carbamylating activity is in determining the toxicity of compounds which may be manifested as side effects [2]. The isocyanate intermediates formed by the breakdown of lomustine react with the lysine residues in protein leading to post translational modification of proteins [13]. This could result in partial or complete loss of protein function [14].

The DNA protective enzyme MGMT is known to play a critical role in the defense against alkylating compounds which produce the O^6 alkylguanine lesion. Repair of the O^6 alkylguanine adduct via MGMT is a rapid single step process in which the offending alkyl group is transferred to the cysteine residue of MGMT thereby restoring the affected DNA [5,15,16]. The MGMT level is highly variable among individuals and also among the various tissues in the same individual [17]. A long term study of MGMT in peripheral blood mononuclear cells (PBMC) from healthy human subjects showed that there is a 7 fold variation in MGMT activity between subjects with very little change over time [18].

Due to its functional role in DNA repair, MGMT may have a significant impact on the outcome of cancer therapy with alkylating agents. Certain tumors that are high expressers of MGMT were found to be less sensitive to treatment with nitrosoureas while tumors that were deficient in MGMT or showed relatively low expression responded better to nitrosourea therapy [17]. MGMT levels in normal tissues may also have significant impact on the choice of therapy to be used. A dose limiting side effect of most nitrosourea compounds is myelotoxicity, and it is thought that this could be due to the low MGMT expression in bone marrow cells [16,19]. There is data indicating that MGMT expression is inducible (via transcriptional activation) by alkylating agents, X-ray or other DNA damaging agents [20]. Studies in rat liver cells have shown a 2–5 fold MGMT gene induction with maximum induction happening around 24 to 48 h after exposure to X-ray or the alkylating agent, methylnitronitrosoguanidine (MNNG) [20,21].

In our previously published cytotoxicity study [22], lomustine and its metabolites showed similar degree of cell killing in the canine lymphoid cell lines 17–71 and GL-1, and canine hepatocytes. As alkylation is thought to be the main reason for the cytotoxic effects of these drugs [3], we wanted to investigate if the compounds have similar pattern of alkylation. It is believed that the concentration of an internal dosimeter such as DNA adducts is a more accurate measure of the amount of mutagen reaching the target site than the applied dose [7]. In a recent study published, it was shown that N^7 hydroxyethyl guanine and O^6 hydroxyethyldeoxyguanosine are some of the main DNA alkylation products formed after exposure to chloroethylating agents [23]. It is reported that the cis-4 and trans-4 metabolites of lomustine may have reduced toxic effects relative to lomustine [24] and therefore the metabolites might have advantage over lomustine for clinical use [25]. Carbamylation of proteins is believed to contribute to the side effects seen with lomustine [2].

The aim of this study was to compare the alkylation and carbamylation potential of lomustine and its trans-4 and cis-4 metabolites in canine lymphoma cell lines and hepatocytes. The secondary aim was to evaluate the MGMT expression and enzyme activity in canine lymphoid cell lines and primary canine hepatocytes as we tried to correlate the MGMT levels with the cytotoxicity of lomustine and its metabolites in these cells and also the level of DNA adducts formed by these compounds.

2. Materials and Methods

2.1. DNA Adduct Detection Assay

The O^6 hydroxyethyldeoxyguanosine and N^7 hydroxyethylguanine adducts were measured in canine lymphoid cell lines 17–71 and GL-1 [26,27] and primary canine hepatocytes (isolated from six dogs that were euthanized at the Champaign county animal control facility) after exposure to lomustine, trans-4 and cis-4 by the LC/MS/MS method as mentioned below. The cell lines were grown and maintained at 37 °C in 5% CO_2, and cultures were passaged as necessary to maintain high cell viability (above 90%) in culture media Dulbecco's modified Eagle medium (DMEM) supplemented with 10% fetal bovine serum (FBS) and 1% penicillin/streptomycin.

2.1.1. Isolation of Canine Hepatocytes

Isolation of canine hepatocytes was performed as previously described [28] with few modifications. Liver samples (25 gms) from freshly euthanized dogs were placed in PBS containing 1% penicillin/streptomycin, finely minced, washed a couple of times with PBS, and transferred into 100 mL of cold collagenase solution (Collagenase II, 300 units/mg, 500 ng/mL in hank's balanced salt solution (HBSS)-Hepes buffer) and stirred for 10 min. At the end of incubation, 10 mL of FBS and 50 mL of ice cold HBSS were added. The suspension was filtered through a cell strainer (100 micron pore size) and the filtrate was centrifuged at 50 *g* for 5 min at 4 °C. The pellet was washed twice with PBS with 1% penicillin/streptomycin and centrifuged twice at 150 *g* for 2 min each and resuspended in 5 mL PBS. The cell suspension was layered over 15 mL cushion of 60% Percoll in PBS and centrifuged at 70 *g* at 4 °C for 5 min. The pellet was washed again with PBS and cell viability was determined by Trypan blue dye exclusion test. The cells were then suspended in DMEM (supplemented with 10% FBS and 1% penicillin/streptomycin) at a density of 0.6 million/mL and incubated at 37 °C for 48 h to acclimatize and form a monolayer. After 48 h the media was replaced by hepatocyte maintenance media (Triangle Research, NC, USA). The maintenance media was changed every day.

2.1.2. Sample Preparation

For this experiment, 10^6 cells were used per sample. The cells were exposed to fresh media (hepatocyte maintenance media for the canine hepatocytes and DMEM supplemented with 10% FBS and 1% penicillin/streptomycin for the canine cell lines 17–71 and GL-1) containing varying concentrations of lomustine, trans-4 or cis-4 metabolites (300, 1000, 3000, 10,000 and 50,000 ng/mL) for 4 h. At the end of 4 h, the DNA was isolated using Qiagen blood mini kit (Qiagen). The extracted DNA was lyophilized and concentrated to 100 µg and then digested as follows: per 50 µL DNA, 10 µL of 0.5 M Tris (pH 7.3), 2 µL of 1 M $MgCl_2$, 10 µL DNAse I (5 mg/mL, 2303 units/mg, Worthington), 10 µL of snake venom phosphatase (5 mg/mL, 36 units/mg, Worthington) and 4 µL of bacterial alkaline phosphatase (5 mg/mL, 35 units/mg, Worthington) was added final volume adjusted to 150 µL with deionized water. The mixture was incubated overnight at 37 °C and then heated to 100 °C for 90 s to inactivate the enzymes. The samples were briefly centrifuged to sediment the proteins and the supernatant was analyzed by LC/MS/MS. For the cell lines, the experiment was done two separate times, with two technical replicates each. For the canine hepatocytes, the experiment was done once with duplicate samples.

The 4 h time point for measuring adducts after drug exposure was based on a published study that looked at DNA alkylation products after exposure to lomustine and adducts were measured between 1 and 6 h. The published results showed that the adducts were formed rapidly and were detected at 1 h after drug exposure [23]. In our initial experimentation, the 1 h samples showed very low adduct level at the 10,000 ng and 50,000 ng concentrations and no adducts were detected at the lower drug concentrations. Even in the 4 h samples, the adducts were only detected at the 10,000 ng and 50,000 ng but the response was greater compared to the 1 h samples. Hence we chose to detect the adducts at 4 h. The N^7 adduct was detected at the concentration of 10,000 ng/mL and above while the mutagenic adduct O^6 hydroxyethyldeoxyguanosine was only detected at 50,000 ng/mL drug concentration. Therefore the 10,000 ng/mL and 50,000 ng/mL concentrations were used to compare the adducts formed by the three drugs.

2.2. LC/MS/MS Method for Detection of DNA Adducts

An LC/MS/MS method was developed to quantify the O^6 hydroxyethyldeoxyguanosine and N^7 hydroxyethylguanine adducts in the DNA samples.

2.2.1. Standards Preparation

Pure standards of O^6 hydroxyethyldeoxyguanosine and N^7 hydroxyethylguanine were purchased from Toronto research company (Toronto, ON, Canada). Deuterated O^6 methylguanine (D3-O^6 methylguanine) was used as internal standard (Sigma Aldrich, St. Louis, MO, USA). Standards were dissolved in methanol to prepare stock solutions. Standard curve range was 0.1–10 ng for each compound and 50 ng of internal standard was added to each sample. The final volume was adjusted to 150 µL with water.

2.2.2. LC/MS/MS Conditions

Samples were analyzed with the QTRAP 5500 LC/MS/MS system (AB Sciex, Foster City, CA, USA) with the 1200 series HPLC system (Agilent Technologies, Santa Clara, CA, USA) including a degasser, an autosampler, and a binary pump. The LC separation was performed on an Agilent SB-Aq column (4.6 mm × 50 mm, 5 µ) (Santa Clara, CA, USA) with mobile phase A (0.1% formic acid in water) and mobile phase B (0.1% formic acid in acetonitrile). The flow-rate was 0.35 mL/min. The linear gradient was as follows: 0–1 min, 100% A; 8–11 min, 25% A; 12–18 min, 100% A.

The autosampler was set at 5 °C and the injection volume is 5 µL. Positive mass spectrometry was achieved with electrospray ionization (ESI). The ion spray voltage was 5500 V. The source temperature was 400 °C. The curtain gas, ion source gas 1, and ion source gas 2 were 32, 65, and 50, respectively. Multiple reaction monitoring (MRM) was used to quantify O^6 hydroxyethyldeoxyguanosine (m/z 312.2 àm/z 110.1), N^7 hydroxyethylguanine (m/z 196.1 àm/z 110.1), and the internal standard deuterated O^6 methylguanine (m/z 169.1 àm/z 70.1) (Figure 1).

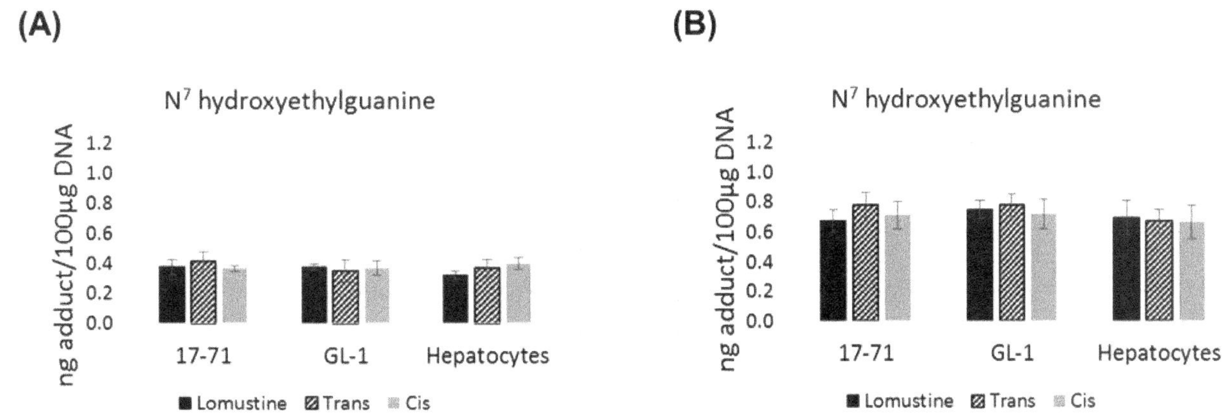

Figure 1. Graphs showing the N^7 hydroxyethylguanine adduct formed after treatment with lomustine, trans-4-hydroxylomustine and cis-4-hydroxylomustine metabolites at 10,000 ng/mL (**A**) and 50,000 ng/mL (**B**) concentration in 17–71 and GL-1 cells and hepatocytes from 6 dogs ($n = 6$).

2.3. Carbamylation Assay

Carbamylation was measured in primary hepatocytes harvested from six dogs euthanized at the Champaign county animal control facility (hepatocyte isolation procedure as mentioned above) and canine cell lines 17–71 and GL-1 after treatment with lomustine and its metabolites using Oxyselect™ carbamylation ELISA kit.

Cells were counted and 10^6 cells were used per sample. The cells were exposed to fresh media (hepatocyte maintenance media for the canine hepatocytes and DMEM supplemented with 10% FBS and 1% penicillin/spreptomycin for the canine cell lines 17-71 and GL-1) containing varying concentrations of lomustine, trans-4 or cis-4 metabolites (300, 1000, 3000 and 10,000 ng/mL). Carbamylation was measured at 4 h after exposure to drugs as per the ELISA kit instructions. Carbamylation is a rapid process occurring within a few minutes and previously published studies have measured carbamylation at similar time points (2, 19). Initial experimentation did not show any carbamylation at 300, 1000 and 3000 ng/mL drug concentration. Thus 10,000 ng/mL concentration was used to compare the carbamylation effects of the three drugs. For the cell lines, the experiment was done two separate times, with two technical replicates each. For the canine hepatocytes, the experiment was done once with duplicate samples.

2.4. MGMT mRNA Expression in 17–71 and GL-1 Cells and Canine Primary Hepatocytes

The canine cell lines 17–71 and GL-1 were grown and maintained at 37 °C in 5% CO_2, and cultures were passaged as necessary to maintain high cell viability (above 90%) in culture media DMEM supplemented with 10% FBS and 1% penicillin/streptomycin. For the MGMT gene induction study, MGMT gene expression was measured in canine cells at 6, 12, 24 and 48 h after exposure to varying concentrations of lomustine (1000, 3000 and 12,000 ng/mL) to study MGMT induction. The cells were only treated with 12,000 ng/mL concentration of trans-4 and cis-4, based on the initial results obtained after lomustine treatment study. Untreated samples were used to measure basal MGMT mRNA expression in these cells. Hepatocytes were isolated from six dogs euthanized at the Champaign county animal control facility.

MGMT mRNA Expression Assay

The total RNA from samples was extracted using RNeasy mini kit (Qiagen). Relative expression levels of the MGMT gene was carried out using Taqman Real-Time quantitative real-time polymerase chain reaction (RT-PCR (QPCR)) analysis on an ABI Prism 7500 thermal cycler. An ABI canine MGMT specific Taqman probe (cf02626419_m1) spanning the exon 1/2 junction was used for all analyses. HPRT-1 was used as internal reference for normalization (ABI Taqman probe cf02626258_m1). For this analysis, 1 µg aliquot of total RNA from a given sample was converted to cDNA using Superscript III first strand synthesis system (Life technologies, Carlsbad, CA, USA). The resulting cDNA was used in separate Taqman QPCR analyses, each including triplicate technical repeats. Expression comparisons was made between treated and untreated (control) samples and also between different cell types. The mRNA expression was measured two separate times in all samples (canine cell lines and hepatocytes) with two technical replicates each time. In order to ascertain that the Taqman assay is able to detect the gene expression correctly, MGMT gene expression was measured in three canine glioma cell lines J3T-Bg, SDT-3 and G06A.

2.5. MGMT Enzyme Activity in 17–71 and GL-1 Cells and Canine Hepatocytes

A fluorometric oligonucleotide assay was used for measuring MGMT enzyme activity [29]. The following 18 base pair (bp) 5'hexachlorofluoroscein phosphoramitide (HEX) labelled oligonucleaotide (oligo) containing O^6-methylguanine lesion within a *Pvu*II restriction site and its complementary oligo were custom made (Sigma Aldrich).

Hex labeled oligo: 5'HEX-GCCCGGCCAGCTGCAGTT
Complementary oligo: 3'-CGGGCCGGTCGACGTCAA

*Pvu*II restriction site

G = O^6 methylguanine

Oligonucleotide strands were annealed to complementary strands in 10 mM Tris–HCl, 1 mM EDTA, 33 mM NaCl, pH 8.0, by heating to 90 °C for 2 min to denature and cooling to room temperature overnight. The 17–71 and GL-1 cells and hepatocytes were maintained in culture media as mentioned above. Cells (10^6) were harvested and resuspended in serum-containing culture medium (DMEM), then centrifuged at 1500 *g* for 5 min.

The cells were washed with 10 mL of PBS and recentrifuged, then resuspended in 0.5 mL assay buffer (50 mM Tris–HCl, 1 mM DTT, 0.5 mM EDTA, 5% glycerol, pH 8.0) and kept on ice. Protein from cells was extracted by pulse-sonication on ice five times for 5 seconds each, then centrifuged at 14,000 *g* at 4 °C for 30 min. The total protein was quantitated by measuring absorbance at 595 nm using the Pierce bicinchoninic acid (BCA) kit reagent. To measure the MGMT activity the 200 fmols of HEX labeled oligo was incubated with cell protein (500 µg) at 37 °C for 2 h. The oligo was extracted by phenol:chloroform:isoamyl alcohol (25:24:1) extraction and using sodium acetate and ethanol with tRNA (10 μg) as a carrier. This was vortex mixed for 5 s and then centrifuged at 12,000 g for 5 min at room temperature. The upper aqueous phase was transferred to a new tube and the purified oligo was digested with a restriction enzyme *Pvu*II (Promega) for 2 h in a total reaction mixture of 20 μL following manufacturer's instructions. *Pvu*II cleaves the oligo at the O^6-methylguanine lesion producing two short fragments (10 bp and 8 bp). After adding formamide loading buffer (10 μL), the samples were denatured by heating at 95 °C for 5 min. Sample solutions (15 μL) were applied to a pre-warmed 20% polyacrylamide gel containing 8 M urea in 1× Tris–borate EDTA (TBE) buffer and run at 50 mA for 15 min. Detection and quantitation of the fluorescent HEX labeled oligonucleotides was done by using a fluorescent imaging system (Typhoon 9410 Variable Mode Imager).

The MGMT enzyme activity was quantified by comparing the intensity of the bands (18 bp) between the *Pvu*II treated and *Pvu*II nontreated (control) samples. The MGMT activity was calculated by comparing the intensity (density volume obtained from the fluorescent reader) of the top band (18 bp) in the samples with that in the controls. The density of the control band was considered as 100%. The deficit in intensity in the sample bands compared to the control bands represents the amount of cleavage which corresponds to the MGMT enzyme activity. For the cell lines and hepatocytes, the experiment was done with duplicate samples.

For measuring the lower limit of detection (LOD) and limit of quantitation (LOQ) of the method, serial dilution of the HEX labelled oligo was made from 1–200 fmols in deionized water and the fluorescent intensity was measured and plotted against the oligo concentration. The lowest concentration showing 3 times the fluorescent intensity compared to the blank sample was chosen as the LOD and the lowest concentration with CV less than or equal to 15% was chosen as the LOQ of the method.

3. Statistical Analysis

Statistical analysis was done using SPSS (IBM, Armonk, NY, USA). Descriptive statistics were produced for all continuous variables. Mean and standard deviation were calculated. Normality of data was assessed using the Shapiro-Wilks test. For alkylating and carbamylation assays, paired *t*-tests were performed to evaluate differences between technical repeats of each drug and one way ANOVA and Tukey's post hoc test were performed to evaluate the between drug differences. Kruskal-Wallis one way ANOVA was used to compare the means of the drug treated and non-treated groups at different time points in the MGMT gene induction study. Correlation between MGMT mRNA expression and enzyme activity was evaluated by Pearson's correlation. The p value was set at 0.05.

4. Results

There is no statistically significant difference in the levels of N^7 hydroxyethylguanine and O^6 hydroxyethyldeoxyguanosine adducts formed by lomustine, trans-4 or cis-4. The N^7 hydroxyethylguanine adduct was detected at similar level in 17–71, GL-1 and the hepatocytes from six dogs after exposure to lomustine, trans-4 and cis-4 at 10,000 ng/mL and 50,000 ng/mL concentration (Figure 1). However the mutagenic adduct O^6 hydroxyethyldeoxyguanosine was detected at a significantly lower level in the hepatocytes (2–3 fold) as compared to the cell lines when treated with the three drugs at 50,000 ng/mL concentration (Figure 2).

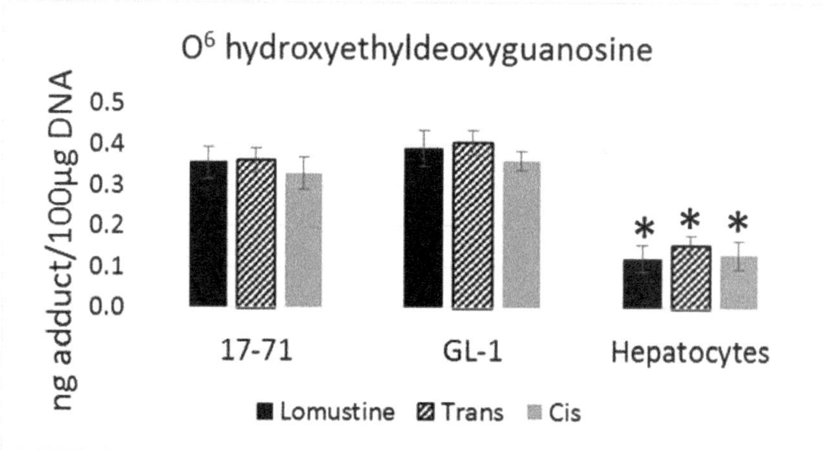

Figure 2. Graph showing the O^6 hydroxyethyldeoxyguanosine adduct formed after treatment with lomustine, trans-4-hydroxylomustine and cis-4-hydroxylomustine metabolites at 50,000 ng/mL concentration in 17–71 and GL-1 cells and hepatocytes from six dogs ($n = 6$). * denotes statistical significance as compared to the 17–71 and GL-1 cells. $p = 0.05$.

In the canine cell lines 17–71 and GL-1 and in the canine hepatocyte samples, lomustine caused significantly greater carbamylation as compared to its metabolites (Figure 3). Both the metabolites showed similar carbamylation levels. In all the six canine hepatocyte samples tested, the carbamylation caused by all the three drugs was 1.5–2 fold greater than that seen in 17–71 and GL-1 cells. Among the six dog hepatocyte samples, two dogs showed about 2 fold higher level of carbamylation compared to the others with lomustine, trans-4 and cis-4.

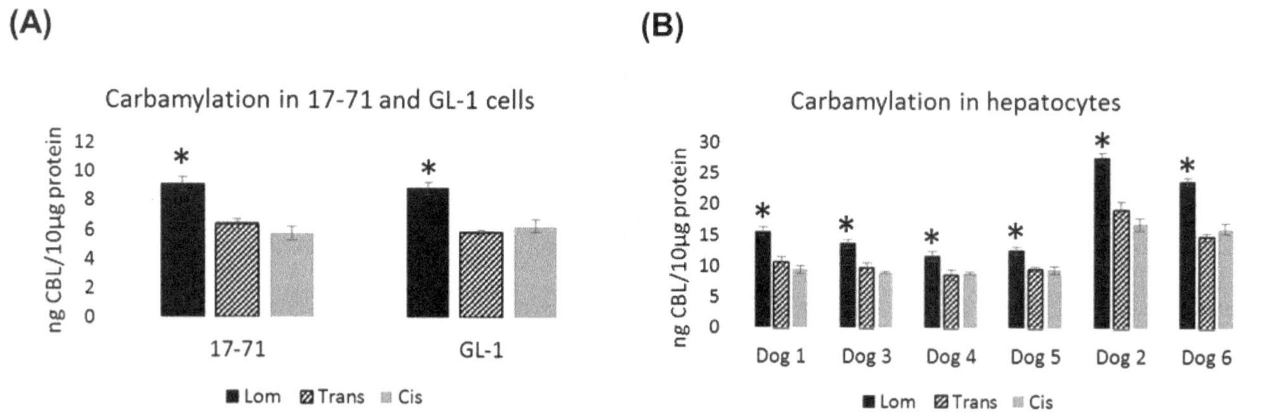

Figure 3. Graphs showing the carbamylation induced by lomustine, trans-4-hydroxylomustine and cis-4-hydroxylomustine at 10,000 ng/mL concentration in 17–71 and GL-1 cells (**A**) and hepatocytes from six dogs (**B**). * indicates statistical significance compared to trans-4-hydroxylomustine and cis-4-hydroxylomustine. $p = 0.05$.

GL-1 cells did not show any MGMT mRNA expression in untreated samples. When GL-1 samples were treated with lomustine, trans-4 and cis-4 at 1000, 3000 and 12,000 ng/mL and incubated for 12, 24 and 48 h, still no MGMT mRNA expression was detected. In the 17–71 cells, a low basal level of MGMT expression was seen in the untreated samples (Figure 4). Upon treatment with various concentrations of lomustine, trans-4 and cis-4 and incubated for different time points, no statistically significant difference was seen in any of the drug treated samples at any time point as compared to the vehicle control (Figures 4 and 5).

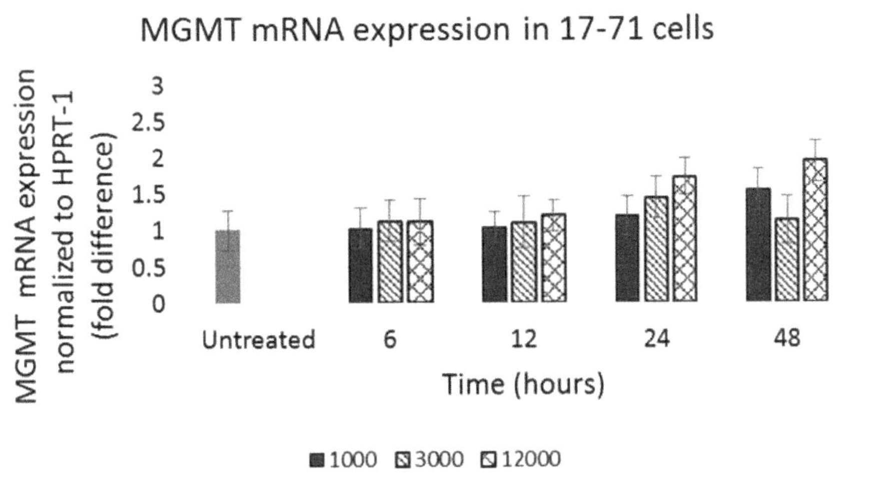

Figure 4. Graph showing MGMT mRNA expression in 17–71 cells before (untreated) and after treatment with lomustine at 1000, 3000 and 12,000 ng/mL and incubated for 6, 12, 24 and 48 h.

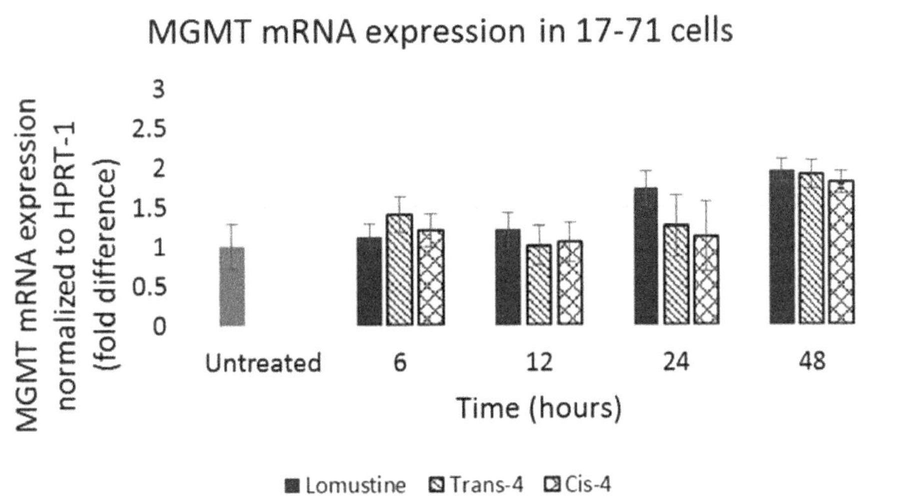

Figure 5. Graph showing MGMT mRNA expression in 17–71 cells before (untreated) and after treatment with trans-4-hydroxylomustine and cis-4 hydroxylomustine at 12,000 ng/mL concentration and incubated for 6, 12, 24 and 48 h.

The MGMT gene expression measured in the hepatocytes of the six dogs was 2-3 fold greater than that seen in the 17–71 cells (Figure 6). The variation in MGMT mRNA expression among the six dogs was low except for one dog which showed a lower MGMT level. Two of the glioma cell lines SDT-3 and J3G-Bg showed high MGMT mRNA expression (see supplemental data). The results show that the Taqman qPCR assay is able to detect higher transcript levels of MGMT gene and that the previously measured low MGMT gene expressions in 17–71 cells are indeed true values.

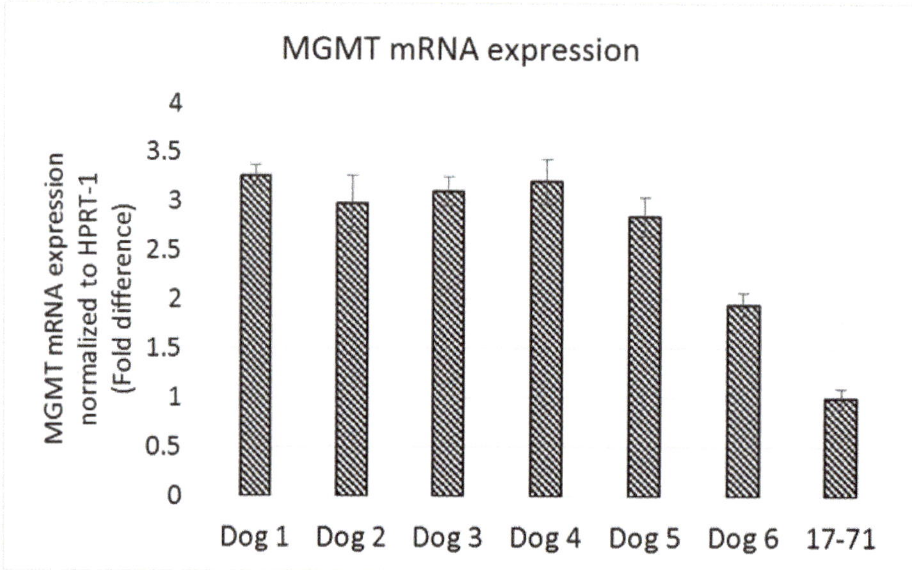

Figure 6. Graphs showing the MGMT mRNA expression in canine lymphoma cell line 17–71 cells and primary hepatocytes from six dogs.

The LOD of the fluorometric MGMT enzyme activity assay was 5 fmols while the LOQ was 10 fmols (see supplemental data). For GL-1 and 17–71 cell line, using 100 µg and 200 µg of cell protein did not show any MGMT activity. In order to ascertain the functionality of the assay, human recombinant MGMT (Cayman chemicals) was used as a positive control. The results showed that with increasing concentration of MGMT, greater cleavage of the oligo was seen (see supplemental data). Thus the protein amount in the assay was increased to 500 µg and in the 17–71 samples showed visible cleavage of the oligo (Figure 7A). The GL-1 cell lines did not show any MGMT enzyme activity even when 500 µg cell protein was used for the assay.

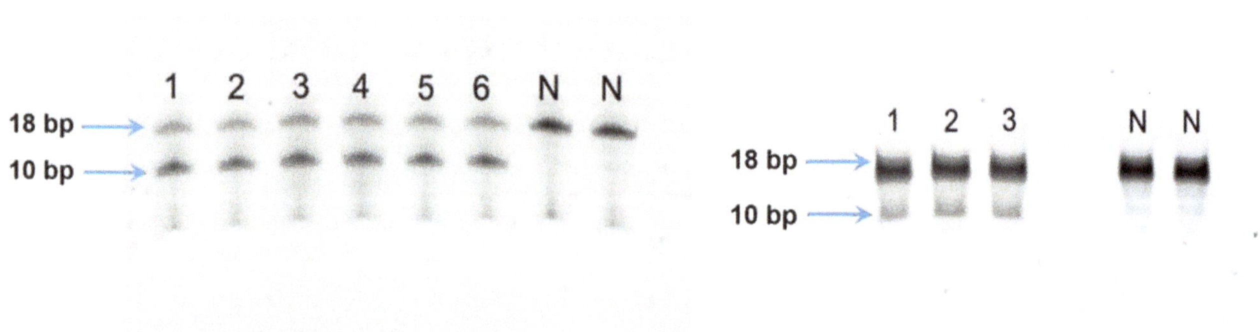

(A) (B)

Figure 7. (**A**) MGMT activity in canine lymphoma cell line 17–71: lanes 1–3 represent replicate oligo samples treated with 500 µg cell protein from 17–71 cells. Lanes labeled "N" are untreated oligo samples (control). Upper and lower bands represent 18 bp substrate and 10 bp cleavage product, respectively; (**B**) MGMT activity in primary hepatocytes obtained from six dogs: lanes 1–6 represent oligo samples treated with 500 µg cell protein from hepatocytes obtained from six dogs. Lanes labeled "N" are untreated oligo samples (control). Upper and lower bands represent 18 bp substrate and 10 bp cleavage product, respectively.

The MGMT activity in the 17–71 cells was about 90 fmols/mg protein (range 83–96 fmols/mg protein, SD 10.11). In the GL-1 cell line, as no MGMT gene expression was detected, consequently, MGMT enzyme activity was also absent. The enzyme activity measured in the hepatocytes was greater than in 17–71 cells, proportional to the mRNA levels. The MGMT enzyme activity measured in canine hepatocytes is about 250–350 fmols/mg protein (Figures 7B and 8). There was good correlation between MGMT gene expression and enzyme activity in the 17–71 and the canine hepatocytes (Figure 9).

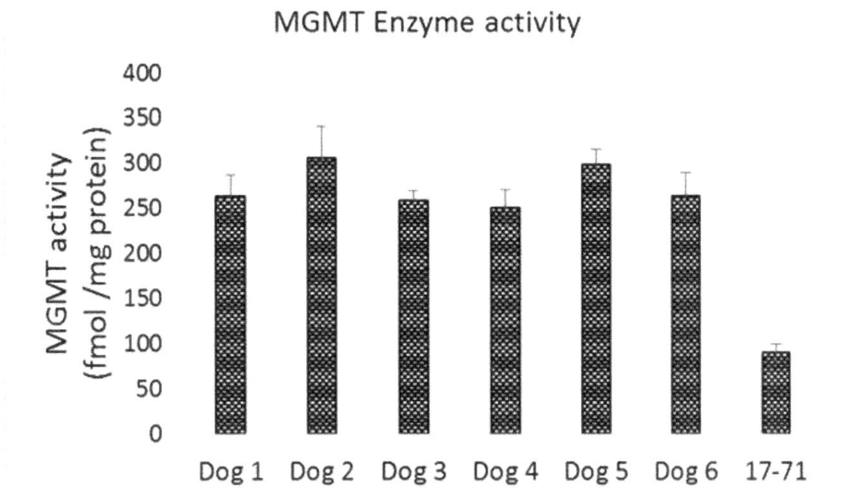

Figure 8. Graph showing MGMT enzyme activity in the primary hepatocytes obtained from six dogs and in the canine lymphoma cell line 17–71.

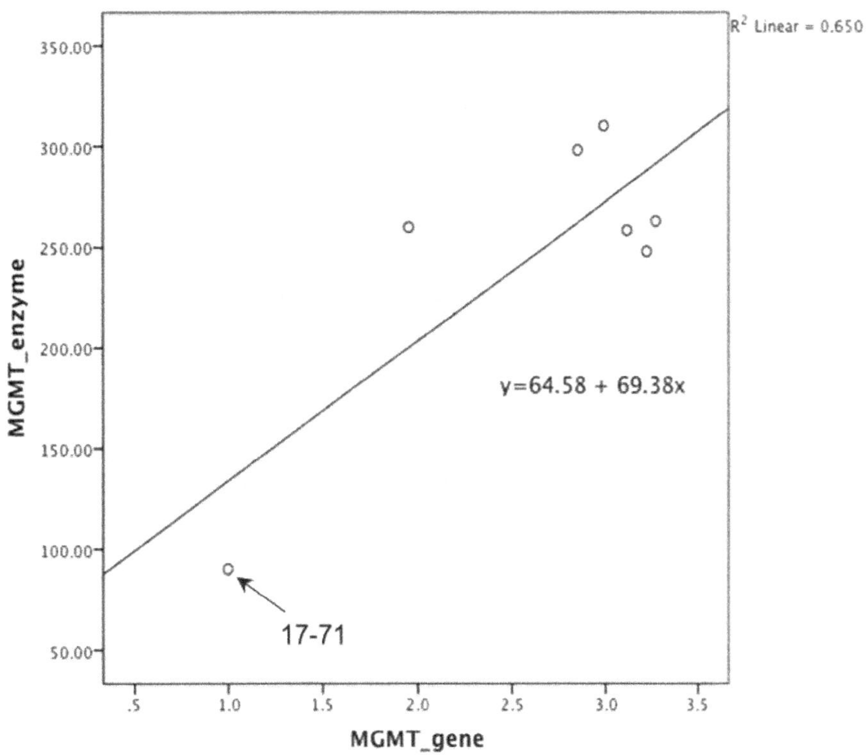

Figure 9. Graph showing correlation between MGMT gene expression and enzyme activity in canine lymphoma cell line 17–71 and the hepatocytes obtained from six dogs. Pearson's correlation was 0.806 which was highly significant with *p* value of 0.028. (*p* value set at 0.05).

5. Discussion

In our study we found no significant difference in the N^7 hydroxyethylguanine and O^6 hydroxyethyldeoxyguanosine adduct level formed by lomustine, trans-4 and cis-4 which correlates with the similar cytotoxicity of these compounds. The mutagenic O^6 adduct was higher in the canine cell lines 17–71 and GL-1 as compared to the hepatocytes which may indicate either lower adduct formation or rapid repair in canine hepatocytes. Rapid repair may be a possibility since all the canine hepatocyte samples showed greater MGMT level. It can be speculated that as MGMT is a DNA repair enzyme, an enhanced repair of O^6 adducts could contribute to the reduced sensitivity of hepatocytes to the alkylating action of lomustine and its metabolites.

It should however be noted that we have only detected the levels of two individual adducts after drug exposure. The cell killing action of nitrosoureas may be orchestrated by the formation and cumulative action of multiple adducts that these drugs are capable of forming. Also, in case of chloroethylating agents like lomustine, cross linking of DNA is known to be harmful lesion that can lead to double stand breaks and ultimately apoptosis [13]. Thus in our alkylation study, measuring the two adducts can act only as a molecular dosimeter of therapeutic response and not a measure of the full extent of alkylation caused by the drugs.

Carbamylation was measured in the canine lymphoma cell lines and hepatocytes by an ELISA kit. The assay measures the amount of CBL in the samples. Our results show that lomustine causes greater carbamylation as compared to its metabolites in canine cell lines and hepatocytes. All the three compounds caused greater carbamylation in hepatocytes as compared to the canine cell lines. Also hepatocyte samples from two dogs showed greater carbamylation following treatment with lomustine and its metabolites compared to the others. But it should be noted that all of the dog hepatocyte samples showed no cytotoxicity to lomustine or its metabolites up to six days of incubation. Hence it is unlikely that greater carbamylation in the hepatocytes in the two dogs would lead to cell death in our experiments, although it may be inhibiting various proteins in these cells. The same would also hold true for the cell lines 17–71 and GL-1 where we see lower carbamylation but greater cytotoxicity after treatment with the drugs.

Even though the hepatocyte samples showed greater carbamylation than the cell lines it is not known if this is of clinical relevance with regards to hepatotoxicity caused by lomustine since carbamylation levels have not been measured in dogs that show hepatotoxicity after lomustine treatment. Carbamylation of proteins may interfere with the proper functioning or replication of the cells which may not necessarily result in cell death. It has also been shown that nitrosoureas which form isocyanates are particularly able to inhibit the polymerization of purified brain tubulin in a dose dependent manner [30]. In a study where rats were given lomustine by oral gavage at 50 mg/kg dose, and sacrificed at different time points, the hepatocytes remained normal at early time points although the bile canaliculi became dilated and contained bile thrombi [31]. In another study in rats that were administered lomustine at 20 mg/kg, hepatocytes were not markedly altered with normal nuclei and cell organelles. The main alteration of the parenchymal cells occurred after the 6th day with modification of the cytoskeletal components and reduction in number of microtubules [32]. It is suggested that the isocyanates carbamylate tubulin in hepatocytes leading to mitotic spindle inhibition and G2 cell cycle arrest or may cause disruption of secretory functions such as bile secretion which in turn results in cholestasis and secondary hepatic injury [32,33]. Thus carbamylation of proteins may not necessarily manifest as immediate cell killing.

For the MGMT gene expression studies, HPRT-1 was used as an endogenous control. Before measuring the MGMT expression, we studied the suitability of HPRT-1 as endogenous control in the canine cell lines and liver samples based on the cycle number (cT). HPRT-1 was always measured within 0.5 cT. We understand that the most accurate way of testing HPRT-1 would be by using another endogenous control and that the cT values may be affected by pipetting errors. However, HPRT-1 has a high cT value (above 26), and so these errors would have minimal effect on the cT value.

The canine lymphoma cell line 17–71 showed low MGMT mRNA expression and enzyme activity (about 90 fmols/mg protein). MGMT activity data from humans show that similar level of activity is seen in brain tissue (about 100 fmols/mg protein) which is one of the organs expressing the lowest level of MGMT activity in the body [17]. The GL-1 cells did not show any detectable MGMT mRNA expression or enzyme activity. It has been reported that while MGMT is expressed in all normal human cell types and tissues, 20%–30% of human tumor or more than 50% of virally transformed cell lines are completely deficient in MGMT expression [33,34]. It is not clear yet if the process of immortalization may be leading to loss of MGMT expression [35]. It is known that lack of expression is not due to deletion of the gene [36] and may possibly be an epigenetic event [37,38].

MGMT induction is known to result from transcriptional activation of the MGMT gene in response to DNA damage [39]. In our gene induction study, the 17–71 cells did not show any significant increase in gene expression after 48 h of exposure to lomustine and its metabolites, while the GL-1 cells still did not show any detectable gene expression at all. Time dependent expression of MGMT gene has been measured after exposure to different types of DNA damages including X-ray treatment and methylating agents, and the maximum induction (2–5 fold) was seen at 24 to 72 h [37]. A major limitation of our MGMT gene expression study is the lack of appropriate positive and negative controls. However we believe that this limitation may be offset by the multiple number of technical replicates used and independent experiments performed.

The hepatocytes obtained from the six dogs showed a 2–3 fold greater MGMT mRNA expression as compared to the canine cell line 17–71. The MGMT enzyme activity measured in the hepatocytes is about 250–350 fmol/mg protein as compared to 90 fmol/mg protein in 17–71 cells. This indicates a positive correlation between the MGMT mRNA expression and the enzyme activity in the canine cell lines and the hepatocytes. In Figure 9, it can be noted that the positive correlation between MGMT gene expression and enzyme activity is due mostly to the point corresponding to the 17–71 cells. This data should be considered as preliminary and the correlation can be strengthened by studying the MGMT levels in more dogs/canine cells. Data from humans also suggest that MGMT activity corresponds with the MGMT protein and RNA level [17]. The average MGMT activity in human liver is reported to be around 600 fmol/mg protein, however there is wide inter-individual variation [17,40]. In our MGMT activity assay in hepatocytes, there was over 70% enzymatic cleavage of the substrate oligo (Figure 7). This may indicate a sub-optimal enzyme-substrate ratio which could lead to a lower rate of reaction. It is suggested that enzyme reactions be conducted under initial rate conditions with total consumption of substrate less than 20% [41]. Hence it is possible that the MGMT activity measured in the canine hepatocytes in our study is lower than the actual values.

In our previous study, we have shown that lomustine and its metabolites showed a time and concentration dependent toxicity in canine lymphoma cell lines 17–71 and GL-1 [22]. However the canine hepatocytes did not show any detectable cell killing even 6 days after exposure to the drugs. When the toxic O^6

guanine adduct was measured in the cells after exposure to lomustine and the metabolites, the canine cell lines showed higher levels of the adduct as compared to the hepatocytes. It is known that MGMT directly repairs the O^6 adducts in a rapid stoichiometric reaction. In our MGMT study, we saw that the hepatocytes had 2–3 fold greater enzyme activity compared to the 17–71 cell line. Correlating all this data together it is plausible that higher MGMT enzyme activity may be a reason for the lower levels of O^6 adducts detected in the hepatocyte samples. The higher level of MGMT may cause repair of adducts, and hence contributing to the lower cytotoxicity of lomustine and its metabolites in hepatocytes. However this interpretation must be viewed with caution, as no significant difference in the O^6 adduct levels between 17–71 cells and GL-1 cells was noted even though we were unable to detect any MGMT activity in the GL-1 cells. Also lomustine and its metabolites form multiple adducts at the O^6 guanine position out of which we chose the O^6 hydroxyethyldeoxyguanosine as a marker or indicator of the genotoxic potential of the compounds. It should be noted that MGMT is only one of the several ways in which alkylation damage in DNA is repaired by the cell. Other pathways such as base excision repair and mismatch repair are also known to repair damaged DNA depending on the stage and type of the damage. Thus it may also be possible that the lower O^6 hydroxyethyldeoxyguanosine measured in the hepatocytes may be due to lower formation or a DNA repair mechanism other than MGMT.

6. Conclusions

In this study, we show that lomusine and its metabolites form similar levels of the DNA adducts N^7 hydroxyethylguanine and O^6 hydroxyethyldeoxyguanosine which corresponds to the similar cytotoxicity of these compounds. In terms of carbamylation, lomustine showed greater carbamylation in the canine hepatocytes and lymphoma cell lines. Thus if carbamylation of proteins is indeed one of the reasons for the side effects of lomustine, then using the metabolites instead may be a better therapeutic option. Additionally, we also show that MGMT mRNA expression in 17–71 cells and canine hepatocytes correlates with the MGMT enzyme activity in these cells.

Acknowledgment

This study was supported by the University of Illinois at Urbana-Champaign Research Board as the Arnold O. Beckman Research Award.

Authors Contributions

All the authors included in this study contributed to study design, data analysis, sample collection and manuscript preparation.

Abbreviations

BCA	Bicinchoninic acid
bp	Base pair
CBL	Carbamylated lysine
Cis-4	Cis-4-hydroxylomustine
DMEM	Dulbecco's modified Eagle medium
ELISA	Enzyme-linked immunosorbent assay

FBS	Fetal bovine serum
HEX	Hexachloro-fluorescein
LC/MS/MS	Liquid chromatography-tandem mass spectrometry
MGMT	O^6methylguanine DNA methyltransferase
MRM	Multiple reaction monitoring
Oligo	Oligonucleaotide
PBMC	Peripheral blood mononuclear cells
PBS	Phosphate buffered saline
RT-PCR	Real time polymerase chain reaction
SD	Standard deviation
Trans-4	Trans-4-hydroxylomustine

Conflict of Interest

The authors declare no conflict of interest.

References

1. Montgomery, J.; James, R.; McCaleb, G.; Johnston, T. The modes of decomposition of 1,3-bis(2-chloroethyl)-1-nitrosourea and related compounds. *J. Med. Chem.* **1967**, *10*, 668–674.
2. Wheeler, G.; Bowdon, B.; Grimsley, J.; Lloyd, H. Interrelationships of some chemical, physicochemical, and biological activities of several 1-(2-haloethyl)-1-nitrosoureas. *Cancer Res.* **1974**, *34*, 194–200.
3. Ludlum, D. DNA alkylation by the haloethylnitrosoureas—Nature of modifications produced and their enzymatic repair or removal. *Mutat. Res.* **1990**, *233*, 117–126.
4. Boysen, G.; Pachkowski, B.F.; Nakamura, J.; Swenberg, J.A. The formation and biological significance of N7-guanine adducts. *Mutat. Res. Genet. Toxicol. Environ. Mutagen.* **2009**, *678*, 76–94.
5. Sedgwick, B. Repairing DNA-methylation damage. *Nat. Rev. Mol. Cell Biol.* **2004**, *5*, 148–157.
6. Rinne, M.L.; He, Y.; Pachkowski, B.F.; Nakamura, J.; Kelley, M.R. *N*-methylpurine DNA glycosylase overexpression increases alkylation sensitivity by rapidly removing non-toxic 7-methylguanine adducts. *Nucleic Acids Rese.* **2005**, *33*, 2859–2867.
7. Beranek, D. Distribution of methyl and ethyl adducts following alkylation with monofunctional alkylating-agents. *Mutat. Res.* **1990**, *231*, 11–30.
8. Singer, B. *In vivo* formation and persistence of modified nucleosides resulting from alkylating agents. *Environ. Health Perspect.* **1985**, *62*, 41.
9. Kaina, B. DNA damage-triggered apoptosis: Critical role of DNA repair, double-strand breaks, cell proliferation and signaling. *Biochem. Pharmacol.* **2003**, *66*, 1547–1554.
10. Colvin, M.; Brundrett, R.; Cowens, W.; Jardine, I.; Ludlum, D. A chemical basis for the antitumor activity of chloroethylnitrosoureas. *Biochem. Pharmacol.* **1976**, *25*, 695.
11. Weinkam, R.; Liu, T.; Lin, H. Protein mediated chemical-reactions of chloroethylnitrosoureas. *Chem. Biol. Interact.* **1980**, *31*, 167–177.
12. Wheeler, G.; Bowdon, B.; Struck, R. Carbamoylation of amino acid, peptides, and proteins by nitrosoureas. *Cancer Res.* **1975**, *35*, 2974.

13. Lemoine, A.; Lucas, C.; Ings, R.M.J. Metabolism of the chloroethylnitrosoureas. *Xenobiotica* **1991**, *21*, 775–791.
14. Jaisson, S.; Pietrement, C.; Gillery, P. Carbamylation-derived products: Bioactive compounds and potential biomarkers in chronic renal failure and atherosclerosis. *Clin. Chem.* **2011**, *57*, 1499–1505.
15. Kaina, B.; Christmann, M.; Naumann, S.; Roos, W.P. MGMT: Key node in the battle against genotoxicity, carcinogenicity and apoptosis induced by alkylating agents. *DNA Repair* **2007**, *6*, 1079–1099.
16. Gerson, S. Clinical relevance of MGMT in the treatment of cancer. *J. Clin. Oncol.* **2002**, *20*, 2388–2399.
17. Christmann, M.; Verbeek, B.; Roos, W.P.; Kaina, B. O-6-methylguanine-DNA methyltransferase (MGMT) in normal tissues and tumors: Enzyme activity, promoter methylation and immunohistochemistry. *Biochim. Biophys. Acta-Rev. Cancer* **2011**, *1816*, 179–190.
18. Janssen, K.; Eichhorn-Grombacher, U.; Schlink, K.; Nitzsche, S.; Oesch, F.; Kaina, B. Long-time expression of DNA repair enzymes MGMT and APE in human peripheral blood mononuclear cells. *Arch. Toxicol.* **2001**, *75*, 306–312.
19. Maze, R.; Carney, J.P.; Kelley, M.R.; Glassner, B.J.; Williams, D.A.; Samson, L. Increasing DNA repair methyltransferase levels via bone marrow stem cell transduction rescues mice from the toxic effects of 1,3-bis(2-chloroethyl)-1-nitrosourea, a chemotherapeutic alkylating agent. *Proc. Natl. Acad. Sci. USA* **1996**, *93*, 206–210.
20. Grombacher, T.; Kaina, B. Constitutive expression and inducibility of O6-methylguanine-DNA methyltransferase and *N*-methylpurine-DNA glycosylase in rat liver cells exhibiting different status of differentiation. *Biochim. Biophys. Acta (BBA)* **1995**, *1270*, 63–72.
21. Grombacher, T.; Mitra, S.; Kaina, B. Induction of the alkyltransferase (MGMT) gene by DNA damaging agents and the glucocorticoid dexamethasone and comparison with the response of base excision repair genes. *Carcinogenesis* **1996**, *17*, 2329–2336.
22. Chakkath, C.; Lavergne, S.N.; Fan, T.M.; Bunick, D.; Dirikolu, L. Preliminary metabolism of lomustine in dogs and comparative cytotoxicity of lomustine and its major metabolites in canine cells. *Vet. Sci.* **2014**, *1*, 159–173.
23. Bodell, W.J. DNA alkylation products formed by 1-(2-chloroethyl)-1-nitrosourea as molecular dosimeters of therapeutic response. *J. Neuro Oncol.* **2009**, *91*, 257–264.
24. Wheeler, G.; Johnston, T.; Bowdon, B.; McCaleb, G.; Hill, D.; Montgomery, J. Comparison of the properties of metabolites of CCNU. *Biochem. Pharmacol.* **1977**, *26*, 2331.
25. Heal, J.M.; Fox, P.A.; Doukas, D.; Schein, P.S. Biological and biochemical properties of 2-hydroxyl metabolites of 1–2-chloroethyl)-3-cyclohexyl-1-nitrosourea. *Cancer Res.* **1978**, *38*, 1070–1074.
26. Nakaichi, M.; Taura, Y.; Kanki, M.; Mamba, K.; Momoi, Y.; Tsujimoto, H.; Nakama, S. Establishment and characterization of a new canine B-cell leukemia cell line. *J. Vet. Med. Sci.* **1996**, *58*, 469–471.
27. Steplewski, Z.; Jeglum, K.A.; Rosales, C.; Weintraub, N. Canine lymphoma-associated antigens defined by murine monoclonal antibodies. *Cancer Immunol. Immunother.* **1987**, *24*, 197–201.
28. Spotorno, V.G.; Hidalgo, A.; Barbich, M.; Lorenti, A.; Zabal, O. Culture of bovine hepatocytes: A non-perfusion technique for cell isolation. *Cytotechnology* **2006**, *51*, 51–56.

29. Kreklau, E.; Limp-Foster, M.; Liu, N.; Xu, Y.; Kelley, M.; Erickson, L. A novel fluorometric oligonucleotide assay to measure O-6-methylguanine DNA methyltransferase, methylpurine DNA glycosylase, 8-oxoguanine DNA glycosylase and abasic endonuclease activities: DNA repair status in human breast carcinoma cells overexpressing methylpurine DNA glycosylase. *Nucleic Acids Res.* **2001**, *29*, 2558–2566.
30. Ducastelle, T.; Raguenezviotte, G.; Fouinfortunet, H.; Matysiak, M.; Hemet, J.; Fillastre, J. The hepatotoxicity of 1-(2-chloroethyl)-3-cyclohexyl-1-nitrosourea (CCNU) in rats—Ultrastructural evidence of a delayed microtubular toxicity. *Cancer Chemother. Pharmacol.* **1988**, *22*, 153–162.
31. Day, R.; Ziolkowski, C.; Scudiero, D.; Meyer, S.; Lubiniecki, A.; Girardi, A.; Bynum, G. Defective repair of alkylated DNA by human-tumor and Sv40-transformed human cell strains. *Nature* **1980**, *288*, 724–727.
32. Tsujimura, T.; Zhang, Y.; Fujio, C.; Chang, H.; Watatani, M.; Ishizaki, K.; Ikenaga, M. O-6-methylguanine methyltransferase activity and sensitivity of japanese tumor-cell strains to 1-(4-amino-2-methyl-5-pyrimidinyl)methyl-3-(2-chloroethyl)-3-nitrosourea hydrochloride. *Jpn. J. Cancer Res.* **1987**, *78*, 1207–1215.
33. Harris, L.; vonWronski, M.; Venable, C.; Remack, J.; Howell, S.; Brent, T. Changes in O-6-methylguanine-DNA methyltransferase expression during immortalization of cloned human fibroblasts. *Carcinogenesis* **1996**, *17*, 219–224.
34. Tano, K.; Shiota, S.; Collier, J.; Foote, R.; Mitra, S. Isolation and structural characterization of a cDNA clone encoding the human DNA-repair protein for O-6-alkylguanine. *Proc. Natl. Acad. Sci. USA* **1990**, *87*, 686–690.
35. Cairnssmith, S.; Karran, P. Epigenetic silencing of the DNA repair enzyme O(6)-methylguanine-DNA methyltransferase in Mex- human-cells. *Cancer Res.* **1992**, *52*, 5257–5263.
36. Vonwronski, M.; Brent, T. Effect of 5-azacytidine on expression of the human DNA-repair enzyme O-6-methylguanine-DNA methyltransferase. *Carcinogenesis* **1994**, *15*, 577–582.
37. Grombacher, T.; Eichhorn, U.; Kaina, B. p53 is involved in regulation of the DNA repair gene O^6-methylguanine-DNA methyltransferase (MGMT) by DNA damaging agents. *Oncogene* **1998**, *17*, 845–851.
38. Kroes, R.; Erickson, L. The role of messenger-rna stability and transcription in O-6-methylguanine DNA methyltransferase (MGMT) expression in Mer(+) human tumor-cells. *Carcinogenesis* **1995**, *16*, 2255–2257.
39. Pegg, A. Formation and metabolism of alkylated nucleosides: Possible role in carcinogenesis by nitroso compoundsand alkylating agents. In *Advances Cancer Research*; Klein, G., Weinhouse, S., Eds.; Academic Press: New York, NY, USA, 1977; p. 195.
40. Margison, G.P.; Povey, A.C.; Kaina, B.; Santibanez Koref, M.F. Variability and regulation of O6-alkylguanine-DNA alkyltransferase. *Carcinogenesis* **2003**, *24*, 625–635.
41. Wenham, D.; Illy, C.; St. Pierre, J.A.; Bouchard, N. Development of high throughput screening assays for kinase drug targets using Alphascreen technology. In *Handbook of Assay Development in Drug Discovery*; Manor, L.K., Ed.; Academic Press CRC: London, UK, 2006; p. 56.

16

Review of Animal Models of Prostate Cancer Bone Metastasis

Jessica K. Simmons [1], Said M. Elshafae [1], Evan T. Keller [2], Laurie K. McCauley [3] and Thomas J. Rosol [1,*]

[1] Department of Veterinary Biosciences, The Ohio State University, 1925 Coffey Road, Columbus, OH 43210, USA; E-Mails: simmons.379@osu.edu (J.K.S.); elshafae.1@osu.edu (S.M.E.)

[2] Department of Pathology and Unit for Laboratory Animal Medicine, School of Medicine, University of Michigan, Ann Arbor, MI 48109, USA; E-Mail: etkeller@med.umich.edu

[3] Department of Periodontics & Oral Medicine, School of Dentistry, University of Michigan, 1011 N University Avenue, Ann Arbor, MI 48109, USA; E-Mail: mccauley@umich.edu

* Author to whom correspondence should be addressed; E-Mail: rosol.1@osu.edu;

Abstract: Prostate cancer bone metastases are associated with a poor prognosis and are considered incurable. Insight into the formation and growth of prostate cancer bone metastasis is required for development of new imaging and therapeutic strategies to combat this devastating disease. Animal models are indispensable in investigating cancer pathogenesis and evaluating therapeutics. Multiple animal models of prostate cancer bone metastasis have been developed, but few effectively model prostatic neoplasms and osteoblastic bone metastases as they occur in men. This review discusses the animal models that have been developed to investigate prostate cancer bone metastasis, with a focus on canine models and also includes human xenograft and rodent models. Adult dogs spontaneously develop benign prostatic hyperplasia and prostate cancer with osteoblastic bone metastases. Large animal models, such as dogs, are needed to develop new molecular imaging tools and effective focal intraprostatic therapy. None of the available models fully reflect the metastatic disease seen in men, although the various models have provided important insight into the metastatic process. As additional models are developed and knowledge from the different models is combined, the molecular mechanisms of prostate cancer bone metastasis can be deciphered and targeted for development of novel therapies and molecular diagnostic imaging.

Keywords: prostate cancer; bone metastasis; animal models

1. Introduction

Prostate cancer is the most common newly diagnosed cancer in men in the United States and it is estimated to have resulted in 10% of all cancer deaths in men in 2013 [1]. Between 70% and 100% of patients that die due to prostate cancer have bone metastases [2,3]. Patients with skeletal metastases have a five-year survival rate of 25% and median survival of 40 months [4]. The most common sites of bone metastasis in prostate cancer are pelvic bones, vertebral column, ribs, and long bones (primarily femur and humerus) [5,6]. Bone metastases in prostate cancer are primarily osteoblastic, or bone-forming lesions. These metastases result in pain, fractures and nerve compressions that reduce quality of life and represent incurable disease to clinicians [7].

In vivo animal models are the key to understanding the pathogenesis of prostate cancer bone metastasis to develop better therapeutics. The perfect model would include a species with a prostate structurally and functionally similar to humans, have slowly developing disease that progresses through prostatic intra-epithelial neoplasia (PIN), locally invasive carcinoma and late-stage osteoblastic metastasis to the pelvis, vertebrae, ribs, and long bones [8]. No model exists at this time that perfectly recapitulates human disease; however, each available model has its applicability towards particular aspects of bone metastasis. As new models are developed that more fully encompass the spectrum of human prostate cancer bone metastasis, novel strategies for palliative and curative treatments can be developed.

In an effort to accurately replicate different stages of tumor progression and metastasis, multiple injection models have been developed. These include subcutaneous, orthotopic, intracardiac, tail vein, and bone (Figure 1). The injection models can be controversial because they fail to fully recapitulate human disease by eliminating the early stages of carcinogenesis; however, they remain one of the most widely used investigative techniques of cancer until more complete models are developed.

2. Prostate Cancer in Dogs

The dog is the only species other than man to spontaneously develop benign prostatic hyperplasia (BPH) and prostate cancer at a significant incidence [9]. However, even though intact adult male dogs have a high incidence of BPH, they have a low incidence of spontaneous prostate cancer compared to men. One study reported the incidence of prostate cancer to be 0.2% in dogs and 12% in men [10]. Unlike the single-lobed architecture of the human prostate, the canine prostate is bilobed and lacks the differential regions or zones that are characteristic of the human prostate gland (peripheral, transitional, and central zones) [11,12]. All aged, intact male dogs will develop benign prostatic hyperplasia to a variable degree [11]. BPH can be severe enough to cause clinical disease, which includes dorsal compression of the colon and dyschezia. Dysuria is not a typical clinical problem in dogs with BPH compared to men. BPH does not appear to be a preneoplastic condition of the prostate in dogs, similar to men.

Figure 1. Different injection models of prostate cancer to investigate cancer progression and metastasis. The metastatic cascade involves the local invasion of tumor cells from the prostate, intravasation into a blood or lymph vessel, extravasation out of the circulation, and survival and growth at a secondary site (distant metastasis). At this time, metastasis models are not able to recapitulate this process from cancer initiation to metastatic disease. Therefore, different injection models are used to investigate this complex process. Prostatic (orthotopic) injections model invasion, extravasation, and distant metastasis. Intravascular injections (intracardiac, tail vein) model extravasation and metastasis. Tail vein injections tend to favor lung metastases, whereas intracardiac injection of cancer cells into the left ventricle permits cancer cells to localize to any tissue of the body depending on its inherent metastatic phenotype. Finally, intratibial injections model the ability to grow in and modify the bone microenvironment. Together, the different injection models reveal important information about the pathogenesis of the metastatic cascade.

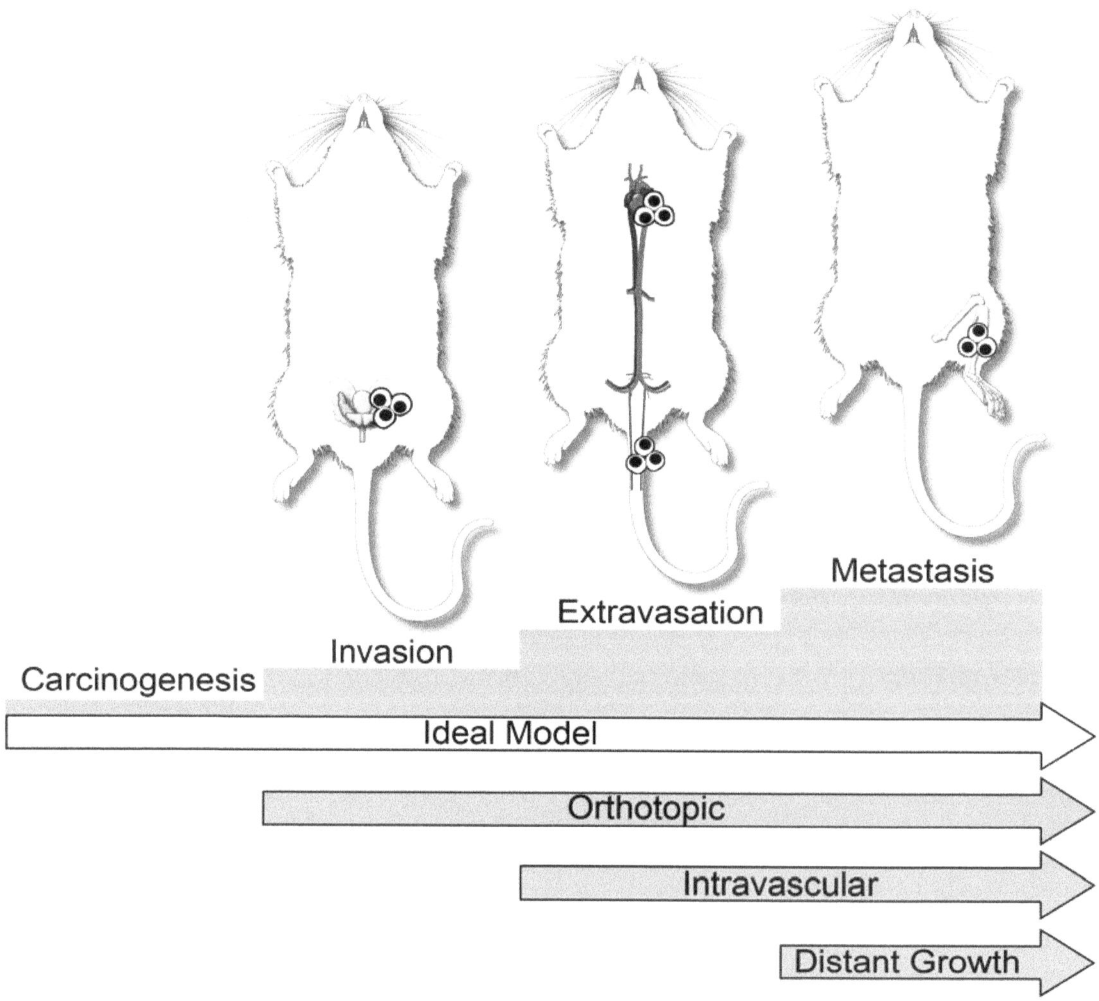

Prostatic intra-epithelial neoplasia (PIN) has been reported in dogs with or without invasive carcinoma [13]. The incidence of PIN in the clinically normal canine prostate gland has been reported to be approximately 3%; however, the incidence increased to 69% in glands that also had invasive carcinoma [14]. However, the role of PIN in dogs has not been thoroughly investigated. PIN may be a preneoplastic condition in dogs, but it has not been commonly reported. It may be that the incidence of both PIN and prostate carcinoma are lower in dogs compared to men. It is common practice in some countries to neuter pet dogs. Interestingly, the incidence of prostate cancer is similar or greater in neutered dogs compared to intact dogs [15]. This suggests that prostate cancer in dogs may develop from androgen-independent stem cells that are present in the atrophied ducts of the prostate glands of neutered dogs [16]. An alternative theory is that non-testicular sources of androgen in the body may be sufficient to provide androgen activity on the prostate cells.

A striking difference between men and dogs is the role of androgens in prostate cancer pathogenesis. Androgens play a prominent role in the development and function of male accessory sex organs, and the androgen signaling pathway is considered essential to the development of prostate cancer in men [17]. Androgen deprivation therapy is an established early therapy for androgen-dependent prostate cancer in men, and even after progression to androgen-resistance the androgen signaling pathway is still the primary target of many therapeutics [18]. In dogs, the androgen receptor is present in normal prostatic tissue, is important for normal accessory sex organ maintenance and function, and necessary for the development of BPH in adult intact male dogs. In contrast to humans, most dogs with prostate cancer have absent expression of the androgen receptor (AR) [19]. Since castration of dogs does not decrease the incidence of prostate cancer and androgen receptor expression is not present in canine prostate cancer, it is possible that the AR does not play a central role in the pathogenesis of canine prostate cancer. Interestingly, secretory cells of the prostatic acini are androgen dependent; however, the prostatic ducts and urothelium of the prostatic urethra are maintained independent of androgen [20]. This suggests that canine prostate cancer may originate from prostatic ductular epithelium rather than the acini as occurs in men.

In men, immunohistochemical markers are often used to distinguish between prostatic and urothelial carcinoma. A prominent example is prostate specific antigen (PSA), which is found in prostatic epithelial cells, but not transitional cells of the urothelium [21]. PSA is not produced in dogs, but instead a related kallikrein enzyme, arginine esterase, is considered to be the main secretory product of the canine prostate [22]. Unfortunately, arginine esterase does not differentiate between prostatic or urothelial origin of canine prostate cancer [23]. Another marker used often in men is prostate specific membrane antigen (PSMA). In the past it has been reported that PSMA was not expressed in the canine prostate; however, recent work has shown it to be present in at least two canine prostate cancer cell lines (Ace-1 and Leo) [24,25]. Prostatic acid phosphatase has also been used in men as a prostate lineage specific marker; yet investigation of its use in canine prostate cancer has not been extensively pursued [26,27]. In men, keratin 7 expression is also used for differentiating urothelial carcinoma from prostatic adenocarcinoma. Studies have shown that keratin 7 does not differentiate between these two tumors types in dogs, making it an unsuitable marker [23,28]. At this time, there is no definitive marker in dogs that can confidently differentiate between prostate tumors originating from the acinar secretory cells and the ductular epithelium or urothelium.

Prostate cancer affects older dogs (mean age of 10 years old) and the tumors can be heterogeneous. The most common diagnosis is prostatic adenocarcinoma, but as many as 53% of canine prostate carcinomas show mixed morphologic features [12,29]. The most common pattern of growth is intra-alveolar, where the cells form papillary or cribiform projections of epithelium filling dilated ducts or alveoli [30]. The second pattern is acinar, in which one to two layers of cuboidal to columnar cells line acini (though in some cases, acini can be completely filled with a solid mass of cells) [30]. Unlike in men, grading is not routine. All canine prostate cancers are considered malignant with a high metastatic potential, and no survival difference has been found for the different histologic subtypes [31]. At the time of necropsy, it has been reported that up to 80% of dogs with a primary prostate carcinoma will have gross metastases with skeletal metastases (predominantly in the axial skeleton) present in approximately 20% of cases [29]. Greater than 75% of canine prostate cancer skeletal metastases are osteoblastic or mixed osteoblastic/osteolytic in nature, similar to men [31,32].

3. Dogs in Prostate Cancer Research

Prostate Tissue–Bone Interaction *in vivo*: Since a unique characteristic of prostate cancer bone metastasis is the ability to cause dramatic new bone formation, methods of investigating the tissue-specific mechanisms responsible for the osteoblastic phenotype are vital to understanding its pathogenesis. Dogs have proven to be an excellent model for these investigations. A novel approach was utilized to investigate the prostate-specific effects on bone [33]. Canine prostate, kidney, urinary bladder, spleen, and skeletal muscle were implanted adjacent to the calvaria of immunodeficient mice *in vivo*. Only the prostatic tissue resulted in significant rapid new bone formation (Figure 2). A possible mechanism for the new bone formation was discovered through *in vitro* studies co-culturing rat calvaria with homogenates of normal canine prostate. These experiments revealed that osteoblasts are activated by the canine prostatic tissue through an endothelin-dependent mechanism [34]. The importance of this work is highlighted by the fact that endothelin has become an important target in human prostate cancer metastases in the last five years [35–39]. This particular model has the advantage of providing an easily manipulated system for investigating prostate-specific mechanisms of new bone formation. Another benefit is the use of prostatic tissue rather than a cell line, which may more closely represent the complex microenvironment of metastases. Canine prostate, in particular, is uniquely useful since it is known to produce bioactive factors (such as endothelin and parathyroid hormone-related peptide) that are also produced in the human prostate and are thought to be important in the pathogenesis of osteoblastic metastases [40,41].

Canine Prostate Cancer Cell Lines: In order to model human prostate carcinoma bone metastasis, multiple canine cell lines have been created and utilized *in vivo*. There are six canine prostate cancer cell lines that have been reported: DPC-1 [42], CPA-1 [43], Ace-1 [44], Leo [45], CT-1258 [46] and Probasco. To date, only DPC-1, Ace-1, Leo, and Probasco cells have been used to study bone metastasis (Table 1).

DPC-1: DPC-1 originated from an 11-year-old Doberman Pinscher with a poorly differentiated prostatic adenocarcinoma [42]. The DPC-1 cells are tumorigenic in both immunosuppressed mice (subcutaneous injection) and dogs (orthotopic injection). In studies where the cells were injected into the prostate glands of immunosuppressed dogs, it was found that they metastasized to the pelvic bones in two out of 12 dogs, forming mixed osteoblastic/osteolytic metastases [42,47].

Figure 2. Effects of canine prostatic tissue implanted adjacent to murine calvaria *in vivo.* (**A**) Decalcified calvarium with prostate tissue implanted between the skin and calvarium (above and out of the plane of the image). Note pre-existing calvaria (**C**) and marked periosteal thickening caused by dramatic new bone formation (arrowheads) (H&E). (**B**) Undecalcified calcein-labeled prostate-implanted calvaria. Calcein is a green fluorescent calcium-binding dye that is taken up at sites of active bone mineralization. Note calcein fluorescence in mineralized periosteal new bone (arrowheads). Pre-existing calvaria (**C**) had minimal fluorescence (Unstained).

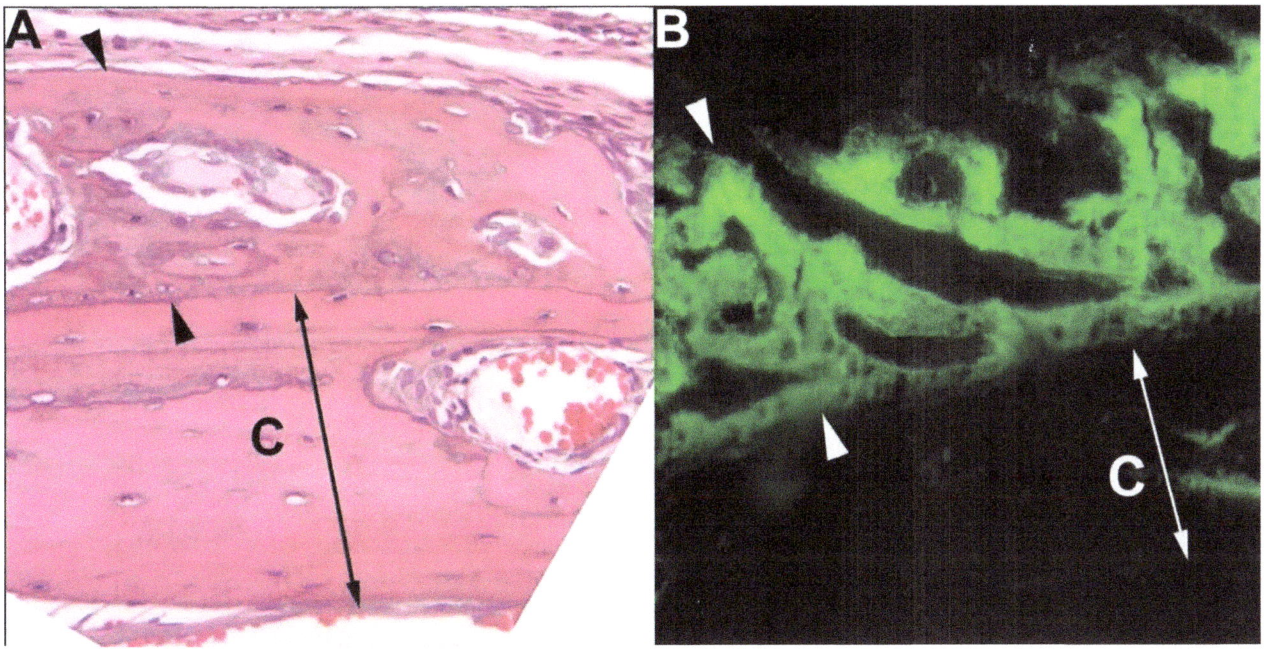

Table 1. Canine Cell Lines that Metastasize to Bone.

Cell Line	Models	Notes
DCP-1	Subcutaneous xenograft in mice Orthotopic allograft in dogs	Mixed osteoblastic/osteolytic metastases to pelvic bones in allograft model
Ace-1	Subcutaneous, intratibial, intracardiac, and intra-vossicle xenografts in mice Orthotopic allograft in dogs	Mixed osteoblastic/osteolytic tumors in intratibial, intracardiac and intra-vossicle models. Metastasis to long bones, ribs and vertebrae in intracardiac model Metastasis to lymph nodes and bone in allograft model
Leo	Subcutaneous, intratibial and intracardiac xenografts in mice	Osteolytic tumors in intratibial and intracardiac models. Metastasis primarily to brain and spinal cord, but also long bones in intracardiac model
Probasco	Subcutaneous, intratibial and intracardiac xenografts in mice	Osteoblastic tumors in intratibial and intracardiac models. Metastasis primarily to long bones

Figure 3. Intraprostatic Ace-1 tumor in an immunosuppressed dog. Ace-1 cells formed poorly demarcated masses (right side of image) that invaded the prostatic glands and ducts. The cells were polygonal to mildly spindle-shaped (epithelial-mesenchymal transition) and formed nests and papillary projections, frequently filling acini. Larger papillary projections were associated with coagulation necrosis. Lymphoplasmacytic inflammation and desmoplasia surrounded the affected acini and between the border of the invasive neoplastic cells into the normal prostatic tissue to the left. The left side of the image is composed of numerous variably sized, hypercellular glands lined by tall columnar to cuboidal epithelium and occasional prominent intra-luminal papillary projections (benign prostatic hyperplasia) (H&E).

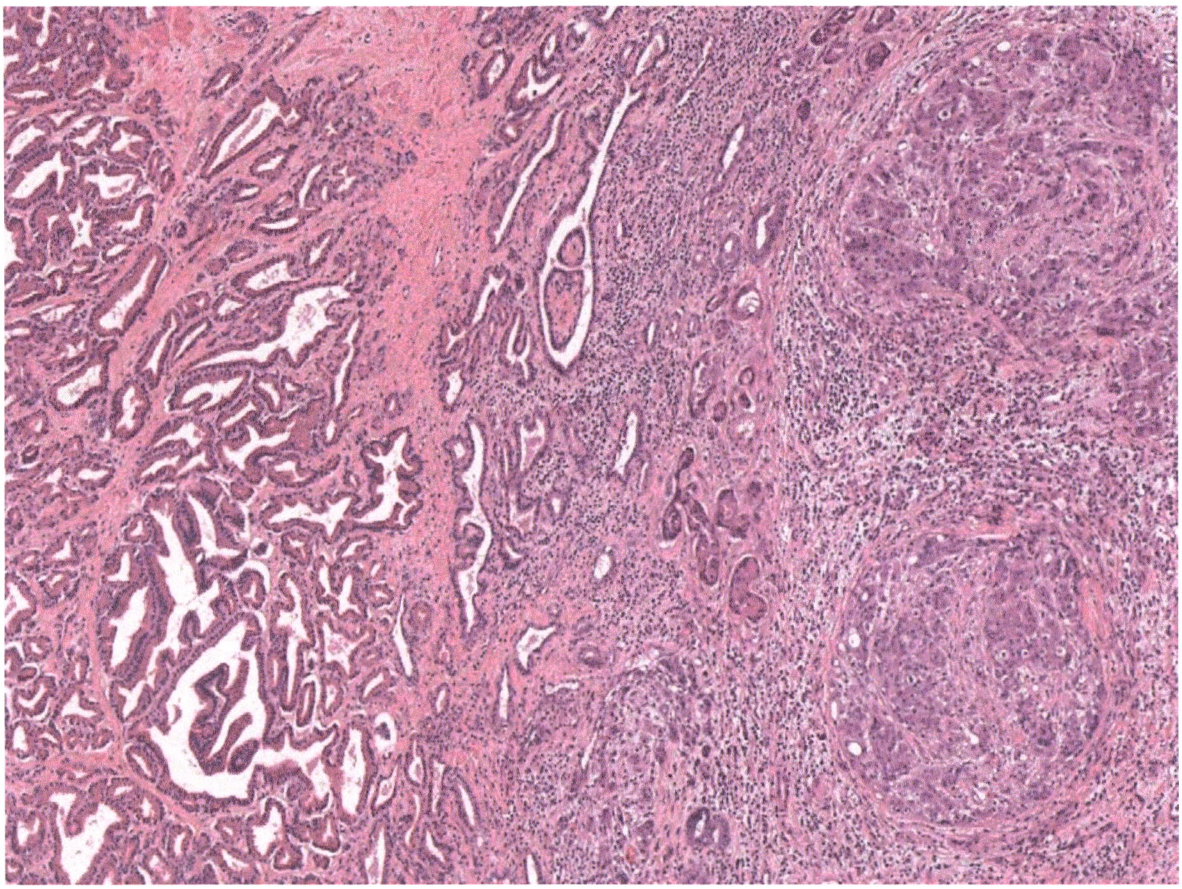

Ace-1: The Ace-1 cell line was developed from a primary prostatic carcinoma (intra-alveolar type) of an eight-year-old male castrated Labrador Retriever. The cells are tumorigenic in immunocompromised mice and rats and form mixed osteoblastic/osteolytic metastases after intratibial, intracardiac, and intra-vossicle injection in nude mice [44,48–50]. In bone, the cells initially induce the formation of new woven bone on metaphyseal trabecular bone and then on periosteal surfaces in areas with osteoclastic bone resorption of cortical bone. After intracardiac injection in mice, affected bones included humeri, femurs, tibias, ribs, and lumbar vertebrae. The Ace-1 cells have also been injected orthotopically in immunosuppressed dogs to develop an experimental model of prostate cancer (Figure 3) [51]. The Ace-1 cells are versatile and have been used both for metastasis studies and also as a model of tumor-induced bone pain [52,53]. The Ace-1 cells are very permissive to transfection and transduction. They have been stably transduced with yellow fluorescent protein (YFP) and luciferase (luc) to enable bioluminescent imaging for easier *in vivo* monitoring of metastasis and growth. Ace-1 cells have also been stably transfected with human Dickkopf-1 (Dkk-1) to determine the role of Wnt signaling in prostate cancer bone metastasis [54]. It was found that Dkk-1 upregulated non-canonical Wnt/JNK signaling and increased tumor growth and the number of metastases *in vivo*. Ace-1 cells have also been transfected with parathyroid hormone-related peptide (PTHrP) and it was found that PTHrP expression resulted in increased subcutaneous tumor growth and increased osteoclastogenesis, osteoblastogenesis, and angiogenesis in vossicles (neonatal murine vertebrae; Figure 4) transplanted in nude mice [49]. Ace-1 cells have proven to be a valuable model of mixed osteoblastic/osteolytic prostate cancer metastasis.

Figure 4. Nude mouse subcutaneously transplanted vertebral vossicle with canine Ace-1 tumor cells (T). The vossicle has cortical and trabecular bone with normal bone marrow (BM) hematopoietic cells (darkly stained cells). Note the new trabecular bone formation (arrowhead) induced by the Ace-1 tumor cells that surrounds the tumor cells. The image on the right is a magnification of the hyperplastic trabecular bone (arrowheads) induced by the Ace-1 tumor cells (T) (H&E).

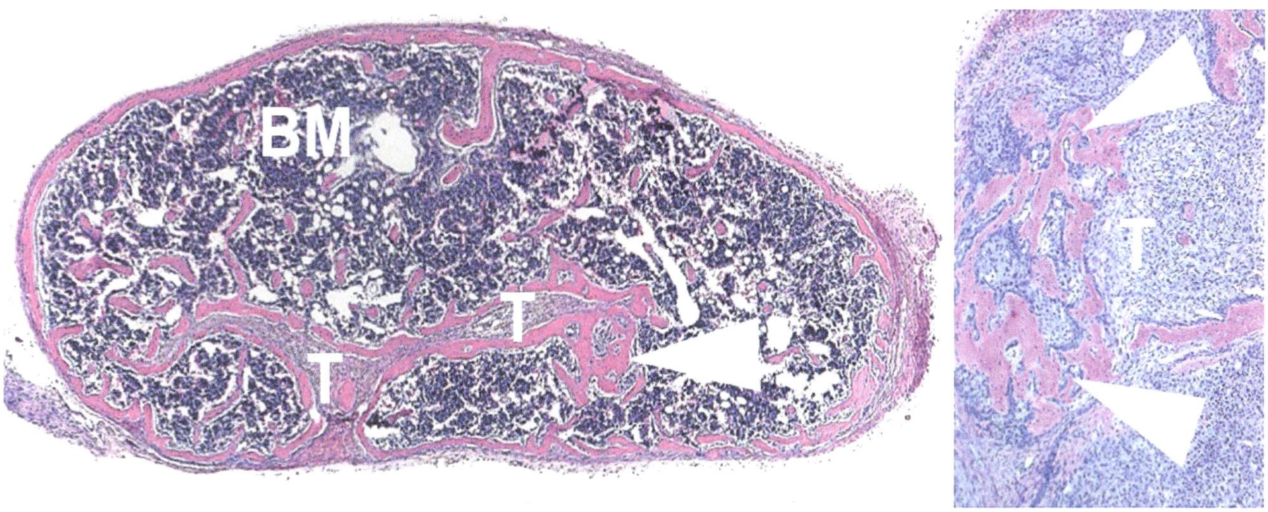

Leo: The Leo cell line originated from a primary prostate carcinoma from a five-year-old mixed breed dog. Similar to Ace-1, these cells have been transduced with YFP/Luc to allow for *in vivo* bioluminescent imaging. After intra-cardiac injection into nude mice, the most common site of metastasis was the brain and spinal cord followed by metastases to long bones [45]. Bone metastases were characterized by loss of cortical and trabecular bone. Brain metastasis in prostate cancer is rare, and there are few models available to study its pathogenesis. This unique cell line has the potential to contribute to this field.

Probasco: The Probasco cells came from the primary prostate carcinoma of a 10.5-year-old castrated mixed-breed dog that had been previously treated with palliative radiation therapy and metronomic chemotherapy (piroxicam, cyclophosphamide, toceranib phosphate, and chlorambucil) [55]. Similar to the Ace-1 and Leo cell lines, this cell line was also developed in the laboratory of Thomas Rosol. Like the Ace-1 cells, these cells have been transduced with YFP/Luc and are very permissive to transduction or transfection. Following intracardiac injection, Probasco cells metastasized primarily to the appendicular skeleton, and both intratibial and intracardiac injections produced markedly osteoblastic tumors in bone (Figure 5). Metastases had extensive new bone formation on both the endosteal and periosteal surfaces. In the early intra-tibial lesions (three weeks post-injection), the new woven bone was confined to the endosteal surfaces and marrow spaces. At six weeks post-injection, the Probasco cells penetrated the cortical bone and induced marked periosteal new bone formation. The overall effect on the bone was markedly osteoblastic, with mild osteolysis. These cells have been transfected with PTHrP and it was found to increase osteolysis and tumor growth *in vivo*. The osteoblastic nature and ease of transfection/transduction make these cells useful for studying bone metastasis pathogenesis and osteoblastic metastases.

Figure 5. Intratibial Probasco tumor in a nude mouse. (**A**) Micro-computed tomography (μCT) and of a nude mouse tibia injected with Probasco cells (right) and control tibia (left) at three weeks. Tibias in the Probasco-injected group had dramatic new bone formation signified by the increased radio-opacity in the diaphyseal region compared to the control bone; (**B**) Photomicrograph of intratibial tumor. Densely packed large polygonal neoplastic cells formed sheets and irregular glands with surrounding large irregular trabeculae of induced woven bone. Numerous polygonal to cuboidal osteoblasts line the trabecular bone and in some areas there is apposition of the prostate cancer cells to the new woven bone surfaces. Mitotic figures are frequent (H&E).

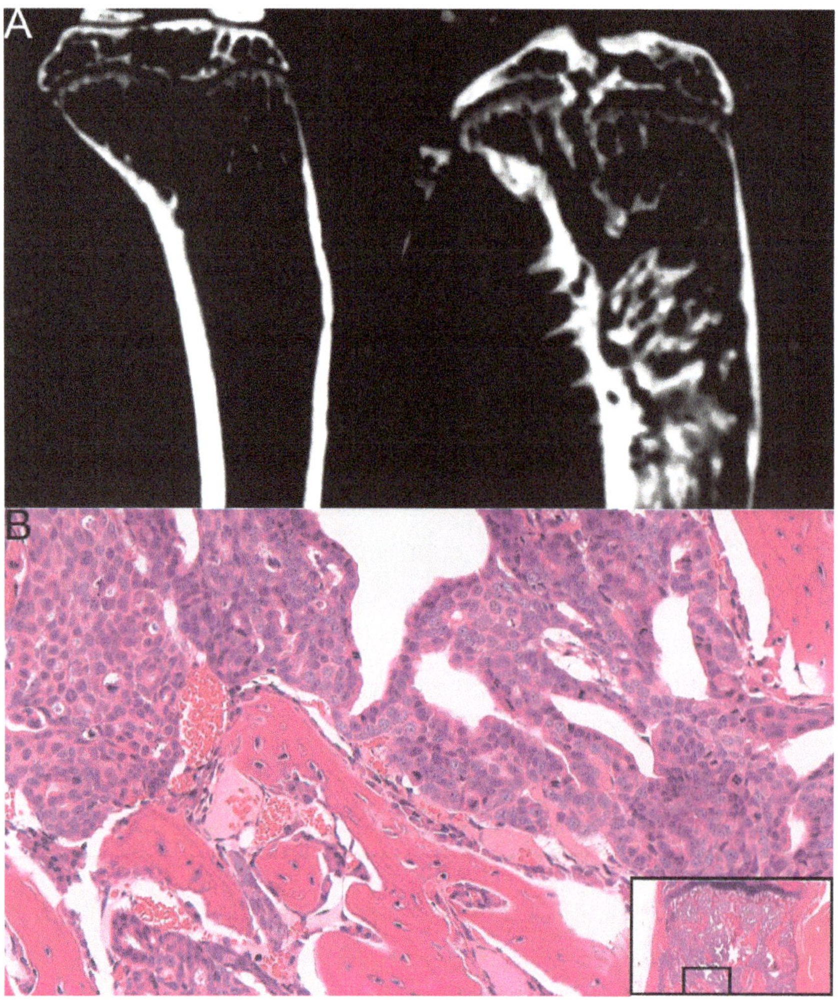

Canine Cell Lines in Immunocompromised Dogs: Dogs provide a useful large animal model for prostate cancer because they share several anatomic and physiologic similarities with men. The larger size of dogs also makes them helpful to investigate new molecular diagnostics for imaging and surgical procedures that cannot be performed readily in mice. However, the genetic heterogeneity of dogs as well as their cost can make them a challenging research model [56]. Canine cell lines have been injected orthotopically in immunosuppressed dogs to investigate their growth and metastasis *in vivo* and response to histotripsy. The Ace-1 cells formed prostate neoplasms in all injected dogs and metastases to the lungs and regional lymph nodes occurred in four out of 10 dogs. No bone metastases were present at the time of euthanasia; however, the experimental time course was relatively short (2–6 weeks). The tumors could be imaged by transrectal ultrasound and PET [57]. It was shown that histotripsy was effective in causing necrosis of the tumor tissue [51]. The DPC-1 cells have also been successfully implanted in dogs using a CT-guided transperitoneal approach with subsequent metastasis to lymph nodes (9/12), lungs (5/12) and bones (mixed osteoblastic/osteolytic metastasis) in two out of 12 dogs after 3–4 months [47].

4. Human Prostate Cancer Xenografts in Immunocompromised Mice

Much research on prostate cancer bone metastasis is performed with human prostate cancer xenografts. The most commonly used cell lines are PC3 (derived from a bone metastasis), DU145 (derived from a brain metastasis), and LNCaP (derived from a lymph node metastasis). The PC3 and LNCaP cell lines and their sublines have been widely used to study bone metastasis, as well as several less commonly used cell lines. The DU145 cell lines do not metastasize or grow in bone *in vivo.* Of the human prostate cancer cell lines available, PC3, PC3M, LAPC-4, LAPC-9, LNCaP, LNCaPC4-2, MDA PCa 2b, Wish-pc2, CL-1, CWR22R and ARCaP have been shown to produce bone metastases *in vivo* (Table 2).

PC3 and PC3M: PC3 cells are androgen insensitive and form osteolytic metastases after orthotopic, intra-cardiac and intratibial injection [58–60]. After orthotopic or intra-cardiac injection, sites of bone metastasis include the skull, ribs, pelvis, femur and tibia, mandible, and occasionally the brain and spinal cord. PC3 cells will also form osteolytic metastases in human fetal and adult bones implanted subcutaneously after tail vein injection of neoplastic cells [61,62] and when cells are injected adjacent to adult human bone implanted subcutaneously in immunocompromised mice [58]. This cell line has been transduced with green fluorescent protein (GFP) and luciferase (luc), allowing for more efficient imaging of metastases. A variant of PC3 which has a higher incidence of metastasis, PC3M, also forms osteolytic metastases (frequently within the mandible) after orthotopic and intracardiac injection [63,64]. Mandibular metastases in prostate cancer (and cancer in general) is an uncommon, but devastating event [65].

LAPC-4 and LAPC-9: Both LAPC-4 and LAPC-9 were derived from a femoral metastasis and are androgen dependent [66]. LAPC-4 produced mixed osteoblastic/osteolytic bone tumors when injected either orthotopically or adjacent to subcutaneously implanted fragments of adult human bone [67,68]. LAPC-9, a more recently developed cell line, has been shown to produce predominantly osteoblastic tumors after intratibial injection [58]. Since osteoblastic tumors are unusual in human cell lines, the LAPC-9 model should prove to be a valuable tool to investigate the pathogenesis of osteoblastic metastasis. For both cell lines, severely immunocompromised mice (such as NOD/SCID) must be used to allow for tumor growth *in vivo*.

Table 2. Human Cell and Tumor Lines used to Model Bone Metastasis in Mice.

Cell line	Models	Notes
PC3	Orthotopic, intratibial, and intracardiac injection Human fetal and adult bone with tail vein injection	Osteolytic tumors Metastasizes to skull, ribs, pelvis, femur and tibia after orthotopic or intracardiac injection
PC3M	Orthotopic and intracardiac injection	Osteolytic tumors with metastasis primarily to mandible
LAPC-4	Orthotopic injection Human adult bone with adjacent injection	Mixed osteoblastic/osteolytic tumors
LAPC-9	Intratibial injection	Osteoblastic tumors
LNCAP	Human adult bone with intra-bone or tail vain injection	Mixed osteoblastic/osteolytic tumors
LNCaP C4-2	Subcutaneous, orthotopic, and intracardiac injection	Vertebral osteolytic metastases
LNCaP C4-2B_4	Intrafemoral	Mixed osteoblastic/osteolytic tumors
LNCaP CL-1	Orthotopic injection	Osteolytic tumors Direct invasion and metastasis to skull, rib, pelvis, femur and tibia
MDA PCa 2b	Intrafemoral injection Injected human adult bone	Osteoblastic tumors
CWR22R	Subcutaneous injection	LacZ-positive bone micro-metastases Metastases not histologically confirmed
ARCaP	Orthotopic injection	Mixed osteoblastic/osteolytic tumors
LuCap 35	Intratibial injection Orthotopic injection	Osteolytic tumors in intratibial injections Bone marrow PSA positive sites after orthotopic injection (not histologically confirmed)
LuCaP 23.1	Intratibial injection	Osteoblastic tumors
Wish-pc2	Intrafemoral or intratibial injection	Osteolytic tumors

LNCaP and Sublines: The LNCap cell line and two of its sublines, LNCaP C4-2 and CL-1, have been used to study prostate cancer bone metastasis *in vivo*. LNCaP is androgen dependent and has been shown to form mixed osteoblastic/osteolytic tumors in subcutaneously implanted human adult bone after either direct injection into human bone or tail vein injection in immunocompromised mice [62,69]. Interestingly, LNCaP does not metastasize to murine bone after orthotopic, intracardiac, or tail vein injection [63]. The LNCaP cell line has been transfected with luciferase for bioluminescent imaging [70,71]. The subline LNCaP C4-2 is castration resistant and has been reported to metastasize to vertebrae and form mixed bone metastases after subcutaneous, orthotopic, and intracardiac injection [59,72]. The LNCaP C4-2B_4 cell line was derived from a LNCaP C4-2 bone metastasis [72]. The LNCaP C4-2B4 cell line is also castration-resistant and forms mixed osteoblastic/osteolytic metastases after intra-femoral injection [59]. The CL-1 subline is also castration resistant and has been reported to directly invade and induce lysis of the lumbar vertebral column after orthotopic injection. Metastases to bone after orthotopic injection have been reported using green fluorescent protein (GFP) expression, although these were not confirmed histologically [60,73]. A potential disadvantage of LNCaP cells is that they can be challenging to work with *in vivo* since they are slow growing and require the use of severely immunocompromised mice (such as NOD/SCID) and/or the use of the basement membrane product, Matrigel™ (Corning, Tewksbury, MA), with the cell injections.

MDA PCa 2b: The MDA PCa 2b cells were derived from a prostate cancer vertebral bone metastasis and demonstrate androgen-sensitive growth [56,74]. The MDA PCA 2b line forms predominantly osteoblastic tumors when injected into mouse long bones (femurs and tibias) or when directly injected into subcutaneously implanted human adult bone [75,76]. This cell line has been used extensively to investigate androgen signaling and progression to androgen independence [77–80].

CWR22R: The CWR22R cells were derived from a primary prostatic carcinoma and are castration resistant [81]. Transfection of the CWR22R cell line with lacZ allowed for visualization of micro-metastases after subcutaneous injection; however, histology was not used to confirm the metastases and no bone pathology was reported [82].

ARCaP: ARCaP cells were derived from the ascites fluid of a man diagnosed with metastatic prostate carcinoma. Mixed osteoblastic/osteolytic metastases were reported when the cells were injected orthotopically [83]. The cell line is unique in that they are characterized by an androgen-repressed phenotype (growth is suppressed when exposed to androgens).

LuCaP 23.1 and LuCaP35: Both LuCaP 23.1 and 35 are serially transplantable, prostate specific antigen-producing tumor lines that do not grow *in vitro* and were developed from prostate cancer lymph node metastases [84,85]. Both are androgen sensitive; however, LuCaP 35 can transition to androgen independence [84]. When injected intra-tibially, LuCaP 35 forms osteolytic metastases, while LuCaP 23.1 produces predominantly osteoblastic lesions [86]. After orthotopic implantation there was PSA mRNA detected in the bone marrow by real-time polymerase chain reaction (RT-PCR), suggesting micrometastases were present [87]. A challenge with the tumor lines is the lack of *in vitro* capacity for propagation and hence an inability to perform *in vitro* assays to investigate molecular mechanisms of pathogenesis.

Wish-pc2: The Wish-pc2 tumor line was developed from a poorly differentiated prostate carcinoma. These cells are castration resistant and considered to be prostatic neuroendocrine cells and represent a model for small cell carcinoma of the prostate. Intraosseous (femur or tibia) injection of the cells into mice results in primarily osteolytic tumors [88].

5. Prostate Cancer in Mice

The prostate gland of the mouse is significantly different to men and dogs. The anatomy of the murine prostate consists of four grossly and histologically distinct lobes (ventral, dorsal, lateral, and anterior) unlike the single lobe of the human prostate. The ventral lobe of the mouse prostate has no human counterpart. In the past, the dorsal and lateral lobes were considered analogous to the peripheral zone of the human prostate, and the anterior lobe is similar to the central zone in men; however, a 2004 consensus report determined that there was no evidence for a direct relationship between the mouse prostate lobes and human prostate zones [89,90]. Wild-type mice rarely develop spontaneous prostate cancer; therefore, transgenic mice have been developed to study particular mutations or transgenes in prostate cancer pathogenesis and treatment. A potential limitation in the use of transgenic mice is that few mutations can be studied concurrently, which does not reflect spontaneous invasive and metastatic prostate cancer. However, transgenic models do permit investigations on the interactions between neoplastic cells and the surrounding stroma and the role of stroma in cancer progression. Another challenge to developing a useful transgenic mouse model for prostate cancer research is that very few develop bone metastases. Most mouse models of prostate cancer do not progress beyond the stage of invasive carcinoma [91]. This is unfortunate, since most morbidity and complications in prostate cancer are due to advanced or metastatic disease, which cannot be treated surgically. However, transgenic models can be useful to study chemoprevention of prostate cancer [92–94]. Only the TRAMP, LPB-Tag/PB-hepsin, CR2-T-Ag, and 12T-7f transgenic models have been reported to develop metastasis to bone, albeit infrequently.

TRAMP: Transgenic adenocarcinoma of the mouse prostate (TRAMP) mice are considered a model of neuroendocrine prostate carcinoma [95]. Bone metastasis has been infrequently reported in transgenic adenocarcinoma of the mouse prostate (TRAMP) mice and only in the FVB background strain. Uncommon skeletal metastasis (one study reported 5/20 mice) has been reported to occur at approximately 23 weeks of age in the [TRAMP X FVB] F1strain, although histology revealed only minimal osteolytic/osteoblastic response to the presence of the neoplastic cells [96–99].

LPB-Tag/PB-Hepsin: Femoral metastases were found in a small percentage of LPB-Tag/PB-hepsin mice by 21 weeks; however, there was no associated osteolysis or new bone formation [100]. It is important to note that only femoral bones were examined.

CR2-T-Ag: Similar to TRAMP mice, Cryptdin-2/sv40 T (CR2-T-Ag) transgenic mice are considered a model of neuroendocrine prostate carcinoma and are reported to occasionally develop bone metastases by 24 weeks, though associated bone pathology was not described [101]. Similarly to the LPB-Tag/PB-hepsin study, only femurs were examined for metastases.

12T-7f: 12T-7f/MT-DNIIR and 12T-7f mice are two additional models of neuroendocrine prostate carcinoma and both rarely develop bone metastases, although no associated bone pathology has been described [102]. Only lumbar spine was evaluated.

G3/4 LSL-mTert PB-Pten/p53: These mice were generated by crossing p53/Pten conditional knockout mice with LSL-mTert mice that have Cre-mediated telomerase reactivation [103]. By 24 weeks of age, 25% of mice develop lumbar spine metastases. The osteoblastic or osteolytic nature of these metastases was not characterized.

Pten/p53/Smad4: These mice were generated by crossing p53/Pten double null mice with a Smad4 conditional knockout model [103]. By 17 weeks of age, approximately 12% of Pten/P53/Smad4 mice developed lumbar spine metastases. Similar to the G3/4 LSL-mTert PB-Pten/p53 model, the osteoblastic or osteolytic nature of these metastases was not characterized.

There are other transgenic mice that are reported to have bone metastases; however, this was based on positive PCR from bone marrow or from areas of bone remodeling without histologic confirmation of neoplastic cells. These include the prostate-specific PTEN knockout mouse [104] and the *Gγ/T-15* stains [105]. These mice were not included in this review as their usefulness in studying the pathogenesis of bone metastases is limited by the lack of histologically confirmed disease.

6. Mouse Prostate Reconstitution Model

The basic concept of the mouse prostate reconstitution model is to combine prostate cells (neoplastic or non-neoplastic) with urogenital sinus mesenchyme cells (rat or mouse) and implantation of the cells beneath the renal capsule of an immunodeficient mouse [32,106]. This model has been used to study the differentiation of putative prostate cancer stem cells, the significance of carcinogenic genes that cannot be investigated with whole-animal knockouts, as well as epithelial and mesenchymal interactions in prostate cancer [107–109]. One model that developed frequent micrometastases to bone is mouse prostate tissue over-expressing both *ras* and *myc* co-implanted with p53 knockout mouse urogenital sinus cells [110]. While the mouse prostate reconstitution model provides a fascinating avenue to further explore the genetic pathogenesis of prostate cancer progression and metastasis, its use is limited by the complexity and high technical skill required to isolate and implant the tissue.

7. End-Stage Mouse Models of Tumor/Bone Interactions

The ability to address specific questions regarding how tumors interact with the bone microenvironment is critical to understanding the cellular and molecular mechanisms of prostate cancer skeletal morbidity. Despite the fact that bone homing and the prostate cancer metastatic cascade in mice is quite different from dogs and humans, tissue reconstitution models can address specific mechanistic questions. The intratibial injection model has the advantage of direct placement of tumor cells into bone [111]. A disadvantage is that the trauma associated with injecting the tumor cells represents an atypical metastatic dissemination with wound healing consequences that are dramatic in bone. In addition, intra-tibial injection may force some of the tumor cells directly into bone marrow sinusoids and mimic an intravenous injection. Another novel model termed the "vossicle model" involves co-implantation of tumor cells and neonatal vertebral bodies [111]. This relatively simple model allows combinations of tumor cells or explants with murine bone. Isolated vertebral bones can be isolated from different types of genetically modified mice and/or luciferase-expressing mice in order to determine the impact of altering a gene in bone alone without systemic impact and to monitor tumor and/or bone growth over time.

8. Prostate Cancer in Rats

Similar to mice, the incidence of spontaneous prostate cancer in rats is rare in most strains. Some strains of rats, however, have a notable incidence of prostate cancer. As many as 30% and 16% of aged Lobund-Wistar and ACI/Seg rats, respectively, develop prostate carcinoma, although bone metastases do not occur [112]. To increase prostate tumorigenicity in Lobund-Wistar rats, intravenous injection of N-methyl-N-nitrosourea (MNU) with or without subcutaneous implantation of testosterone proprionate pellets has been shown to produce more rapid and consistent development of prostate cancer with metastasis to the lung and lymph nodes; however, bone metastases were not reported [113]. Most prostate cancer bone metastasis research performed is limited to two rat models: the MATLyLu subline and the PA-III cell line.

MATLyLu: This subline was developed from an original prostate carcinoma from a 22-month-old inbred Copenhagen male rat and the designation MATLyLu is an abbreviation for Metastatic Anaplastic Tumor Metastasizing to Lymph node and Lungs. This subline is considered a poorly differentiated carcinoma, is androgen insensitive and has been used to produce osteoclastic or, with variant R3327, osteoblastic bone metastases in Copenhagen rats after tail vein, intracardiac, and intraosseous injection [114–118]. The "osteoblastic" bone metastases represented osteolytic tumors with secondary periosteal bone proliferation due cortical bone erosion. Blomme *et al.* have reported that the bone metastases that occur with MATLyLu cells are predominantly osteolytic (Figure 6) [117].

PA-III: The PA-III cell line was derived from a spontaneous prostate carcinoma from a Lobund-Wistar rat. Similar to MayLyLu, this line is considered androgen insensitive and has been used to produce mixed osteolytic/osteoblastic lesions when implanted over the calvaria or scapula after periosteal disruption [112,119].

Figure 6. MatLyLu vertebral metastasis in a Copenhagen rat. There is marked replacement of hematopoietic cells with anaplastic carcinoma cells with dramatic loss of the medullary bone. The surfaces of the remaining trabecular bone are scalloped and eroded and they have severely eroded endosteal surfaces due to osteoclastic bone resorption (H&E). Inset: Numerous multinucleated osteoclasts line the scalloped surface of an eroded trabeculae (H&E).

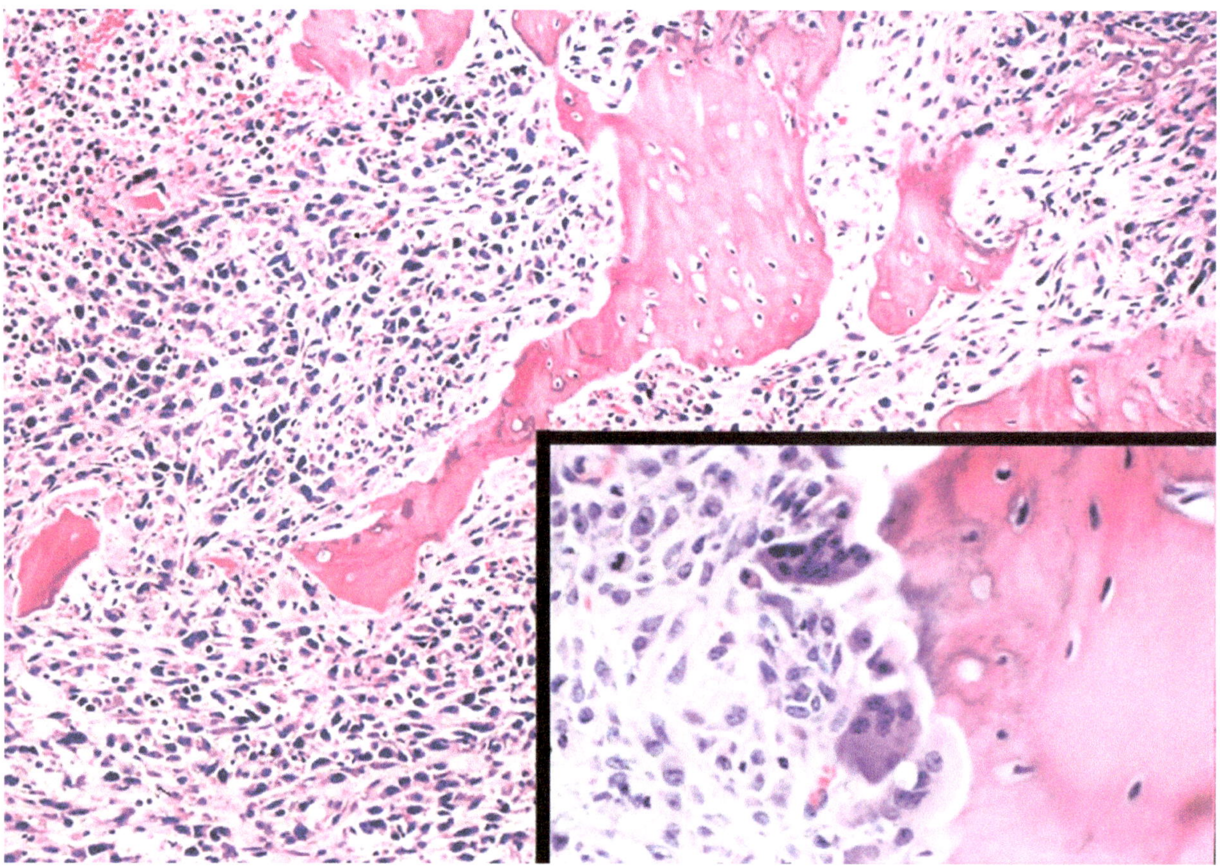

9. Conclusions

There are a considerable number of prostate cancer models available for scientific studies although relatively few of them can be used to consistently model osteoblastic bone metastases as occurs in men. Since bone metastasis represents end-stage disease, it is important that useful animal models are available to investigate novel prevention and treatment strategies. Specific animal models should be carefully chosen for individual experimental designs so that they have the pathogenic characteristics to enable them to test hypotheses that are relevant to human prostate cancer. The canine and human osteoblastic prostate cancer lines have the greatest utility for *in vivo* experiments; however, no model fully recapitulates the disease as it occurs in men.

While there is no perfect animal model of prostate cancer, a few better represent prostate cancer skeletal metastasis. In the author's opinion, the most representative model available is the LAPC-9 human cell line. It is one of the few available cell lines that was derived from a bone metastasis, and one of the very few that form osteoblastic metastases when injected in bone. It can be used for *in vitro* experiments, unlike the LuCaP 23.1 and 35 tumor lines. However, as most prostate cancer bone metastases are castration-resistant in men, the androgen-dependent nature of the LAPC-9 cell line does makes it less representative of the condition in men. The canine cell lines Ace-1 and Probasco are also valuable model systems since they grow well *in vivo* and *in vitro*, are easily transfectable and transducible, form bone metastases after intracardiac injection, and form osteoblastic (Probasco) or mixed osteoblastic/osteolytic (Ace-1) metastases. These two canine cell lines are exceptional model systems for the pathogenesis of bone metastasis and tumor-induced new bone formation; however, the lack of androgen receptor expression does limit their value in the investigation of drugs that inhibit the AR.

Recent breakthroughs in therapeutics have come from targeting metastatic prostate cancer with radiopharmaceuticals such as radium-223 [120]. The success of these therapies in slowing metastatic disease and improving survival indicate a need for increased research in this area, and may result in a future where bone metastases are considered curable. Animal models that best recapitulate human metastatic disease are essential for the development of these novel therapies. The characterization of novel large animal models, such as experimental dogs with orthotopic implantation of canine prostate cancer cells lines, will be helpful to develop and assess new molecular imaging tools and effective intraprostatic therapies. It is hoped that additional animal models are continually developed and critically evaluated as compared to human prostate cancer so the tools are available to effectively target prostate cancer to prevent, slow, or even reverse metastatic disease.

Acknowledgments

This work was funded in part by NCI F32 CA165689, NCI P01 CA093900 and The Ohio State University College of Veterinary Medicine Canine Research Funds. The authors thank Alan Flechtner and Anne Saulsbery for tissue processing and preparation of slides; Shelly Haramia for slide scanning; and Tim Vojt for assistance with figures.

Conflicts of Interest

The authors declare no conflict of interest.

References

1. Siegel, R.; Naishadham, D.; Jemal, A. Cancer statistics, 2013. *CA: Cancer J. Clin.* **2013**, *63*, 11–30.
2. Coleman, R.E. Clinical features of metastatic bone disease and risk of skeletal morbidity. *Clin. Cancer Res.* **2006**, *12*, 6243s–6249s.
3. Mehra, R.; Kumar-Sinha, C.; Shankar, S.; Lonigro, R.J.; Jing, X.; Philips, N.E.; Siddiqui, J.; Han, B.; Cao, X.; Smith, D.C.; *et al.* Characterization of bone metastases from rapid autopsies of prostate cancer patients. *Clin. Cancer Res.* **2011**, *17*, 3924–3932.
4. Sturge, J.; Caley, M.P.; Waxman, J. Bone metastasis in prostate cancer: Emerging therapeutic strategies. *Nat. Rev. Clin. Oncol.* **2011**, *8*, 357–368.
5. Heidenreich, A. Bisphosphonates in the management of metastatic prostate cancer. *Oncology* **2003**, *65*, 5–11.
6. Weilbaecher, K.N.; Guise, T.A.; McCauley, L.K. Cancer to bone: A fatal attraction. *Nat. Rev. Cancer* **2011**, *11*, 411–425.
7. Morgans, A.K.; Smith, M.R. Bone-targeted agents: Preventing skeletal complications in prostate cancer. *Urol. Clin. North Am.* **2012**, *39*, 533–546.
8. Langdon, S.P. Animal modeling of cancer pathology and studying tumor response to therapy. *Curr. Drug Targets* **2012**, *13*, 1535–1547.
9. Waters, D.J.; Hayden, D.W.; Bell, F.W.; Klausner, J.S.; Qian, J.; Bostwick, D.G. Prostatic intraepithelial neoplasia in dogs with spontaneous prostate cancer. *Prostate* **1997**, *30*, 92–97.
10. Gamlem, H.; Nordstoga, K.; Glattre, E. Canine neoplasia—Introductory paper. *APMIS. Suppl.* **2008**, *125*, 5–18.
11. Rosol, T.J.; Tannehill-Gregg, S.H.; LeRoy, B.E.; Mandl, S.; Contag, C.H. Animal models of bone metastasis. *Cancer* **2003**, *97*, 748–757.
12. Smith, J. Canine prostatic disease: A review of anatomy, pathology, diagnosis, and treatment. *Theriogenology* **2008**, *70*, 375–383.
13. Waters, D.J.; Bostwick, D.G. Prostatic intraepithelial neoplasia occurs spontaneously in the canine prostate. *J. Urol.* **1997**, *157*, 713–716.
14. Madewell, B.R.; Gandour-Edwards, R.; DeVere White, R.W. Canine prostatic intraepithelial neoplasia: Is the comparative model relevant? *Prostate* **2004**, *58*, 314–317.
15. Teske, E.; Naan, E.C.; van Dijk, E.M.; van Garderen, E.; Schalken, J.A. Canine prostate carcinoma: Epidemiological evidence of an increased risk in castrated dogs. *Mol. Cell. Endocrinol.* **2002**, *197*, 251–255.
16. Moulay, M.; Liu, W.; Willenbrock, S.; Sterenczak, K.A.; Carlson, R.; Ngezahayo, A.; Murua Escobar, H.; Nolte, I. Evaluation of stem cell marker gene expression in canine prostate carcinoma- and prostate cyst-derived cell lines. *Anticancer Res.* **2013**, *33*, 5421–5431.
17. Sharifi, N. Mechanisms of androgen receptor activation in castration-resistant prostate cancer. *Endocrinology* **2013**, *154*, 4010–4017.
18. Derleth, C.L.; Yu, E.Y. Targeted therapy in the treatment of castration-resistant prostate cancer. *Oncology (Williston Park)* **2013**, *27*, 620–628.

19. Gallardo, F.; Mogas, T.; Baro, T.; Rabanal, R.; Morote, J.; Abal, M.; Reventos, J.; Lloreta, J. Expression of androgen, oestrogen alpha and beta, and progesterone receptors in the canine prostate: Differences between normal, inflamed, hyperplastic and neoplastic glands. *J. Comp. Pathol.* **2007**, *136*, 1–8.
20. Leav, I.; Schelling, K.H.; Adams, J.Y.; Merk, F.B.; Alroy, J. Role of canine basal cells in postnatal prostatic development, induction of hyperplasia, and sex hormone-stimulated growth; and the ductal origin of carcinoma. *Prostate* **2001**, *48*, 210–224.
21. Genega, E.M.; Hutchinson, B.; Reuter, V.E.; Gaudin, P.B. Immunophenotype of high-grade prostatic adenocarcinoma and urothelial carcinoma. *Mod. Pathol.* **2000**, *13*, 1186–1191.
22. Gobello, C.; Castex, G.; Corrada, Y. Serum and seminal markers in the diagnosis of disorders of the genital tract of the dog: A mini-review. *Theriogenology* **2002**, *57*, 1285–1291.
23. LeRoy, B.E.; Nadella, M.V.; Toribio, R.E.; Leav, I.; Rosol, T.J. Canine prostate carcinomas express markers of urothelial and prostatic differentiation. *Vet. Pathol.* **2004**, *41*, 131–140.
24. Aggarwal, S.; Ricklis, R.M.; Williams, S.A.; Denmeade, S.R. Comparative study of psma expression in the prostate of mouse, dog, monkey, and human. *Prostate* **2006**, *66*, 903–910.
25. Wu, L.Y.; Johnson, J.M.; Simmons, J.K.; Mendes, D.E.; Geruntho, J.J.; Liu, T.; Dirksen, W.P.; Rosol, T.J.; Davis, W.C.; Berkman, C.E. Biochemical characterization of prostate-specific membrane antigen from canine prostate carcinoma cells. *Prostate* **2014**, *74*, 451–457.
26. Paner, G.P.; Luthringer, D.J.; Amin, M.B. Best practice in diagnostic immunohistochemistry: Prostate carcinoma and its mimics in needle core biopsies. *Arch. Pathol. Lab. Med.* **2008**, *132*, 1388–1396.
27. McEntee, M.; Isaacs, W.; Smith, C. Adenocarcinoma of the canine prostate: Immunohistochemical examination for secretory antigens. *Prostate* **1987**, *11*, 163–170.
28. LeRoy, B.; Painter, A.; Sheppard, H.; Popiolek, L.; Samuel-Foo, M.; Andacht, T.M. Protein expression profiling of normal and neoplastic canine prostate and bladder tissue. *Vet. Comp. Oncol.* **2007**, *5*, 119–130.
29. Chen, Y.; Scher, H.I. Prostate cancer in 2011: Hitting old targets better and identifying new targets. *Nat. Rev. Clin. Oncol.* **2012**, *9*, 70–72.
30. Meuten, D.J. *Tumors in Domestic Animals*, 4th ed.; Wiley-Blackwell: Ames, IA, USA, 2002.
31. Cornell, K.K.; Bostwick, D.G.; Cooley, D.M.; Hall, G.; Harvey, H.J.; Hendrick, M.J.; Pauli, B.U.; Render, J.A.; Stoica, G.; Sweet, D.C.; *et al.* Clinical and pathologic aspects of spontaneous canine prostate carcinoma: A retrospective analysis of 76 cases. *Prostate* **2000**, *45*, 173–183.
32. Valkenburg, K.C.; Williams, B.O. Mouse models of prostate cancer. *Prostate Cancer* **2011**, *2011*, doi:10.1155/2011/895238.
33. LeRoy, B.E.; Bahnson, R.R.; Rosol, T.J. New bone formation in nude mouse calvaria induced by canine prostate tissue. *Mol. Cell. Endocrinol.* **2002**, *197*, 257–263.
34. LeRoy, B.E.; Sellers, R.S.; Rosol, T.J. Canine prostate stimulates osteoblast function using the endothelin receptors. *Prostate* **2004**, *59*, 148–156.
35. Heidegger, I.; Massoner, P.; Eder, I.E.; Pircher, A.; Pichler, R.; Aigner, F.; Bektic, J.; Horninger, W.; Klocker, H. Novel therapeutic approaches for the treatment of castration-resistant prostate cancer. *J. Steroid Biochem. Mol. Biol.* **2013**, *138*, 248–256.

36. Rove, K.O.; Crawford, E.D. Evolution of treatment options for patients with CRPC and bone metastases: Bone-targeted agents that go beyond palliation of symptoms to improve overall survival. *Oncology (Williston Park)* **2011**, *25*, 1362–1370, 1375–1381, 1387.
37. Pinto, A.; Merino, M.; Zamora, P.; Redondo, A.; Castelo, B.; Espinosa, E. Targeting the endothelin axis in prostate carcinoma. *Tumour Biol.* **2012**, *33*, 421–426.
38. Roh, M.; Abdulkadir, S.A. Targeting the endothelin receptor in prostate cancer bone metastasis: Back to the mouse? *Cancer Biol. Ther.* **2010**, *9*, 615–617.
39. Shao, N.; Wang, Y.; Jiang, W.Y.; Qiao, D.; Zhang, S.G.; Wu, Y.; Zhang, X.X.; Wang, J.L.; Ding, Y.; Feng, N.H. Immunotherapy and endothelin receptor antagonists for treatment of castration-resistant prostate cancer. *Int. J. Cancer.* **2013**, *133*, 1743–1750.
40. Ishizaka, K.; Azuma, H.; Matsubara, O.; Kitahara, S.; Oshima, H. Production of endothelin by canine prostatic epithelial cells and its stimulatory effects on their growth. *J. Androl.* **1999**, *20*, 529–536.
41. Blomme, E.A.; Sugimoto, Y.; McCauley, L.K.; Lin, Y.C.; Capen, C.C.; Rosol, T.J. Stromal and epithelial cells of the canine prostate express parathyroid hormone-related protein, but not the pth/pthrp receptor. *Prostate* **1998**, *36*, 110–120.
42. Anidjar, M.; Villette, J.M.; Devauchelle, P.; Delisle, F.; Cotard, J.P.; Billotey, C.; Cochand-Priollet, B.; Copin, H.; Barnoux, M.; Triballeau, S.; *et al. In vivo* model mimicking natural history of dog prostate cancer using DPC-1, a new canine prostate carcinoma cell line. *Prostate* **2001**, *46*, 2–10.
43. Eaton, C.L.; Pierrepoint, C.G. Growth of a spontaneous canine prostatic adenocarcinoma *in vivo* and *in vitro*: Isolation and characterization of a neoplastic prostatic epithelial cell line, CPA 1. *Prostate* **1988**, *12*, 129–143.
44. LeRoy, B.E.; Thudi, N.K.; Nadella, M.V.; Toribio, R.E.; Tannehill-Gregg, S.H.; van Bokhoven, A.; Davis, D.; Corn, S.; Rosol, T.J. New bone formation and osteolysis by a metastatic, highly invasive canine prostate carcinoma xenograft. *Prostate* **2006**, *66*, 1213–1222.
45. Thudi, N.K.; Shu, S.T.; Martin, C.K.; Lanigan, L.G.; Nadella, M.V.; Van Bokhoven, A.; Werbeck, J.L.; Simmons, J.K.; Murahari, S.; Kisseberth, W.C.; *et al.* Development of a brain metastatic canine prostate cancer cell line. *Prostate* **2011**, *71*, 1251–1263.
46. Fork, M.A.; Murua Escobar, H.; Soller, J.T.; Sterenczak, K.A.; Willenbrock, S.; Winkler, S.; Dorsch, M.; Reimann-Berg, N.; Hedrich, H.J.; Bullerdiek, J.; *et al.* Establishing an *in vivo* model of canine prostate carcinoma using the new cell line ct1258. *BMC Cancer* **2008**, *8*, doi:10.1186/1471-2407-8-240.
47. Anidjar, M.; Scarlata, E.; Cury, F.L.; Rocha, J.; Hamel, L.; Luz, M.; Chevalier, S. Refining the orthotopic dog prostate cancer (DPC)-1 model to better bridge the gap between rodents and men. *Prostate* **2012**, *72*, 752–761.
48. Li, X.; Liao, J.; Park, S.I.; Koh, A.J.; Sadler, W.D.; Pienta, K.J.; Rosol, T.J.; McCauley, L.K. Drugs which inhibit osteoclast function suppress tumor growth through calcium reduction in bone. *Bone* **2011**, *48*, 1354–1361.
49. Liao, J.; Li, X.; Koh, A.J.; Berry, J.E.; Thudi, N.; Rosol, T.J.; Pienta, K.J.; McCauley, L.K. Tumor expressed pthrp facilitates prostate cancer-induced osteoblastic lesions. *Int. J. Cancer.* **2008**, *123*, 2267–2278.

50. Wise-Milestone, L.; Akens, M.K.; Rosol, T.J.; Hojjat, S.P.; Grynpas, M.D.; Whyne, C.M. Evaluating the effects of mixed osteolytic/osteoblastic metastasis on vertebral bone quality in a new rat model. *J. Orthop. Res.* **2012**, *30*, 817–823.
51. Schade, G.R.; Keller, J.; Ives, K.; Cheng, X.; Rosol, T.J.; Keller, E.; Roberts, W.W. Histotripsy focal ablation of implanted prostate tumor in an ACE-1 canine cancer model. *J. Urol.* **2012**, *188*, 1957–1964.
52. Halvorson, K.G.; Kubota, K.; Sevcik, M.A.; Lindsay, T.H.; Sotillo, J.E.; Ghilardi, J.R.; Rosol, T.J.; Boustany, L.; Shelton, D.L.; Mantyh, P.W. A blocking antibody to nerve growth factor attenuates skeletal pain induced by prostate tumor cells growing in bone. *Cancer Res.* **2005**, *65*, 9426–9435.
53. Halvorson, K.G.; Sevcik, M.A.; Ghilardi, J.R.; Rosol, T.J.; Mantyh, P.W. Similarities and differences in tumor growth, skeletal remodeling and pain in an osteolytic and osteoblastic model of bone cancer. *Clin. J. Pain* **2006**, *22*, 587–600.
54. Thudi, N.K.; Martin, C.K.; Murahari, S.; Shu, S.T.; Lanigan, L.G.; Werbeck, J.L.; Keller, E.T.; McCauley, L.K.; Pinzone, J.J.; Rosol, T.J. Dickkopf-1 (DKK-1) stimulated prostate cancer growth and metastasis and inhibited bone formation in osteoblastic bone metastases. *Prostate* **2011**, *71*, 615–625.
55. Simmons, J.K.; Dirksen, W.P.; Hildreth, B.E., 3rd; Dorr, C.; Williams, C.; Thomas, R.; Breen, M.; Toribio, R.E.; Rosol, T.J. Canine prostate cancer cell line (probasco) produces osteoblastic metastases *in vivo*. *Prostate* **2014**, *PROS-14-178*, in press.
56. Navone, N.M.; Logothetis, C.J.; von Eschenbach, A.C.; Troncoso, P. Model systems of prostate cancer: Uses and limitations. *Cancer Metastasis Rev.* **1998**, *17*, 361–371.
57. Keller, J.M.; Schade, G.R.; Ives, K.; Cheng, X.; Rosol, T.J.; Piert, M.; Siddiqui, J.; Roberts, W.W.; Keller, E.T. A novel canine model for prostate cancer. *Prostate* **2013**, *73*, 952–959.
58. Lee, Y.P.; Schwarz, E.M.; Davies, M.; Jo, M.; Gates, J.; Zhang, X.; Wu, J.; Lieberman, J.R. Use of zoledronate to treat osteoblastic *versus* osteolytic lesions in a severe-combined-immunodeficient mouse model. *Cancer Res.* **2002**, *62*, 5564–5570.
59. Wu, T.T.; Sikes, R.A.; Cui, Q.; Thalmann, G.N.; Kao, C.; Murphy, C.F.; Yang, H.; Zhau, H.E.; Balian, G.; Chung, L.W. Establishing human prostate cancer cell xenografts in bone: Induction of osteoblastic reaction by prostate-specific antigen-producing tumors in athymic and SCID/bg mice using LNCaP and lineage-derived metastatic sublines. *Int. J. Cancer* **1998**, *77*, 887–894.
60. Yang, M.; Jiang, P.; Sun, F.X.; Hasegawa, S.; Baranov, E.; Chishima, T.; Shimada, H.; Moossa, A.R.; Hoffman, R.M. A fluorescent orthotopic bone metastasis model of human prostate cancer. *Cancer Res.* **1999**, *59*, 781–786.
61. Nemeth, J.A.; Harb, J.F.; Barroso, U., Jr.; He, Z.; Grignon, D.J.; Cher, M.L. Severe combined immunodeficient-hu model of human prostate cancer metastasis to human bone. *Cancer Res.* **1999**, *59*, 1987–1993.
62. Yonou, H.; Yokose, T.; Kamijo, T.; Kanomata, N.; Hasebe, T.; Nagai, K.; Hatano, T.; Ogawa, Y.; Ochiai, A. Establishment of a novel species- and tissue-specific metastasis model of human prostate cancer in humanized non-obese diabetic/severe combined immunodeficient mice engrafted with human adult lung and bone. *Cancer Res.* **2001**, *61*, 2177–2182.

63. Pettaway, C.A.; Pathak, S.; Greene, G.; Ramirez, E.; Wilson, M.R.; Killion, J.J.; Fidler, I.J. Selection of highly metastatic variants of different human prostatic carcinomas using orthotopic implantation in nude mice. *Clin. Cancer Res.* **1996**, *2*, 1627–1636.
64. Kozlowski, J.M.; Fidler, I.J.; Campbell, D.; Xu, Z.L.; Kaighn, M.E.; Hart, I.R. Metastatic behavior of human tumor cell lines grown in the nude mouse. *Cancer Res.* **1984**, *44*, 3522–3529.
65. Parkins, G.E.; Klufio, G.O. Prostate cancer metastasis to the mandible: Case report. *East Afr. Med. J.* **2009**, *86*, 251–252.
66. Craft, N.; Chhor, C.; Tran, C.; Belldegrun, A.; DeKernion, J.; Witte, O.N.; Said, J.; Reiter, R.E.; Sawyers, C.L. Evidence for clonal outgrowth of androgen-independent prostate cancer cells from androgen-dependent tumors through a two-step process. *Cancer Res.* **1999**, *59*, 5030–5036.
67. Davies, M.R.; Lee, Y.P.; Lee, C.; Zhang, X.; Afar, D.E.; Lieberman, J.R. Use of a scid mouse model to select for a more aggressive strain of prostate cancer. *Anticancer Res.* **2003**, *23*, 2245–2252.
68. Tsingotjidou, A.S.; Zotalis, G.; Jackson, K.R.; Sawyers, C.; Puzas, J.E.; Hicks, D.G.; Reiter, R.; Lieberman, J.R. Development of an animal model for prostate cancer cell metastasis to adult human bone. *Anticancer Res.* **2001**, *21*, 971–978.
69. Yonou, H.; Kanomata, N.; Goya, M.; Kamijo, T.; Yokose, T.; Hasebe, T.; Nagai, K.; Hatano, T.; Ogawa, Y.; Ochiai, A. Osteoprotegerin/osteoclastogenesis inhibitory factor decreases human prostate cancer burden in human adult bone implanted into nonobese diabetic/severe combined immunodeficient mice. *Cancer Res.* **2003**, *63*, 2096–2102.
70. Dias, S.J.; Li, K.; Rimando, A.M.; Dhar, S.; Mizuno, C.S.; Penman, A.D.; Levenson, A.S. Trimethoxy-resveratrol and piceatannol administered orally suppress and inhibit tumor formation and growth in prostate cancer xenografts. *Prostate* **2013**, *73*, 1135–1146.
71. Scatena, C.D.; Hepner, M.A.; Oei, Y.A.; Dusich, J.M.; Yu, S.F.; Purchio, T.; Contag, P.R.; Jenkins, D.E. Imaging of bioluminescent LNCaP-luc-M6 tumors: A new animal model for the study of metastatic human prostate cancer. *Prostate* **2004**, *59*, 292–303.
72. Thalmann, G.N.; Anezinis, P.E.; Chang, S.M.; Zhau, H.E.; Kim, E.E.; Hopwood, V.L.; Pathak, S.; von Eschenbach, A.C.; Chung, L.W. Androgen-independent cancer progression and bone metastasis in the LNCaP model of human prostate cancer. *Cancer Res.* **1994**, *54*, 2577–2581.
73. Tso, C.L.; McBride, W.H.; Sun, J.; Patel, B.; Tsui, K.H.; Paik, S.H.; Gitlitz, B.; Caliliw, R.; van Ophoven, A.; Wu, L.; *et al.* Androgen deprivation induces selective outgrowth of aggressive hormone-refractory prostate cancer clones expressing distinct cellular and molecular properties not present in parental androgen-dependent cancer cells. *Cancer J.* **2000**, *6*, 220–233.
74. Navone, N.M.; Olive, M.; Ozen, M.; Davis, R.; Troncoso, P.; Tu, S.M.; Johnston, D.; Pollack, A.; Pathak, S.; von Eschenbach, A.C.; *et al.* Establishment of two human prostate cancer cell lines derived from a single bone metastasis. *Clin. Cancer Res.* **1997**, *3*, 2493–2500.
75. Yang, J.; Fizazi, K.; Peleg, S.; Sikes, C.R.; Raymond, A.K.; Jamal, N.; Hu, M.; Olive, M.; Martinez, L.A.; Wood, C.G.; *et al.* Prostate cancer cells induce osteoblast differentiation through a cbfa1-dependent pathway. *Cancer Res.* **2001**, *61*, 5652–5659.
76. Goya, M.; Miyamoto, S.; Nagai, K.; Ohki, Y.; Nakamura, K.; Shitara, K.; Maeda, H.; Sangai, T.; Kodama, K.; Endoh, Y.; *et al.* Growth inhibition of human prostate cancer cells in human adult bone implanted into nonobese diabetic/severe combined immunodeficient mice by a ligand-specific antibody to human insulin-like growth factors. *Cancer Res.* **2004**, *64*, 6252–6258.

77. Zhao, X.Y.; Malloy, P.J.; Krishnan, A.V.; Swami, S.; Navone, N.M.; Peehl, D.M.; Feldman, D. Glucocorticoids can promote androgen-independent growth of prostate cancer cells through a mutated androgen receptor. *Nat. Med.* **2000**, *6*, 703–706.
78. Hara, T.; Nakamura, K.; Araki, H.; Kusaka, M.; Yamaoka, M. Enhanced androgen receptor signaling correlates with the androgen-refractory growth in a newly established MDA PCa 2b-hr human prostate cancer cell subline. *Cancer Res.* **2003**, *63*, 5622–5628.
79. Zhao, X.Y.; Boyle, B.; Krishnan, A.V.; Navone, N.M.; Peehl, D.M.; Feldman, D. Two mutations identified in the androgen receptor of the new human prostate cancer cell line MDA PCa 2a. *J. Urol.* **1999**, *162*, 2192–2199.
80. Liu, X.H.; Kirschenbaum, A.; Yao, S.; Liu, G.; Aaronson, S.A.; Levine, A.C. Androgen-induced wnt signaling in preosteoblasts promotes the growth of MDA-PCa-2b human prostate cancer cells. *Cancer Res.* **2007**, *67*, 5747–5753.
81. Pretlow, T.G.; Wolman, S.R.; Micale, M.A.; Pelley, R.J.; Kursh, E.D.; Resnick, M.I.; Bodner, D.R.; Jacobberger, J.W.; Delmoro, C.M.; Giaconia, J.M.; *et al.* Xenografts of primary human prostatic carcinoma. *J. Natl. Cancer Inst.* **1993**, *85*, 394–398.
82. Holleran, J.L.; Miller, C.J.; Culp, L.A. Tracking micrometastasis to multiple organs with lacZ-tagged CWR22R prostate carcinoma cells. *J. Histochem. Cytochem.* **2000**, *48*, 643–651.
83. Zhau, H.Y.; Chang, S.M.; Chen, B.Q.; Wang, Y.; Zhang, H.; Kao, C.; Sang, Q.A.; Pathak, S.J.; Chung, L.W. Androgen-repressed phenotype in human prostate cancer. *Proc. Natl. Acad. Sci. U.S.A* **1996**, *93*, 15152–15157.
84. Corey, E.; Quinn, J.E.; Buhler, K.R.; Nelson, P.S.; Macoska, J.A.; True, L.D.; Vessella, R.L. LuCaP 35: A new model of prostate cancer progression to androgen independence. *Prostate* **2003**, *55*, 239–246.
85. Ellis, W.J.; Vessella, R.L.; Buhler, K.R.; Bladou, F.; True, L.D.; Bigler, S.A.; Curtis, D.; Lange, P.H. Characterization of a novel androgen-sensitive, prostate-specific antigen-producing prostatic carcinoma xenograft: LuCaP 23. *Clin. Cancer Res.* **1996**, *2*, 1039–1048.
86. Corey, E.; Quinn, J.E.; Bladou, F.; Brown, L.G.; Roudier, M.P.; Brown, J.M.; Buhler, K.R.; Vessella, R.L. Establishment and characterization of osseous prostate cancer models: Intra-tibial injection of human prostate cancer cells. *Prostate* **2002**, *52*, 20–33.
87. Corey, E.; Quinn, J.E.; Vessella, R.L. A novel method of generating prostate cancer metastases from orthotopic implants. *Prostate* **2003**, *56*, 110–114.
88. Pinthus, J.H.; Waks, T.; Schindler, D.G.; Harmelin, A.; Said, J.W.; Belldegrun, A.; Ramon, J.; Eshhar, Z. WISH-PC2: A unique xenograft model of human prostatic small cell carcinoma. *Cancer Res.* **2000**, *60*, 6563–6567.
89. Lee, C.H.; Akin-Olugbade, O.; Kirschenbaum, A. Overview of prostate anatomy, histology, and pathology. *Endocrinol. Metab. Clin. North Am.* **2011**, *40*, 565–575.
90. Shappell, S.B.; Thomas, G.V.; Roberts, R.L.; Herbert, R.; Ittmann, M.M.; Rubin, M.A.; Humphrey, P.A.; Sundberg, J.P.; Rozengurt, N.; Barrios, R.; *et al.* Prostate pathology of genetically engineered mice: Definitions and classification. The consensus report from the bar harbor meeting of the mouse models of human cancer consortium prostate pathology committee. *Cancer Res.* **2004**, *64*, 2270–2305.

91. Kasper, S. Survey of genetically engineered mouse models for prostate cancer: Analyzing the molecular basis of prostate cancer development, progression, and metastasis. *J. Cell. Biochem.* **2005**, *94*, 279–297.
92. Berman-Booty, L.D.; Sargeant, A.M.; Rosol, T.J.; Rengel, R.C.; Clinton, S.K.; Chen, C.S.; Kulp, S.K. A review of the existing grading schemes and a proposal for a modified grading scheme for prostatic lesions in tramp mice. *Toxicol. Pathol.* **2012**, *40*, 5–17.
93. Berman-Booty, L.D.; Chu, P.C.; Thomas-Ahner, J.M.; Bolon, B.; Wang, D.; Yang, T.; Clinton, S.K.; Kulp, S.K.; Chen, C.S. Suppression of prostate epithelial proliferation and intraprostatic progrowth signaling in transgenic mice by a new energy restriction-mimetic agent. *Cancer Prev. Res.* **2013**, *6*, 232–241.
94. Sargeant, A.M.; Klein, R.D.; Rengel, R.C.; Clinton, S.K.; Kulp, S.K.; Kashida, Y.; Yamaguchi, M.; Wang, X.; Chen, C.S. Chemopreventive and bioenergetic signaling effects of PDK1/Akt pathway inhibition in a transgenic mouse model of prostate cancer. *Toxicol. Pathol.* **2007**, *35*, 549–561.
95. Patel, S.J.; Molinolo, A.A.; Gutkind, S.; Crawford, N.P. Germline genetic variation modulates tumor progression and metastasis in a mouse model of neuroendocrine prostate carcinoma. *PLoS One* **2013**, *8*, doi:10.1371/journal.pone.0061848.
96. Gingrich, J.R.; Barrios, R.J.; Morton, R.A.; Boyce, B.F.; DeMayo, F.J.; Finegold, M.J.; Angelopoulou, R.; Rosen, J.M.; Greenberg, N.M. Metastatic prostate cancer in a transgenic mouse. *Cancer Res.* **1996**, *56*, 4096–4102.
97. Hensley, P.J.; Kyprianou, N. Modeling prostate cancer in mice: Limitations and opportunities. *J. Androl.* **2012**, *33*, 133–144.
98. Roy-Burman, P.; Wu, H.; Powell, W.C.; Hagenkord, J.; Cohen, M.B. Genetically defined mouse models that mimic natural aspects of human prostate cancer development. *Endocr.-Relat. Cancer* **2004**, *11*, 225–254.
99. Gupta, S.; Hastak, K.; Ahmad, N.; Lewin, J.S.; Mukhtar, H. Inhibition of prostate carcinogenesis in tramp mice by oral infusion of green tea polyphenols. *Proc. Natl. Acad. Sci. USA* **2001**, *98*, 10350–10355.
100. Klezovitch, O.; Chevillet, J.; Mirosevich, J.; Roberts, R.L.; Matusik, R.J.; Vasioukhin, V. Hepsin promotes prostate cancer progression and metastasis. *Cancer Cell* **2004**, *6*, 185–195.
101. Garabedian, E.M.; Humphrey, P.A.; Gordon, J.I. A transgenic mouse model of metastatic prostate cancer originating from neuroendocrine cells. *Proc. Natl. Acad. Sci. USA* **1998**, *95*, 15382–15387.
102. Tu, W.H.; Thomas, T.Z.; Masumori, N.; Bhowmick, N.A.; Gorska, A.E.; Shyr, Y.; Kasper, S.; Case, T.; Roberts, R.L.; Shappell, S.B.; *et al.* The loss of tgf-beta signaling promotes prostate cancer metastasis. *Neoplasia* **2003**, *5*, 267–277.
103. Ding, Z.; Wu, C.J.; Jaskelioff, M.; Ivanova, E.; Kost-Alimova, M.; Protopopov, A.; Chu, G.C.; Wang, G.; Lu, X.; Labrot, E.S.; *et al.* Telomerase reactivation following telomere dysfunction yields murine prostate tumors with bone metastases. *Cell* **2012**, *148*, 896–907.
104. Wang, S.; Gao, J.; Lei, Q.; Rozengurt, N.; Pritchard, C.; Jiao, J.; Thomas, G.V.; Li, G.; Roy-Burman, P.; Nelson, P.S.; *et al.* Prostate-specific deletion of the murine pten tumor suppressor gene leads to metastatic prostate cancer. *Cancer Cell* **2003**, *4*, 209–221.

105. Perez-Stable, C.; Altman, N.H.; Mehta, P.P.; Deftos, L.J.; Roos, B.A. Prostate cancer progression, metastasis, and gene expression in transgenic mice. *Cancer Res.* **1997**, *57*, 900–906.
106. Cai, Y.; Kregel, S.; Vander Griend, D.J. Formation of human prostate epithelium using tissue recombination of rodent urogenital sinus mesenchyme and human stem cells. *J. Vis. Exp.* **2013**, *22*, doi:10.3791/50327.
107. Buttyan, R. The mouse prostate reconstitution model of prostate diseases. *Prostate* **1997**, *33*, 164–165.
108. Thompson, T.C.; Timme, T.L.; Park, S.H.; Yang, G.; Ren, C. Mouse prostate reconstitution model system: A series of *in vivo* and *in vitro* models for benign and malignant prostatic disease. *Prostate* **2000**, *43*, 248–254.
109. Cunha, G.R.; Hayward, S.W.; Wang, Y.Z. Role of stroma in carcinogenesis of the prostate. *Differentiation* **2002**, *70*, 473–485.
110. Thompson, T.C.; Park, S.H.; Timme, T.L.; Ren, C.; Eastham, J.A.; Donehower, L.A.; Bradley, A.; Kadmon, D.; Yang, G. Loss of p53 function leads to metastasis in ras + myc-initiated mouse prostate cancer. *Oncogene* **1995**, *10*, 869–879.
111. Park, S.I.; Kim, S.J.; McCauley, L.K.; Gallick, G.E. Pre-clinical mouse models of human prostate cancer and their utility in drug discovery. *Curr. Protoc. Pharmacol.* **2010**, doi:10.1002/0471141755.ph1415s51.
112. Blouin, S.; Basle, M.F.; Chappard, D. Rat models of bone metastases. *Clin. Exp. Metastasis* **2005**, *22*, 605–614.
113. Pollard, M.; Suckow, M.A. Hormone-refractory prostate cancer in the lobund-wistar rat. *Exp. Biol. Med.* **2005**, *230*, 520–526.
114. Liepe, K.; Geidel, H.; Haase, M.; Hakenberg, O.W.; Runge, R.; Kotzerke, J. New model for the induction of osteoblastic bone metastases in rat. *Anticancer Res.* **2005**, *25*, 1067–1073.
115. Geldof, A.A.; Rao, B.R. Prostatic tumor (r3327) skeletal metastasis. *Prostate* **1990**, *16*, 279–290.
116. Haq, M.; Goltzman, D.; Tremblay, G.; Brodt, P. Rat prostate adenocarcinoma cells disseminate to bone and adhere preferentially to bone marrow-derived endothelial cells. *Cancer Res.* **1992**, *52*, 4613–4619.
117. Blomme, E.A.; Dougherty, K.M.; Pienta, K.J.; Capen, C.C.; Rosol, T.J.; McCauley, L.K. Skeletal metastasis of prostate adenocarcinoma in rats: Morphometric analysis and role of parathyroid hormone-related protein. *Prostate* **1999**, *39*, 187–197.
118. Tennant, T.R.; Kim, H.; Sokoloff, M.; Rinker-Schaeffer, C.W. The dunning model. *Prostate* **2000**, *43*, 295–302.
119. Koutsilieris, M. PA-III rat prostate adenocarcinoma cells (review). *In Vivo* **1992**, *6*, 199–203.
120. Lorente, D.; de Bono, J.S. Molecular alterations and emerging targets in castration resistant prostate cancer. *Eur. J. Cancer* **2014**, *50*, 753–764.

17

Stimulation with Concanavalin-A Induces IL-17 Production by Canine Peripheral T Cells

Michelle G. Ritt [1,*], Beth A. Lindborg [2], Timothy D. O'Brien [2,3,4], Joseph Bisignano [1] and Jaime F. Modiano [1,3,4,5]

1 Department of Veterinary Clinical Sciences, College of Veterinary Medicine, University of Minnesota, St. Paul, MN 55108, USA; E-Mails: j.bisignano@yahoo.com (J.B.); modiano@umn.edu (J.F.M.)

2 Department of Veterinary Population Medicine, College of Veterinary Medicine, University of Minnesota, St. Paul, MN 55108, USA; E-Mails: ziem0052@umn.edu (B.A.L.); obrie004@umn.edu (T.D.O.B.)

3 Stem Cell Institute, University of Minnesota, Minneapolis, MN 55455, USA

4 Masonic Cancer Center, University of Minnesota, Minneapolis, MN 55455, USA

5 Center for Immunology, University of Minnesota, Minneapolis, MN 55455, USA

* Author to whom correspondence should be addressed; E-Mail: rittx011@umn.edu;

Academic Editors: Duncan C. Ferguson and Margarethe Hoenig

Abstract: The characteristics of canine IL-17-producing cells are incompletely understood. Expression of mRNA encoding orthologs of IL-17 and the IL-17 receptor has been documented in tissues from dogs with arthritis, inflammatory bowel disease, and lymphoma; however, no associations have been found between IL-17 gene expression and disease phenotype in these conditions. Robust assessment of the role of IL-17-producing cells in dogs will require measuring the frequency of these cells in health and disease in balance with other lymphocyte subsets. The aim of this study was to confirm that the T-cell IL-17 response in dogs is evolutionarily conserved. Canine peripheral blood mononuclear cells were stimulated with Concanavalin A with or without polarizing cytokines. We used a canine specific IL-17 ELISA and flow cytometry to identify IL-17-producing T cells. Accumulation of intracellular IL-17 was observed in stimulated CD4 and CD8 T cells. The addition of pro-inflammatory cytokines appeared to enhance polarization of canine CD4 T cells to the Th17 phenotype. Conversely, the addition of IL-2 in the presence of

TGF-β resulted in expansion of Treg cells. We conclude that canine IL-17-producing cells behave similarly to those from humans and mice when stimulated with mitogens and polarized with pro-inflammatory or immune regulatory cytokines.

Key words: canine; cytokine; flow cytometry; T Lymphocytes

1. Introduction

Interleukin-17 (IL-17) is a pro-inflammatory cytokine produced by a subset of T helper cells (Th17). In humans and rodents, these cells act as physiological mediators of inflammation that provide an important counterbalance to the suppressive effects of regulatory T cells (Tregs) [1]. In both of these species, Th17 expansion is favored in the presence of IL-6, IL-1β and transforming growth factor-β (TGF-β), whereas Treg expansion is favored in the presence of IL-2 and TGF-β [1,2]. Excessive and/or inappropriate Th17 responses have been associated with various immune-mediated diseases [3]. However, the identity and function of Th17 cells in dogs and their role in canine autoimmune diseases have yet to be precisely determined [4]. This is at least partly due to the lack of validated reagents to characterize these cells functionally and phenotypically.

IL-17 production is not restricted to Th17 cells. This cytokine also can be produced by a subset of CD8 T cells (Tc17) in humans and mice [5], as well as by a subset of MHC class II-restricted, CD4/CD8 double negative (DN) T cells, at least in mice [6]. Here, we used flow cytometry and an enzyme-linked immunosorbent assay (ELISA) to assess IL-17 production by mitogen-activated canine peripheral blood mononuclear cells (PBMC) and to determine the effect of cytokine polarization on the generation of Th17 and Treg cells. Our results show that IL-17 production is an evolutionarily conserved process that follows predictable patterns upon T-cell activation.

2. Results and Discussion

2.1. Mitogen-Stimulation Promotes IL-17 Production by Canine CD4 and CD8 T Cells

The presence of IL-17 producing cells in dogs was previously inferred from detection of IL-17 mRNA using quantitative real-time reverse-transcriptase polymerase chain reaction or gene expression microarrays [4,7–9]. However, to our knowledge cell-associated expression of canine IL-17 protein and enumeration of IL-17-producing canine T cells have yet to be determined. Thus, we first examined the capability to detect canine IL-17-producing T cells in culture after stimulation by Concanavalin A (ConA) [10,11].

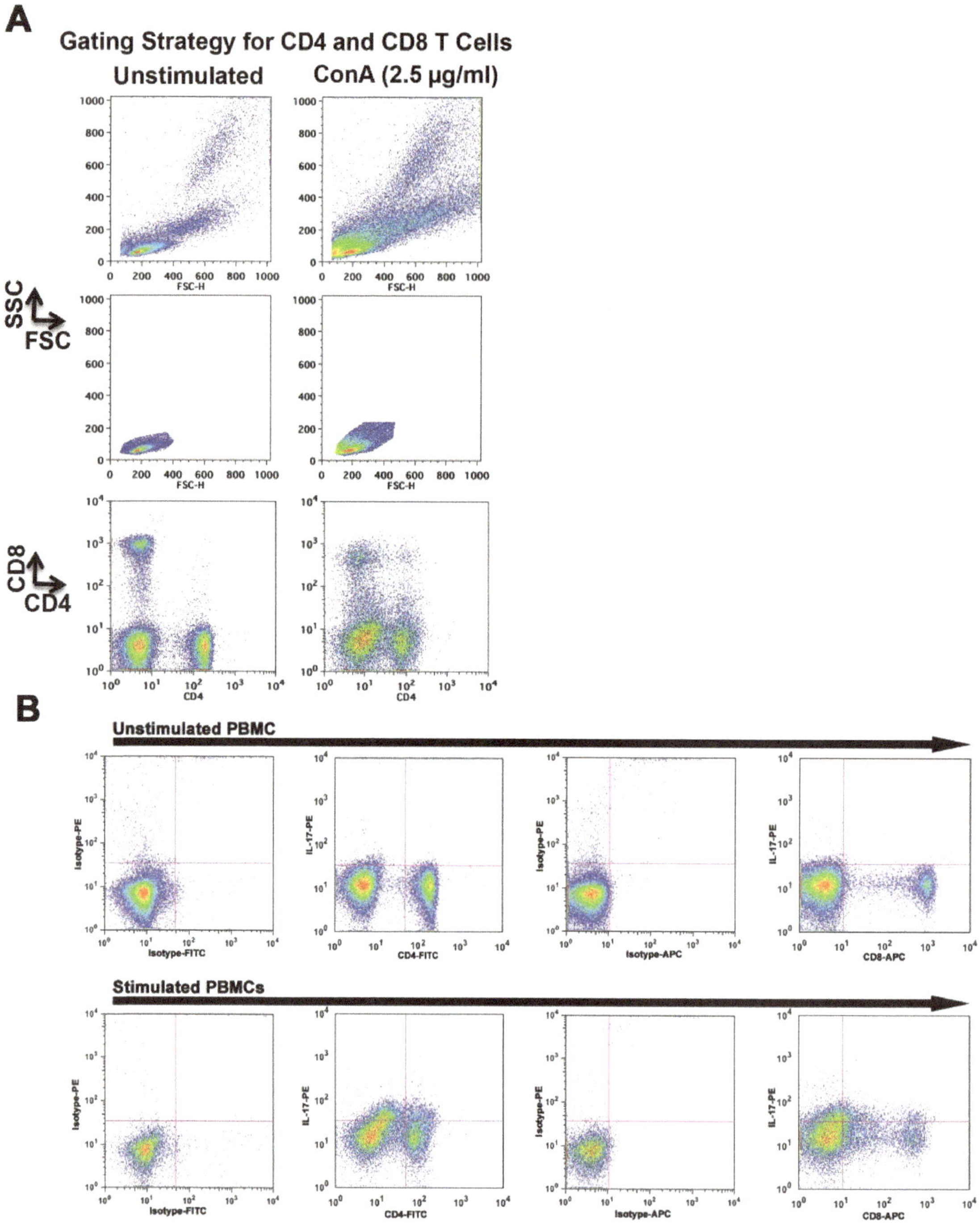

Figure 1. Stimulation of canine peripheral T cells promotes IL-17 production. (**A**) Peripheral T cells were gated from unstimulated (left) or ConA-stimulated (right) PBMCs using light scatter properties to define lymphocyte regions. The top panel shows ungated PBMCs and the middle panel shows the lymphocyte population after the white blood cell population gates were defined. The bottom panel shows separation of $CD4^+$ and $CD8^+$ cells based on immunostaining. (**B**) IL-17 expression was determined by intracellular staining and flow cytometry in the $CD4^+$ and $CD8^+$ subsets from ***a***. Two-dimensional dot plots show staining with isotype control antibodies, as well as staining of CD4 and CD8 cells with anti-IL-17 antibody in unstimulated (top) and ConA-stimulated (bottom) cells. These results represent Dog 1 shown in Table 1. All dogs tested showed expression of IL-17 in at least one T cell subset (see Table 1).

Figure 1A shows the gating strategy used to evaluate intracellular IL-17 in CD4 and CD8 cells from one of four canine PBMC samples (top left panels). The first region (Figure 1A) was created from two-dimensional forward angle (FSC) and right angle (SSC) light scatter dot plots to include cells with properties for lymphocytes and lymphoblasts (middle left panels). CD4 and CD8 subsets were then identified as shown in the bottom left panels and each population was analyzed for intracellular IL-17. Figure 1B shows accumulation of IL-17 was detectable in both CD4 and CD8 T-cells after ConA stimulation. There was a unimodal shift in the mean fluorescence intensity (MFI) in IL-17-stained samples as compared to isotype controls. This shift was consistently greater in the ConA-stimulated population than in the unstimulated population, but in addition, IL-17 staining in these ConA-stimulated populations included a "shoulder" of bright events, likely representing those cells responsible for most of the IL-17 production. This was also observed when $CD4^+$, $CD8^+$, and $CD4^-/CD8^-$ populations were analyzed individually, with an approximate two-fold increase in the MFI observed in CD4+ and in $CD8^+$ cells as compared to $CD4^-/CD8^-$ cells.

Table 1. Percentage of $IL\text{-}17^+$ CD4 and CD8 cells after stimulation with ConA for 6 h [a].

	%IL-17-Producing Cells in ConA Blasts (6 h)	
Dog #	**CD4**	**CD8**
1	12.4	17.6
2	4.5	4.8
3	11	5.2
4	1.0	8.8

[a] PBMCs from four dogs were stimulated as described in Figure 1. The same gating strategy was used, except that the frequency of IL-17 "bright" events was verified in IL-17 (FL2) histograms where the percent positive cells for each population of stimulated cells was determined by considering the top 0.5% of the unimodal control (unstimulated cells) in each dog as the minimum limit for gating.

Table 1 shows a summary of the percentage of IL-17-bright CD4 and CD8 T cells from four different dogs. The demonstrable, albeit modest increase in IL-17-producing cells after stimulation of PBMC is consistent with data obtained after activation of human cells [10]. Tregs ($FoxP3^+/CD25^+$) in unstimulated and stimulated CD4 populations also were quantified for each dog. The percent Treg cells was variable, comprising 0.4%–12% of all CD4 cells. Treg cells showed no change after stimulation in two dogs (2% and 5%, of the $CD4^+$ populations, respectively), a decrease in one dog (4.1% to 0.4%), and an increase in one dog (5.1% to 12%).

2.2. Pro-Inflammatory Cytokines Promote Polarization of Canine T Helper Cells towards the Th17 Phenotype

Experiments using T cells from humans and mice have shown that adding TGF-β, IL-1β, and IL-6 to the stimulation conditions facilitated development of Th17 cells, whereas including TGF-β and IL-2 led to expansion of Tregs [1,2]. To determine if this also occurred in dogs, we cultured canine PBMCs in the presence or absence of ConA as above. After three days, fresh media was replenished to the unstimulated cells and ConA-stimulated cells were divided into groups that received media alone, media supplemented with IL-2 and TGF-β, or media supplemented with IL-1β, IL-6, and TGF-β.

We examined if the effects of polarization were evident using intracellular staining as above. For this, we gated CD4 T cells and evaluated expression of FoxP3 protein and accumulation of intracellular IL-17 to establish the existence of a canine Th17 subset. Figure 2 shows the frequency of IL-17-producing cells and Treg ($FoxP3^+$) cells in the CD4 population from two healthy dogs. The data show modest Treg expansion in five-day ConA-stimulated T cells (compare the U/S and ConA panels) that was further enhanced by addition of IL-2 and TGF-β, but not by addition of IL-1β, IL-6, and TGF-β. Expansion of cells producing IL-17 at this point in five-day ConA-stimulated cells was also modest, with a small shift in MFI similar to that observed in cells during the initial phase of stimulation (Figure 1). The frequency of IL-17-producing CD4 T cells was unaffected by addition of IL-2 and TGF-β, but predictably, addition of IL-1β, IL-6, and TGF-β increased both the MFI of the CD4 T cell population and the frequency of IL-17 "bright" events.

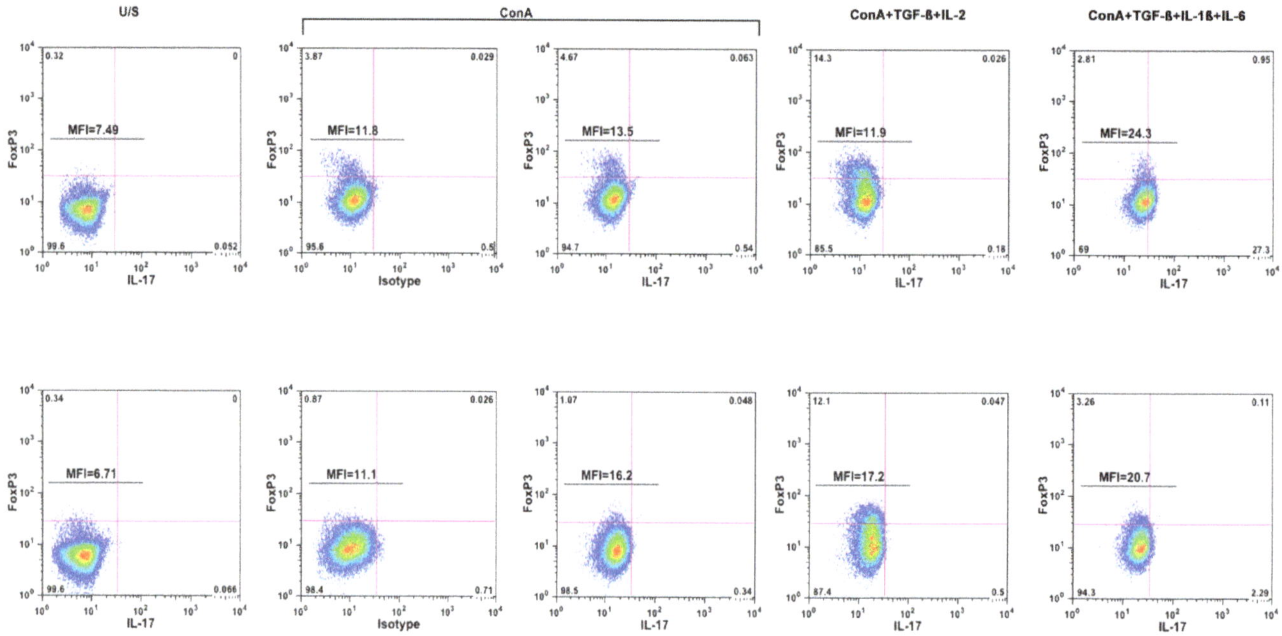

Figure 2. Addition of TGF-β, IL-1β, and IL-6 increases polarization of $CD4^+$ cells toward the Th17 phenotype. PBMCs from two dogs were stimulated as described in the main text and analyzed for polarization of T helper ($CD4^+$) cells toward $FoxP3^+$ (Treg) and $IL\text{-}17^+$ (Th17) phenotypes using flow cytometry. $CD4^+$ cells were identified as described in Figure 1, and stimulation conditions are shown above the top panels, with isotype control staining shown for comparison in the ConA-stimulated samples. Gating was done using isotype control staining for stimulated cells, and MFI was calculated for all $CD4^+$ T cells stained with IL-17 or with the matched isotype control (FL2). The MFI value for unstained cells in both dogs was 5.5.

Generally, these are expected results that mirror what has been shown in humans and mice [12], supporting the evolutionary conservation of this process in dogs, and it is possible that polarization to IL-17 producing cells could be enhanced even further by blockade of Th1 and Th2 cell differentiation [13]. The production of IL-17 in these cultures was confirmed using a canine-specific IL-17 ELISA (Table 2). In the culture supernatants from unstimulated cells, IL-17 was undetectable in samples from one dog, and present at 0.4 (±0.02) ng/mL in samples from the other. Each of the ConA-stimulated samples from both dogs, including those where IL-2 and TGF-β, or IL-1β, IL-6, and TGF-β were added, contained >8.5 ng/mL of IL-17.

Table 2. IL-17 Production by ConA-Stimulated PBMC [a].

Condition	Dog-1	Dog-2
	IL-17 (±S. D.; ng/mL)	
Unstimulated	0 (0)	4.5 (0.8)
ConA	8.3 (0.3)	8.4 (1.7)
ConA+TGF-ß+IL-2	8.4 (1.0)	9.8 (0.4)
ConA+TGF-ß+IL-1ß+IL-6	9.5 (2.7)	9.4 (0.3)

[a] PBMC from two dogs were cultured without stimulation or stimulated by ConA. After 72 h, supernatants were removed and cells were provided with fresh culture media with no additional stimuli, TGF-ß and IL-2, or TGF-ß, IL-1ß, and IL-6 as indicated. Supernatants were recovered 24 h later and IL-17 in each condition was quantified in duplicate with a canine specific IL-17 ELISA. Supernatants were diluted five-fold to ensure values were within the dynamic range of the assay (0–2.0 ng/mL). Values for each sample reflect calibration to the actual concentration.

3. Materials and Methods

Dogs: Six companion dogs were recruited for this study. Dogs belonged to faculty, students, or staff of the University of Minnesota Veterinary Medical Center (St. Paul, MN, USA). In order to be eligible, dogs had to be healthy based on a complete physical exam, and they had to be older than 3 years of age. Samples were obtained under the supervision of the University of Minnesota Institutional Animal Care and Use Committee (protocol 1101A94713) with informed consent from the owners. Whole blood (7–10 mL) was collected using a standard jugular venipuncture approach and evacuated into sterile tubes containing ethylenediaminetetraacetic acid (EDTA) as an anticoagulant. Dogs did not require hospitalization or special housing for the procedure and they were released back to their owners after a short period of observation to ensure neither bleeding nor hematoma formation were evident at the site of venipuncture.

Cells and Cell Culture: Peripheral blood mononuclear cells (PBMCs) were enriched from EDTA-preserved whole blood using a discontinuous Ficoll-Hypaque density gradient [14]. For intracellular IL-17 staining, PBMCs were cultured for 4–6 h in the presence or absence of ConA (2.5 μg/mL, Sigma-Aldrich, St. Louis, MO, USA) with Protein Transport Inhibitor Cocktail reagent (2 μL/mL, eBioscience, San Diego, CA, USA) to prevent protein secretion. For polarization experiments, PBMCs were cultured as above for 3 days, after which fresh media was replenished to the unstimulated cells and ConA-stimulated cells were divided into three groups that received fresh media alone, fresh media supplemented with human recombinant IL-2 (hrIL-2, 10 IU/mL, NCI BMRP, Bethesda, MD, USA) and human TGF-β (5 ng/mL, R&D Systems, Minneapolis, MN, USA), or fresh media supplemented with canine recombinant IL-1β (10 ng/mL, R&D Systems), canine recombinant IL-6 (50 ng/mL, R&D Systems), and TGF-β. Cell-free supernatants were collected 24 hr later to analyze secreted IL-17 using a canine specific IL-17 ELISA, and each culture condition was replenished with media containing the same factors, with Protein Transport Inhibitor Cocktail (2 μL/mL) added for the last 4 h of culture.

Flow Cytometry: Cell handling, antibody staining, and flow cytometric analysis were done as previously described [15]. Antibodies were used to identify T cells (anti-CD5 conjugated to phycoerythrin (PE), eBioscience), B cells (anti-CD22 conjugated to allophycocyanin (APC), Abcam, Cambridge, MA, USA), and monocytes (anti-CD14 conjugated to fluorescein isothiocyanate (FITC), AbD Serotec, Raleigh, NC, USA). Conditions were included to enable further separation of T cells based on expression of CD4 (anti-CD4-FITC), CD8 (anti-CD8-APC), and CD25 (anti-CD25-PE), all of which were obtained from eBioscience. Staining with anti-CD45 antibodies (eBioscience) conjugated to PE, APC, and FITC was used for color compensation. Mouse IgG1 and IgG2a antibodies with irrelevant specificities, conjugated to the appropriate fluorochromes (eBioscience) were used as isotype controls. After the initial staining steps, cells were permeabilized using the Foxp3/Transcription Factor Fixation/Permeabilization Concentrate and Diluent kit (eBioscience) for 45 min followed by intracellular staining for FoxP3 (anti-FoxP3-FITC, eBioscience) and for accumulated IL-17 (anti-mouse IL-17 clone eBio17B7) as recommended by the manufacturer [16]. Similar results were obtained in two samples that were stained concurrently using the anti-mouse IL-17 antibody and anti-human IL-17 (clone eBio64DEC17, eBioscience). Multi-parameter flow cytometry was done using the FACSCalibur instrument platform (BD Biosciences, San Jose, CA, USA), and data were analyzed using FlowJo (Treestar, Ashland, OR, USA).

ELISA: A canine-specific IL-17 ELISA (R&D Systems) was used following the manufacturer's recommendations. The concentration of IL-17 in cell-free supernatants was extrapolated from an IL-17 standard curve based on absorbance values obtained from each undiluted ("neat") sample and from each sample diluted five-fold.

4. Conclusions

In summary, our results show that mitogenic stimulation leads to IL-17 production by both CD4 and CD8 cells, and that anti-inflammatory or pro-inflammatory cytokine signals, respectively, promote expansion of Tregs or Th17 cells. Tc17 cells show species differences: in humans, but not in mice, these cells arise from a unique subset of $CD161^+$ precursors [5]. A similar subset remains to be defined in dogs, so it is not clear if Tc17 cells in this species would be more similar to human or mouse. Considering the importance of IL-17 in autoimmune disease, inflammation and cancer, continued research in this area will help elucidate the role that these important adaptive immune cells play, potentially enabling better treatment options for these conditions.

Acknowledgments

Grant Support: This work was supported in part by a Small Companion Animal Grant from the College of Veterinary Medicine, University of Minnesota.

The authors would like to thank Peggy Just for helpful discussions and manuscript review.

This work was supported in part by a Small Companion Animal Resident Award from the College of Veterinary Medicine Research Office, University of Minnesota. The NIH Comprehensive Cancer Center Support Grant to the Masonic Cancer Center, University of Minnesota (P30 CA077598) provided support for flow cytometry. The authors gratefully acknowledge donations to the Animal Cancer Care and Research Program of the University of Minnesota that helped support this project.

Author Contributions

Michelle G. Ritt: Conceptualization of study, analyzed data, wrote first draft of manuscript, edited and approved manuscript, obtained funding. Beth A. Lindborg: Performed experiments, analyzed data, edited and approved manuscript. Timothy D. O'Brien: Conceptualization of study, analyzed data, edited and approved manuscript, obtained funding. Joseph Bisignano: Performed experiments, analyzed data, edited and approved manuscript, obtained funding. Jaime F. Modiano: Conceptualization of study, performed experiments, analyzed data, co-wrote first draft of manuscript, edited and approved manuscript, obtained funding.

Conflicts of Interest

The authors report no conflicts of interest.

References

1. Awasthi, A.; Kuchroo, V.K. Th17 cells: From precursors to players in inflammation and infection. *Int. Immunol.* **2009**, *21*, 489–498.
2. Gutcher, I.; Donkor, M.K.; Ma, Q.; Rudensky, A.Y.; Flavell, R.A.; Li, M.O. Autocrine transforming growth factor-beta1 promotes *in vivo* th17 cell differentiation. *Immunity* **2011**, *34*, 396–408.
3. Bedoya, S.K.; Lam, B.; Lau, K.; Larkin, J., 3rd. Th17 cells in immunity and autoimmunity. *Clin. Dev. Immunol.* **2013**, doi:10.1155/2013/986789.
4. Schmitz, S.; Garden, O.A.; Werling, D.; Allenspach, K. Gene expression of selected signature cytokines of T cell subsets in duodenal tissues of dogs with and without inflammatory bowel disease. *Vet. Immunol. Immunopathol.* **2012**, *146*, 87–91.
5. Liang, Y.; Pan, H.F.; Ye, D.Q. Tc17 cells in immunity and systemic autoimmunity. *Int. Rev. Immunol.* **2014**, doi:10.3109/08830185.2014.954698.
6. Mou, Z.; Liu, D.; Okwor, I.; Jia, P.; Orihara, K.; Uzonna, J.E. Mhc class II restricted innate-like double negative T cells contribute to optimal primary and secondary immunity to leishmania major. *PLoS Pathog.* **2014**, *10*, e1004396.
7. Jergens, A.E.; Sonea, I.M.; O'Connor, A.M.; Kauffman, L.K.; Grozdanic, S.D.; Ackermann, M.R.; Evans, R.B. Intestinal cytokine mrna expression in canine inflammatory bowel disease: A meta-analysis with critical appraisal. *Comp. Med.* **2009**, *59*, 153–162.
8. Ohta, H.; Takada, K.; Torisu, S.; Yuki, M.; Tamura, Y.; Yokoyama, N.; Osuga, T.; Lim, S.Y.; Murakami, M.; Sasaki, N.; *et al.* Expression of $CD4^+$ T cell cytokine genes in the colorectal mucosa of inflammatory colorectal polyps in miniature dachshunds. *Vet. Immunol. Immunopathol.* **2013**, *155*, 259–263.
9. Frantz, A.M.; Sarver, A.L.; Ito, D.; Phang, T.L.; Karimpour-Fard, A.; Scott, M.C.; Valli, V.E.; Lindblad-Toh, K.; Burgess, K.E.; Husbands, B.D.; *et al.* Molecular profiling reveals prognostically significant subtypes of canine lymphoma. *Vet. Pathol.* **2013**, *50*, 693–703.
10. Lenarczyk, A.; Helsloot, J.; Farmer, K.; Peters, L.; Sturgess, A.; Kirkham, B. Antigen-induced IL-17 response in the peripheral blood mononuclear cells (PBMC) of healthy controls. *Clin. Exp. Immunol.* **2000**, *122*, 41–48.

11. Aprile, J.; Gerhard-Miller, L.; Deeg, H.J. Cluster formation of canine dendritic cells and lymphocytes is calcium dependent and not inhibited by cyclosporine. *Exp. Hematol.* **1990**, *18*, 32–36.
12. Korn, T.; Bettelli, E.; Oukka, M.; Kuchroo, V.K. IL-17 and Th17 cells. *Annu. Rev. Immunol.* **2009**, *27*, 485–517.
13. Lexberg, M.H.; Taubner, A.; Forster, A.; Albrecht, I.; Richter, A.; Kamradt, T.; Radbruch, A.; Chang, H.D. Th memory for interleukin-17 expression is stable *in vivo*. *Eur. J. Immunol.* **2008**, *38*, 2654–2664.
14. Helfand, S.C.; Modiano, J.F.; Nowell, P.C. Immunophysiological studies of interleukin-2 and canine lymphocytes. *Vet. Immunol. Immunopathol.* **1992**, *33*, 1–16.
15. Ito, D.; O'Brien, T.D.; Modiano, J.F. Exclusion of cytoplasmic fragments in flow cytometric analysis of lymph node samples from dogs with lymphoma using membrane-permeable violet laser-excitable DNA-binding fluorescent dye (dyecycle violet). *Vet. Clin. Pathol.* **2010**, *39*, 494–498.
16. Sun, Y.L.; Lin, G.G.; Zhang, K.; Wang, L.N.; Li, J.M. Application and effects of mouse foxp3 antibody and fixation/permeabilization buffer on the detection of $CD4^+$ regulatory T cells in various mammal species. *Genet. Mol. Res.* **2013**, *12*, 6535–6545.

18

Comparative Aspects of Human, Canine, and Feline Obesity and Factors Predicting Progression to Diabetes

Margarethe Hoenig

Department of Veterinary Clinical Medicine, College of Veterinary Medicine, University of Illinois at Urbana-Champaign, 1008 W. Hazelwood Drive, Urbana, IL 61802, USA;
E-Mail: mhoenig@illinois.edu

Abstract: Obesity and diabetes mellitus are common diseases in humans, dogs and cats and their prevalence is increasing. Obesity has been clearly identified as a risk factor for type 2 diabetes in humans and cats but recent data are missing in dogs, although there is evidence that the unprecedented rise in canine obesity in the last decade has led to a rise in canine diabetes of similar magnitude. The insulin resistance of obesity has often been portrayed as major culprit in the loss of glucose control; however, insulin resistance alone is not a good indicator of progression to diabetes in people or pets. A loss of beta cell function is necessary to provide the link to impaired fasting and post-prandial plasma glucose. Increased endogenous glucose output by the liver is also a prerequisite for the increase in fasting blood glucose when non-diabetic obese humans and pets develop diabetes. This may be due to decreased hepatic insulin sensitivity, decreased insulin concentrations, or a combination of both. While inflammation is a major link between obesity and diabetes in humans, there is little evidence that a similar phenomenon exists in cats. In dogs, more studies are needed to examine this important issue.

Keywords: diabetes; obesity; beta cells; gluconeogenesis; glycolysis; cytokines; adiponectin; leptin; insulin; fructosamine

---

1. Introduction

Obesity is the most common nutritional disorder in dogs and cats and has been shown to be a risk factor for the development of type 2 diabetes in cats and humans. More recent epidemiological studies examining if obesity is a risk factor for diabetes in dogs as well are missing, although obesity has also been reported to have increased dramatically in dogs in the last decade and the increase was paralleled by an increase in diabetes of similar magnitude suggesting a cause/effect relationship [1]. Obesity leads to insulin resistance, which, if not accompanied by an appropriate increase in insulin concentrations, sets the path for glucose intolerance and eventually overt diabetes. In the veterinary literature, especially when primary data from pets are missing, it is not uncommon to find attempts to project from the human data connecting obesity to diabetes. Rather than do this, this review will examine the evidence available for similarities and differences among these three species. Specifically, we will examine insulin secretion, regulation of endogenous glucose production by the liver, and the role of inflammation.

2. Obesity-Associated Changes in Insulin Secretion: A Risk Factor for Diabetes Mellitus in Dogs and Cats?

It was shown in a hallmark study by Kealy and coworkers over a decade ago that higher food intake and body fat is detrimental for a dog's health and longevity and leads to changes in lipid and glucose metabolism [2]; however, there are no recent epidemiological studies examining if obesity in the dog also leads to overt diabetes. The fact that data from a large Swedish retrospective study of the prevalence of diabetes, which was carried out from 2000 to 2003, showed that 55% of dogs were overweight or obese at first diagnosis of diabetes compared to 20% of normal-weight dogs of the same age group suggests that obesity may be a risk factor in dogs [3]. A connection between obesity and diabetes was also implied by a recent summary by Banfield Hospitals, in which it was reported that the large increase in canine obesity, which they observed from 2007 to 2012, was accompanied by an equally large increase in diabetes [1], strongly suggesting that obesity might be causing the increase in diabetes. That a form of diabetes similar to type 2 diabetes in humans is present in some dogs has already been shown four decades ago by Kaneko and coworkers who were able to distinguish a group of obese diabetic dogs from lean diabetic dogs based on their insulin and glucose profiles [4]. The obese diabetic dogs were characterized by high glucose and high fasting insulin concentrations but were unable to mount an appropriate insulin response when challenged with high glucose concentrations.

It was suggested in a recent study of a small number of obese non-diabetic dogs which had normal fasting plasma glucose (FPG) and normal glucose tolerance that obese dogs do not develop a type of diabetes similar to type 2 seen in humans because they increase insulin output, including first phase, in response to obesity, whereas people do not [5]. However, such statement about a difference between dog and human insulin secretion is not supported by evidence from human clinical studies. It has been known for decades that in people obesity by itself leads to a robust response in insulin secretion of both phases [6–8]. Results from a large Finnish study showed that obese subjects with an approximately 40% reduction in insulin sensitivity, but FPG and 2 h plasma glucose (2-h PG) concentrations within the reference categories had increases of over 50% in early and late phase insulin secretion [9]. This has been called the Stage 1 or compensation phase of obesity [10] and results from an increase in β-cell mass [10–12]. Insulin sensitivity decreased further when subjects developed impaired fasting glucose and impaired glucose tolerance. However, early-phase insulin release only reached a substantial decrease in those subjects in whom FPG and 2-h PG increased into the diabetic range. This indicates that a decrease in early (first) phase insulin secretion would not be expected in a dog or person with normal FPG and normal glucose tolerance. Instead, non-diabetic obese dogs or people with normal FPG have higher early and late phase insulin secretion compared to lean subjects in this compensation phase, and one can conclude that glucose tolerant people and dogs compensate well for the increase in insulin resistance.

Over 80% of obese insulin-resistant humans remain euglycemic and do not progress to type 2 diabetes [13]. It is not known how many obese dogs progress to diabetes, although, as stated above, new evidence suggests that it is an important risk factor. It was shown in a recent study that several prerequisites have to be present for an insulin-resistant dog to progress to diabetes [14]. In that study, diet-induced obesity led to a decrease in peripheral insulin sensitivity, which was perfectly met by an increase in insulin concentrations. Hepatic insulin sensitivity was maintained and glucose tolerance remained normal, as would be expected in a non-diabetic obese dog. It was not until beta cell mass was greatly reduced by the administration of various doses of the beta cell toxin streptozotocin, that insulin secretion decreased in a dose dependent manner, and impaired fasting glucose and diabetes ensued. It can be seen from that study that insulin resistance alone elicited the appropriate regulatory responses: Insulin concentrations increased to counteract the peripheral resistance, allowing normal glucose control. The loss in beta cells had to be severe before a deterioration of FPG and glucose tolerance was seen. In fact, when fasting blood glucose increased and glucose tolerance became abnormal, insulin concentrations had decreased by 90%.

The compensatory hyperinsulinemia, which is seen in obese non-diabetic dogs, has been thought to be the result of upregulation of beta cell sensitivity to glucose and subsequent increase in insulin secretion. However, based on recent data from a large number of dogs with varying fat mass, it was proposed that changes in insulin clearance resulting in higher insulin levels feed back onto insulin action of peripheral and hepatic tissues and are the primary cause for the hyperinsulinemia of obesity [15].

Figure 1. Area under the curve for insulin during a low dose intravenous glucose tolerance test (0.5 g/kg body weight; Mean ± SEM; 1B) in 20 adult neutered cats (equal gender distribution) at 0%–60% weight increases and in 12 cats at 100%. Identical superscripts indicate significant differences (reprinted with permission from Obesity [21]).

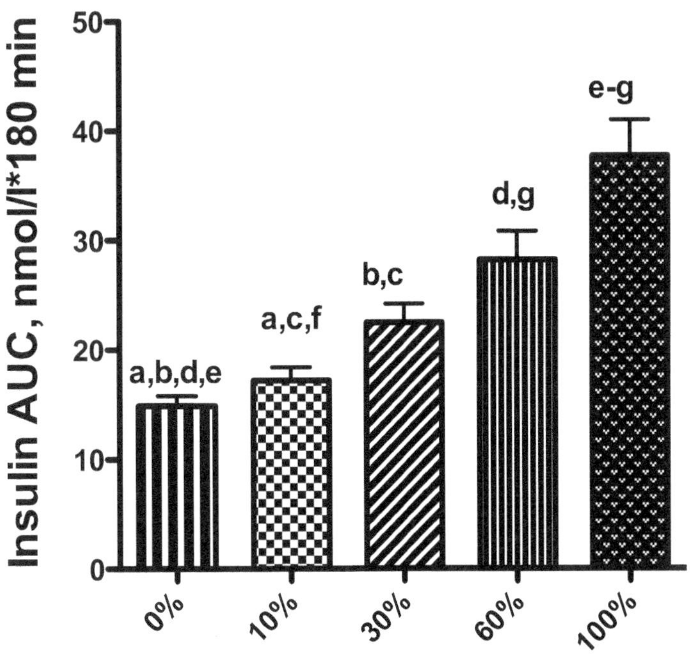

Using the gold-standard method to evaluate insulin sensitivity, the euglycemic hyperinsulinemic clamp, we found that in cats obesity leads to a decrease in glucose effectiveness and an increase in insulin resistance, similar to what has been shown in people and dogs [16,17]. Development of obesity in cats is not associated with a change in FPG, even when obesity is severe [18–20]. This was recently shown in a longitudinal study, where 20 cats were fed ad libitum and became obese [21]. Even with an increase in fat mass of 100%, fasting glucose concentrations remained normal. Early phase and total insulin concentrations increased until 100% increase in fat mass was reached (Figure 1), when a blunting of early insulin secretion and altered glucose clearance was seen, indicating that under extreme conditions (high degree of resistance and high glucose dose), the response of the beta cell to glucose becomes abnormal. These results are similar to those described in people by Matsumoto and coworkers, who compared glucose tolerance, insulin secretion, and insulin sensitivity in a large number of non-obese and obese Japanese subjects [22]. They found a blunted early phase of insulin secretion only in those obese people who had impaired glucose tolerance, and suggested that impaired early phase insulin release may be the initial abnormality in the development of glucose intolerance. The worsening from impaired glucose tolerance to diabetes in their study was associated with a greater decrease in early-phase insulin secretion, a significant decrease in total insulin secretion, and a significant increase in insulin resistance. There is no long-term longitudinal study in obese cats, which has examined if results from intravenous glucose tolerance testing can be used as biomarkers for progression to diabetes. It is questionable if intravenous glucose tolerance testing is appropriate to answer this question. This skepticism is supported by the fact that a difference in glucose tolerance, characterized by a lower glucose clearance, could not be seen between lean and obese cats until a supramaximal dose of glucose (1.3 g/kg) was administered [18]. This suggests that testing beta cells with high glucose concentrations is indicated to evaluate their maximal secretory capacity but the same test might not be a good indicator of an animal's or person's beta cell function during their normal daily routine. One needs to appreciate that glucose values seen during IV glucose tolerance testing with high glucose doses are never seen after a meal in a cat or dog and represent an extreme challenge for the endocrine pancreas, as well as for peripheral tissues and the liver, and results are likely not good indicators of progression. Intravenous glucose tolerance tests are rarely used in human medicine to examine factors that lead to a deterioration of glucose control and the dose is much lower (0.3 g/kg) than that used in cats. In people, glucose tolerance is usually tested with a dose of orally administered glucose (75 g), which leads to blood glucose concentrations not too dissimilar to what a person experiences after normal food intake. This may explain why results from tests in humans are more predictive of progression because the abnormality is already present at lower levels of glucose, *i.e.*, levels that are actually present in a person under normal physiological conditions. It is glucose concentrations seen under those conditions, which influence beta cell function long-term. We were unable to show a difference between lean and obese cats when we followed their daily glucose concentrations with continuous glucose monitoring for 7 days. Only one of the obese cats in that study showed a glucose profile, which fluctuated between the upper and mildly high glucose range after having been severely obese for many years [19]. It would be speculation to make a prediction whether this cat might be a "progressor". It is well known from human subjects that generally about 35% to 50% of those with impaired fasting blood glucose convert to diabetes after 10–20 years of follow-up [23]. While reference values for glucose tolerance tests have been published for client-owned cats, the results vary greatly, even within one and the same laboratory [24–26]. This indicates that these tests are not useful when applied to the general cat population and should only be used in strictly controlled research populations. Clearly, long-term longitudinal studies are needed to examine which biochemical changes might be biomarkers for progression in cats, *i.e.*, healthy cats should be followed until they develop diabetes.

In a recent study of normal-weight, overweight, obese, and diabetic cats, we showed that insulin but not glucose concentrations were significantly higher in overweight and obese non-diabetic cats compared to normal weight non-diabetic cats and were significantly lower in naïve diabetic cats [20], supporting the notion that marked insulin deficiency is necessary for the progression to diabetes. This notion is also supported by the finding that a combination of both insulin resistance and insulin deficiency due to a reduction in beta cell mass were needed for the development of experimental diabetes in cats [27]. In that study, overt diabetes was not seen until insulin secretion was about 80% lower than that seen in healthy cats.

In summary: Insulin resistance alone is not a good indicator of progression to diabetes in people or pets. A loss of beta cell function is necessary to provide the link to impaired fasting and post-prandial plasma glucose.

3. The Role of the Liver in Glucose Control

The liver plays a crucial role in the disposal of exogenous glucose and the control of endogenous glucose production (EGP). As with the evaluation of insulin secretion profiles, one needs to be careful to distinguish obese non-diabetic subjects from obese diabetic subjects when evaluating liver function. Usually, in insulin-resistant obese non-diabetic humans with normal FPG and normal glucose tolerance, the inhibitory effect of insulin on endogenous glucose output is preserved [28,29]. In obese non-diabetic people, the maintenance of euglycemia was found to be due to a reduction in glycogenolysis, whereas gluconeogenesis was increased in both, non-diabetic and diabetic obese people, although more in diabetic subjects. These changes resulted in increased endogenous glucose production in diabetic but not in obese non-diabetic patients [29]. No change in overall glucose production was also seen by Basu and coworkers in obese non-diabetic compared to lean non-diabetic patients [30], although they found that only a change in gluconeogenesis but not glycogenolysis led to the maintenance of euglycemia in obese non-diabetic patients [30]. Progression to impaired glucose tolerance and diabetes was characterized by increased endogenous glucose production and, concomitantly, endogenous glucose production became less suppressible by insulin. No change in endogenous glucose production or suppressibility by insulin occurred in those people, who did not progress to the diabetic state [31].

In our own studies in cats, we found that endogenous glucose production was decreased in obese cats in the fasted and post-prandial state, counteracting the effect of insulin resistance on peripheral glucose uptake and resulting in the maintenance of euglycemia in long-term obese animals [32,33]. In one study of fasted cats, the lower EGP in the obese cats was due to a lower glycogenolysis and gluconeogenesis (Figure 2) [32]. There was a strong negative correlation between plasma insulin concentrations and endogenous glucose production and between endogenous glucose production and girth, as well as body mass index, suggesting that the decreased endogenous glucose production in our long-term obese cats was due to the higher insulin concentrations of obesity. To our knowledge, glucose turnover and metabolic fluxes have not been evaluated in diabetic cats. However, one might expect to also see a progressive loss of insulin sensitivity of the liver and an increase in endogenous glucose production when cats become diabetic, similar to what has been described in humans [31]. However, the switch from normal glucose regulation to diabetes appears to occur quickly in obese cats because there was no difference in fructosamine concentrations, an indicator of glucose control in the previous 2 weeks, among lean, overweight and obese cats [20]. Fructosamine concentrations, which are tightly correlated with blood glucose concentrations (Figure 3), were clearly separated from naïve diabetics and treated diabetics. If progression from the obese to the diabetic state would occur slowly in obese cats, a sliding scale of glucose and fructosamine concentrations would have been expected in this study of client-owned cats.

Figure 2. Mean ± SEM of endogenous glucose production (EGP), glycogenolysis and gluconeogenesis in lean and obese cats. Identical superscripts indicate significant differences (modified from Kley *et al.* Am J Physiol Regul Integr Comp Physiol 296: R936-R943, 2009 [32]).

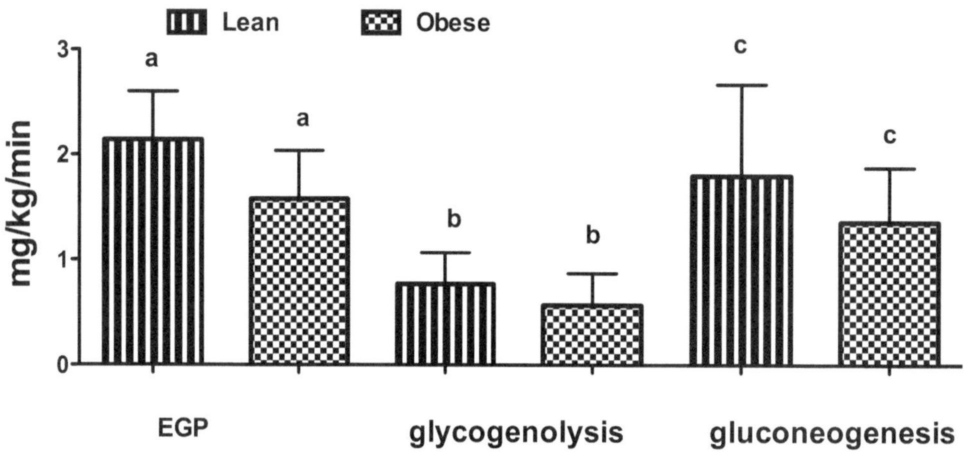

Figure 3. Correlation between serum fructosamine and glucose concentrations in 117 cats (25 normal body condition, 27 overweight, 24 obese, 21 naïve diabetic, and 20 treated diabetic cats) (reprinted with permission from JAVMA [20]).

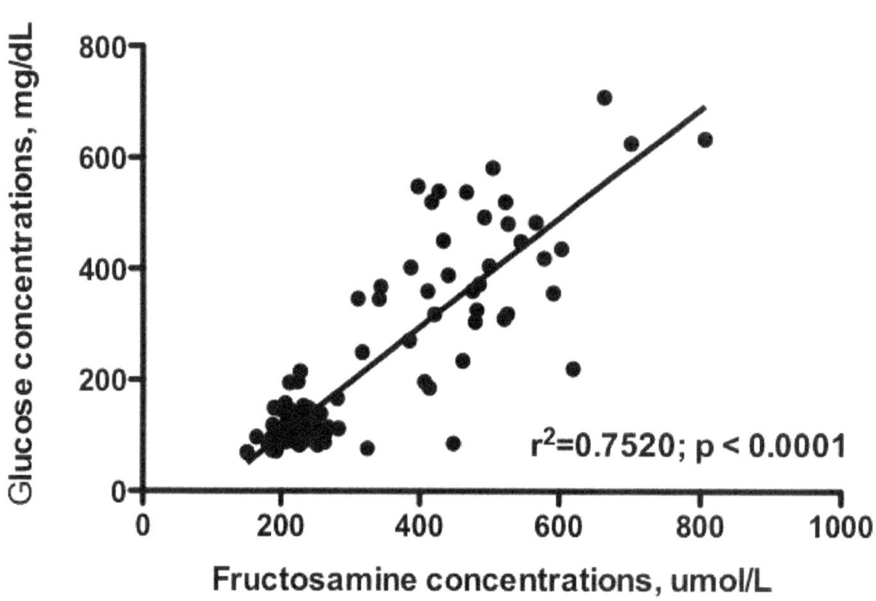

The authors are not aware of a comparison of hepatic metabolism among healthy, obese, and spontaneously diabetic dogs. In 18 hour-fasted lean healthy dogs, glycogenolysis was found to be the major contributor to EGP, and gluconeogenesis accounted for approximately one third of the glucose production [34]. This is different from what has been described in cats and in people for a similar postprandial time period. In both cats and people, gluconeogenesis contributes about two thirds and glycogenolysis contributes about one third to endogenous glucose production [32,33,35]. Glycogenolysis appears to be more sensitive than gluconeogenesis to suppression by insulin in dogs [30,36], whereas both are already suppressed almost completely in lean people by a 50% lower dose of insulin [30]. It is not known what physiological effect this difference might have. Perhaps it should be reflected in a difference in liver glycogen content. It is, however, known, that liver glycogen is similar among the three species. The glycogen content in healthy dogs and people is approximately 4% of liver wet weight [37,38]. We have found that the liver of lean and obese cats contains about 5% of glycogen [33].

It has been suggested that insulin action in the liver is in part determined by the intrahepatic triglyceride content. In people, obesity is associated with an increase in intrahepatic triglycerides, an abnormality known as nonalcoholic fatty liver disease [39]. Its prevalence increases linearly with increasing body mass index but also occurs in about 15% of normal-weight subjects [40]. The amount of triglycerides in the liver was shown in one study not only to correlate with insulin resistance in the liver, but also in muscle and adipose tissue [39]. The mechanism by which hepatic lipids induce hepatic insulin resistance is not well understood and it is unclear if hepatic triglycerides are the cause or effect of insulin resistance. A 2 hits theory has been proposed: The first hit would be lower fatty acid oxidation, higher fatty acid synthesis, and lower VLDL efflux from the liver due to the oversupply of fatty acids because of lower lipoprotein lipase activity and the hyperinsulinemia of obesity. The result would be increased esterification of fatty acids and deposition of triglycerides in the liver. The second hit would be oxidative stress resulting in lipid peroxidation leading to hepatocellular degeneration and necrosis [41].

Traditionally, excessive hepatic triglyceride content, or steatosis, has been defined as exceeding 5% of liver volume or liver weight, or histologically when 5% of hepatocytes contain visible intracellular triglycerides [42]. In a recent study the threshold for a normal amount of intrahepatic triglycerides was reported to be 5.6% of liver volume, whereas others have not found any evidence of an obvious threshold that can be used to define normality [40].

We recently measured liver fat in lean and obese cats using nuclear magnetic resonance spectroscopy. Median liver fat percentages in lean and obese cats were 1.3% and 6.8%, respectively [43]. In a different group of lean and obese cats, we employed a chemical assay with similar results (1.7% for lean cats and 6% for obese cats [43]. A previous publication involving chemical liver triglyceride measurement in wedge biopsies from cats reported a mean liver triglyceride content of 1% for 5 cats of ideal body weight [44]. A 2–3 fold increase in liver fat was also reported in cats after weight gain [45]. This shows that obese cats have higher triglyceride accumulation in the liver compared to lean cats; however, as in the human studies, a cause/effect relationship to insulin sensitivity cannot be established. To our knowledge, liver fat content in obese or diabetic dogs has not been quantified.

Liver steatosis is responsive to thiazolidinediones (TZD) in people. TZDs are agonists of peroxisome proliferator-activated receptor gamma (PPARγ), a nuclear transcription factor that is a key regulator of adipogenesis [46]. The natural ligands for PPARγ are unknown, but the receptor possesses a low affinity for various endogenous fatty acids and eicosanoids [47]. PPARγ is expressed abundantly in adipose tissue, and at low levels in other tissues, including pancreatic β-cells [46,47]. In humans, dogs and cats, TZD administration leads to an increase in whole-body insulin sensitivity [48–50]. It is known that in people this occurs parallel to a reduction of triglyceride content in non-adipose tissues such as liver and skeletal muscle, and lowering of serum triglyceride and/or non-esterified fatty acid concentrations [50]. There are no similar studies in dogs and cats to show if hepatic triglyceride content changes with thiazolidinediones, although one might also expect a reduction in liver steatosis because of the similarities of its positive effect on metabolism and insulin sensitivity in those species.

In summary: Increased endogenous glucose output by the liver is a prerequisite for the increase in fasting blood glucose when non-diabetic obese humans and pets develop diabetes. This may be due to decreased hepatic insulin sensitivity, decreased insulin concentrations, or a combination of both.

4. The Role of Inflammation in Obesity and Diabetes

There is abundant scientific evidence of a link between obesity/diabetes and inflammation in people [51–53]. Inflammatory cells and other markers of inflammation increase with the expansion of fat mass in white adipose tissue and also in the liver in human subjects [39,54]. White adipose tissue secretes a variety of factors, which influence metabolism and are involved in the regulation of inflammation. Some of these, like leptin and adiponectin, are primarily produced by fat tissue. Other cytokines, like TNF-a, MCP-1, and IL-6 are produced by macrophages and other cells involved in the immune response, as well as adipocytes. Lipid accumulation in the adipocyte increases reactive oxygen species (ROS) and cellular stress pathways are activated leading to the secretion of pro-inflammatory cytokines [55]. The increased ROS leads to a decrease in activities of anti-oxidant enzymes, such as glutathione peroxidase, Cu,Zn-superoxide dismutase (SOD), and catalase. When cats were followed longitudinally during the development of obesity in one study, it was shown that there was no change in the anti-oxidant enzymes catalase, glutathione peroxidase, and red blood cell as well as heparin-releasable superoxide dismutase. There was also no change in the inflammatory cytokines, IL-1, IL-6 and TNF-α suggesting that development of obesity in cats does not lead to the same changes in circulating inflammatory markers and activity of antioxidant enzymes that is seen in other species. Urinary isoprostane concentrations were also not different in long-term obese cats and there was no infiltration of white fat with inflammatory cells [21]. Jeusette and coworkers found higher urinary isoprostane concentrations in obese cats compared to lean after both were given ad libitum food for 8 weeks, but no difference in other oxidative stress markers was seen [56]. No difference was also seen before and after successful weight loss of acute phase proteins, and enzymes associated with inflammation (buturylcholinesterase and paraoxonase) [57]. The notion that inflammation does not play a role in the development of insulin resistance with increasing obesity in cats is also supported by results from a study of immune responses in lean and obese cats [58]. In that study, complete blood counts and lymphocyte distribution were examined and immune function was assessed by measuring the proliferative activity of different cellular fractions in response to several polyclonal mitogens. Phagocytosis and natural killer cell cytotoxicity was examined to test innate immune functions. It was shown that a similar immune innate and adaptive immune response was elicited regardless of body condition and concluded that obesity does not alter immune responses in cats. It is unclear why insulin resistance of obesity in cats is not associated with an inflammatory response and a change in immune function. But it may explain the fact that obese cats do not develop cardiovascular disease and clinical hypertension.

Few studies have examined inflammatory cytokines in obese and lean dogs. Anti-oxidant enzyme activity has not been compared between lean and obese dogs, to the author's knowledge. In laboratory dogs, weight loss did not lead to a change in acute phase proteins [59]. The cytokine IL-6 was below the detection limit of the assay in that study. In another study, TNF-α as well as leptin were below the detectable limit in the majority of dogs. Haptoglobin and serum amyloid A were lower after weight loss than before suggesting that obese dogs have higher concentrations but no comparison to normal-weight dogs was included [60]. In both studies, a comparison was not made between lean and obese dogs before weight loss. It appears that a comparison of anti-oxidant enzymes, inflammatory cytokines, and immune function using assays that have been validated for canine serum or plasma are important next steps to elucidate the role of inflammation in obese dogs.

Concentrations of the adipokines, adiponectin and leptin, have been reported in many studies in human subjects and several studies in dogs and cats. Adiponectin, an insulin sensitizing adipokine, has an important role in glucose and lipid metabolism and its expression is regulated by PPAR-γ [57,61,62]. It has anti-inflammatory activity and anti-atherogenic properties, and suppresses NK cytotoxicity. It also inhibits phagocytic activity and TNF-α production, and inhibits lipid accumulation in a variety of cells [63]. In addition, adiponectin has anti-apoptotic effects on beta cells *in vitro*, which appear to be mediated by reduction of ceramide concentrations [64,65]. In people [66] and cats [17,32], fat cells secrete higher amounts of adiponectin in the lean state but concentrations decrease with increasing fat mass. In obese dogs, plasma adiponectin concentrations have been found to be lower [62,67] or unchanged [60,68] compared to lean dogs. In one study, adiponectin was only lower in those obese dogs with metabolic syndrome, *i.e.*, dogs with high glucose and lipid values, systolic blood pressure and body condition scoring but not in obese dogs without signs of metabolic syndrome [69]. In another study, adiponectin levels remained unchanged when dogs lost weight [60]. However, in that study the average adiponectin levels were reported to be very low (10 pg/mL), whereas other studies show adiponectin concentrations in dogs to be several magnitudes higher (ug/mL) and similar to those of other species. This makes the low results questionable.

Leptin is an adipokine, which acts in the hypothalamus and suppresses food intake and increases energy expenditure. Contrary to adiponectin, it is positively correlated with fat mass in humans, dogs, and cats [17,70–72]. Increased circulating leptin in obesity is a marker of leptin resistance. Leptin acts as a positive regulator of immune functions and cytotoxicity of splenic NK cells at physiological concentrations [73]. In human subjects, it stimulates proliferation and cytokine synthesis in peripheral lymphocytes [74]. Plasma levels of leptin and inflammatory markers are positively correlated in people and predict cardiovascular risk [75,76]. In fact, leptin has a structural and functional relation to proinflammatory cytokines [77]. It is not known if high leptin in dogs is associated with an increased cardiovascular risk as it is in people. Obesity has been found to only be a secondary cause of hypertension in dogs in association with other primary diseases in one study [78]. In another study, approximately 10/35 obese dogs had mild hypertension, which only normalized in 2/35 with weight loss [59]. A comparison to normal-weight dogs was not made and the clinical significance is not known. And in yet another study, obese dogs had on average higher systemic blood pressure than lean dogs but their blood pressure fell within the normal canine range and they were only at mild risk for target organ damage. They also had higher left ventricular free wall thickness than lean dogs based on echocardiographic Doppler measurements but not on postmortem examination. The authors concluded that longitudinal studies were needed to examine if obese dogs developed cardiomyopathy over time [79].

In summary: There is abundant scientific evidence of a link between obesity/diabetes and inflammation in people. There is little evidence to support that inflammation plays a role in the pathogenesis of obesity in cats. More controlled studies using validated assays are needed to address this issue in dogs.

5. Conclusions

The pathophysiologies of obesity and its progression to diabetes in people, dogs and cats share similarities, but also show differences. In many instances, information, which is available in humans, is still missing in pets. Researchers should not be content to apply data from humans, but rather seek to fill these gaps. Not only will this lead to crucial comparative information, but it will also aid the design of preventive and therapeutic strategies in domestic animals. Ideally, we would employ large multi-center studies to follow obese dogs and cats longitudinally for many years to find true biomarkers and make accurate assessments about factors involved in the progression from obesity to diabetes.

Conflicts of Interest

The author declares no conflict of interest.

References

1. Howard, B. Banfield sees bump in fat pets. *DVM Newsmag. Vet. Med.* **2012**, *43*, 1.
2. Kealy, R.D.; Lawler, D.F.; Ballam, J.M.; Mantz, S.L.; Biery, D.N.; Greeley, E.H.; Lust, G.; Segre, M.; Smith, G.K.; Stowe, H.D. Effects of diet restriction on life span and age-related changes in dogs. *J. Am. Vet. Med. Assoc.* **2002**, *220*, 1315–1320.
3. Fall, T.; Hamlin, H.H.; Hedhammar, A.; Kampe, O.; Egenvall, A. Diabetes mellitus in a population of 180,000 insured dogs: Incidence, survival, and breed distribution. *J. Vet. Intern. Med.* **2007**, *21*, 1209–1216.
4. Kaneko, J.J.; Mattheeuws, D.; Rottiers, R.P.; Vermeulen, A. Glucose tolerance and insulin response in diabetes mellitus of dogs. *J. Small Anim. Pract.* **1978**, *19*, 85–94.
5. Verkest, K.R.; Fleeman, L.M.; Rand, J.S.; Morton, J.M. Evaluation of beta-cell sensitivity to glucose and first-phase insulin secretion in obese dogs. *Am. J. Vet. Res.* **2011**, *72*, 357–366.
6. Karam, J.H.; Grodsky, G.M.; Forsham, P.H. Excessive insulin response to glucose in obese subjects as measured by immunochemical assay. *Diabetes* **1963**, *12*, 197–204.
7. Polonsky, K.S.; Given, B.D.; Hirsch, L.; Shapiro, E.T.; Tillil, H.; Beebe, C.; Galloway, J.A.; Frank, B.H.; Karrison, T.; van Cauter, E. Quantitative study of insulin secretion and clearance in normal and obese subjects. *J. Clin. Invest.* **1988**, *81*, 435–441.
8. Seino, S.; Shibasaki, T.; Minami, K. Dynamics of insulin secretion and the clinical implications for obesity and diabetes. *J. Clin. Investig.* **2011**, *121*, 2118–2125.

9. Stancakova, A.; Javorsky, M.; Kuulasmaa, T.; Haffner, S.M.; Kuusisto, J.; Laakso, M. Changes in insulin sensitivity and insulin release in relation to glycemia and glucose tolerance in 6414 Finnish men. *Diabetes* **2009**, *58*, 1212–1221.
10. Weir, G.C.; Bonner-Weir, S. Five stages of evolving beta-cell dysfunction during progression to diabetes. *Diabetes* **2004**, *53*, S16–S21.
11. Maclean, N.; Ogilvie, R.F. Quantitative estimation of the pancreatic islet tissue in diabetic subjects. *Diabetes* **1955**, *4*, 367–376.
12. Butler, A.E.; Janson, J.; Bonner-Weir, S.; Ritzel, R.; Rizza, R.A.; Butler, P.C. Beta-cell deficit and increased beta-cell apoptosis in humans with type 2 diabetes. *Diabetes* **2003**, *52*, 102–110.
13. Chan, J.M.; Rimm, E.B.; Colditz, G.A.; Stampfer, M.J.; Willett, W.C. Obesity, fat distribution, and weight gain as risk factors for clinical diabetes in men. *Diabetes Care* **1994**, *17*, 961–969.
14. Ionut, V.; Liu, H.; Mooradian, V.; Castro, A.V.; Kabir, M.; Stefanovski, D.; Zheng, D.; Kirkman, E.L.; Bergman, R.N. Novel canine models of obese prediabetes and mild type 2 diabetes. *Am. J. Physiol. Endocrinol. Metab.* **2010**, *298*, E38–E48.
15. Ader, M.; Stefanovski, D.; Kim, S.P.; Richey, J.M.; Ionut, V.; Catalano, K.J.; Hucking, K.; Ellmerer, M.; van Citters, G.; Hsu, I.R.; *et al*. Hepatic insulin clearance is the primary determinant of insulin sensitivity in the normal dog. *Obesity (Silver Spring)* **2014**, *22*, 1238–1245.
16. Hoenig, M.; Thomaseth, K.; Brandao, J.; Waldron, M.; Ferguson, D.C. Assessment and mathematical modeling of glucose turnover and insulin sensitivity in lean and obese cats. *Domest. Anim. Endocrinol.* **2006**, *31*, 373–389.
17. Hoenig, M.; Thomaseth, K.; Waldron, M.; Ferguson, D.C. Insulin sensitivity, fat distribution, and adipocytokine response to different diets in lean and obese cats before and after weight loss. *Am. J. Physiol. Regul. Integr. Comp. Physiol.* **2007**, *292*, R227–R234.
18. Hoenig, M.; Alexander, S.; Holson, J.; Ferguson, D.C. Influence of glucose dosage on interpretation of intravenous glucose tolerance tests in lean and obese cats. *J. Vet. Intern. Med.* **2002**, *16*, 529–532.
19. Hoenig, M.; Pach, N.; Thomaseth, K.; Devries, F.; Ferguson, D.C. Evaluation of long-term glucose homeostasis in lean and obese cats by use of continuous glucose monitoring. *Am. J. Vet. Res.* **2012**, *73*, 1100–1106.
20. Hoenig, M.; Traas, A.M.; Schaeffer, D.J. Evaluation of routine hematology profile results and fructosamine, thyroxine, insulin, and proinsulin concentrations in lean, overweight, obese, and diabetic cats. *J. Am. Vet. Med. Assoc.* **2013**, *243*, 1302–1309.
21. Hoenig, M.; Pach, N.; Thomaseth, K.; Le, A.; Schaeffer, D.; Ferguson, D.C. Cats differ from other species in their cytokine and antioxidant enzyme response when developing obesity. *Obesity (Silver Spring)* **2013**, *21*, E407–E414.
22. Matsumoto, K.; Miyake, S.; Yano, M.; Ueki, Y.; Yamaguchi, Y.; Akazawa, S.; Tominaga, Y. Glucose tolerance, insulin secretion, and insulin sensitivity in nonobese and obese Japanese subjects. *Diabetes Care* **1997**, *20*, 1562–1568.
23. Dankner, R.; Abdul-Ghani, M.A.; Gerber, Y.; Chetrit, A.; Wainstein, J.; Raz, I. Predicting the 20-year diabetes incidence rate. *Diabetes Metab. Res. Rev.* **2007**, *23*, 551–558.

24. Appleton, D.J.; Rand, J.S.; Priest, J.; Sunvold, G.D. Determination of reference values for glucose tolerance, insulin tolerance, and insulin sensitivity tests in clinically normal cats. *Am. J. Vet. Res.* **2001**, *62*, 630–636.
25. Link, K.R.; Rand, J.S.; Hendrikz, J.K. Evaluation of a simplified intravenous glucose tolerance test and a reflectance glucose meter for use in cats. *Vet. Rec.* **1997**, *140*, 253–256.
26. Link, K.R.; Rand, J.S. Reference values for glucose tolerance and glucose tolerance status in cats. *J. Am. Vet. Med. Assoc.* **1998**, *213*, 492–496.
27. Hoenig, M.; Hall, G.; Ferguson, D.; Jordan, K.; Henson, M.; Johnson, K.; O'Brien, T. A feline model of experimentally induced islet amyloidosis. *Am. J. Pathol.* **2000**, *157*, 2143–2150.
28. Muller, C.; Assimacopoulos-Jeannet, F.; Mosimann, F.; Schneiter, P.; Riou, J.P.; Pachiaudi, C.; Felber, J.P.; Jequier, E.; Jeanrenaud, B.; Tappy, L. Endogenous glucose production, gluconeogenesis and liver glycogen concentration in obese non-diabetic patients. *Diabetologia* **1997**, *40*, 463–468.
29. Gastaldelli, A.; Baldi, S.; Pettiti, M.; Toschi, E.; Camastra, S.; Natali, A.; Landau, B.R.; Ferrannini, E. Influence of obesity and type 2 diabetes on gluconeogenesis and glucose output in humans: A quantitative study. *Diabetes* **2000**, *49*, 1367–1373.
30. Basu, R.; Chandramouli, V.; Dicke, B.; Landau, B.; Rizza, R. Obesity and type 2 diabetes impair insulin-induced suppression of glycogenolysis as well as gluconeogenesis. *Diabetes* **2005**, *54*, 1942–1948.
31. Weyer, C.; Bogardus, C.; Mott, D.M.; Pratley, R.E. The natural history of insulin secretory dysfunction and insulin resistance in the pathogenesis of type 2 diabetes mellitus. *J. Clin. Investig.* **1999**, *104*, 787–794.
32. Kley, S.; Hoenig, M.; Glushka, J.; Jin, E.S.; Burgess, S.C.; Waldron, M.; Jordan, E.T.; Prestegard, J.H.; Ferguson, D.C.; Wu, S.; *et al.* The impact of obesity, sex, and diet on hepatic glucose production in cats. *Am. J. Physiol. Regul. Integr. Comp. Physiol.* **2009**, *296*, R936–R943.
33. Hoenig, M.; Jordan, E.T.; Glushka, J.; Kley, S.; Patil, A.; Waldron, M.; Prestegard, J.H.; Ferguson, D.C.; Wu, S.; Olson, D.E. Effect of macronutrients, age, and obesity on 6- and 24-h postprandial glucose metabolism in cats. *Am. J. Physiol. Regul. Integr. Comp. Physiol.* **2011**, *301*, R1798–R1807.
34. Edgerton, D.S.; Cardin, S.; Emshwiller, M.; Neal, D.; Chandramouli, V.; Schumann, W.C.; Landau, B.R.; Rossetti, L.; Cherrington, A.D. Small increases in insulin inhibit hepatic glucose production solely caused by an effect on glycogen metabolism. *Diabetes* **2001**, *50*, 1872–1882.
35. Rothman, D.L.; Magnusson, I.; Katz, L.D.; Shulman, R.G.; Shulman, G.I. Quantitation of hepatic glycogenolysis and gluconeogenesis in fasting humans with 13C NMR. *Science* **1991**, *254*, 573–576.
36. Chiasson, J.L.; Liljenquist, J.E.; Finger, F.E.; Lacy, W.W. Differential sensitivity of glycogenolysis and gluconeogenesis to insulin infusions in dogs. *Diabetes* **1976**, *25*, 283–291.
37. Sokal, J.E.; Gerszi, K.E. Human liver glycogen levels. *J. Lab. Clin. Med.* **1959**, *53*, 876–881.
38. Fittschen, C.; Bellamy, J.E. Prednisone-induced morphologic and chemical changes in the liver of dogs. *Vet. Pathol.* **1984**, *21*, 399–406.
39. Korenblat, K.M.; Fabbrini, E.; Mohammed, B.S.; Klein, S. Liver, muscle, and adipose tissue insulin action is directly related to intrahepatic triglyceride content in obese subjects. *Gastroenterology* **2008**, *134*, 1369–1375.

40. Fabbrini, E.; Sullivan, S.; Klein, S. Obesity and nonalcoholic fatty liver disease: Biochemical, metabolic, and clinical implications. *Hepatology* **2010**, *51*, 679–689.
41. Hijona, E.; Hijona, L.; Arenas, J.I.; Bujanda, L. Inflammatory mediators of hepatic steatosis. *Mediat. Inflamm.* **2010**, doi:10.1155/2010/837418.
42. Kleiner, D.E.; Brunt, E.M.; van Natta, M.; Behling, C.; Contos, M.J.; Cummings, O.W.; Ferrell, L.D.; Liu, Y.C.; Torbenson, M.S.; Unalp-Arida, A.; *et al.* Design and validation of a histological scoring system for nonalcoholic fatty liver disease. *Hepatology* **2005**, *41*, 1313–1321.
43. Clark, M.H.; Larsen, R.; Lu, W.; Hoenig, M. Investigation of 1H MRS for quantification of hepatic triglyceride in lean and obese cats. *Res. Vet. Sci.* **2013**, *95*, 678–680.
44. Hall, J.A.; Barstad, L.A.; Connor, W.E. Lipid composition of hepatic and adipose tissues from normal cats and from cats with idiopathic hepatic lipidosis. *J. Vet. Intern. Med.* **1997**, *11*, 238–242.
45. Ibrahim, W.H.; Bailey, N.; Sunvold, G.D.; Bruckner, G.G. Effects of carnitine and taurine on fatty acid metabolism and lipid accumulation in the liver of cats during weight gain and weight loss. *Am. J. Vet. Res.* **2003**, *64*, 1265–1277.
46. Lehrke, M.; Lazar, M.A. The many faces of PPARgamma. *Cell* **2005**, *123*, 993–999.
47. Walczak, R.; Tontonoz, P. PPARadigms and PPARadoxes: Expanding roles for PPARgamma in the control of lipid metabolism. *J. Lipid Res.* **2002**, *43*, 177–186.
48. Hoenig, M.; Ferguson, D.C. Effect of darglitazone on glucose clearance and lipid metabolism in obese cats. *Am. J. Vet. Res.* **2003**, *64*, 1409–1413.
49. Ikeda, H.; Taketomi, S.; Sugiyama, Y.; Shimura, Y.; Sohda, T.; Meguro, K.; Fujita, T. Effects of pioglitazone on glucose and lipid metabolism in normal and insulin resistant animals. *Arzneimittelforschung* **1990**, *40*, 156–162.
50. Yki-Jarvinen, H. Thiazolidinediones. *N. Engl. J. Med.* **2004**, *351*, 1106–1118.
51. Bastard, J.P.; Maachi, M.; Lagathu, C.; Kim, M.J.; Caron, M.; Vidal, H.; Capeau, J.; Feve, B. Recent advances in the relationship between obesity, inflammation, and insulin resistance. *Eur. Cytokine Netw.* **2006**, *17*, 4–12.
52. Dandona, P.; Aljada, A.; Bandyopadhyay, A. Inflammation: The link between insulin resistance, obesity and diabetes. *Trends Immunol.* **2004**, *25*, 4–7.
53. Lumeng, C.N.; Saltiel, A.R. Inflammatory links between obesity and metabolic disease. *J. Clin. Investig.* **2011**, *121*, 2111–2117.
54. Shoelson, S.E.; Herrero, L.; Naaz, A. Obesity, inflammation, and insulin resistance. *Gastroenterology* **2007**, *132*, 2169–2180.
55. Houstis, N.; Rosen, E.D.; Lander, E.S. Reactive oxygen species have a causal role in multiple forms of insulin resistance. *Nature* **2006**, *440*, 944–948.
56. Jeusette, I.; Torre, C.; Salas, A.; Iraculis, N.; Compagnucci, M.; Romano, V.; Kirschvink, N. Effects of consuming diets containing various fats or citrus flavanones on plasma lipid and urinary F2-isoprostane concentrations in overweight cats. *Am. J. Vet. Res.* **2010**, *71*, 1039–1044.
57. Tvarijonaviciute, A.; Ceron, J.J.; Holden, S.L.; Morris, P.J.; Biourge, V.; German, A.J. Effects of weight loss in obese cats on biochemical analytes related to inflammation and glucose homeostasis. *Domest. Anim. Endocrinol.* **2012**, *42*, 129–141.

58. Jaso-Friedmann, L.; Leary, J.H., 3rd; Praveen, K.; Waldron, M.; Hoenig, M. The effects of obesity and fatty acids on the feline immune system. *Vet. Immunol. Immunopathol.* **2008**, *122*, 146–152.
59. Tvarijonaviciute, A.; Tecles, F.; Martinez-Subiela, S.; Ceron, J.J. Effect of weight loss on inflammatory biomarkers in obese dogs. *Vet. J.* **2012**, *193*, 570–572.
60. German, A.J.; Hervera, M.; Hunter, L.; Holden, S.L.; Morris, P.J.; Biourge, V.; Trayhurn, P. Improvement in insulin resistance and reduction in plasma inflammatory adipokines after weight loss in obese dogs. *Domest. Anim. Endocrinol.* **2009**, *37*, 214–226.
61. Clark, M.; Thomaseth, K.; Dirikolu, L.; Ferguson, D.C.; Hoenig, M. Effects of pioglitazone on insulin sensitivity and serum lipids in obese cats. *J. Vet. Intern. Med.* **2014**, *28*, 166–174.
62. Gayet, C.; Leray, V.; Saito, M.; Siliart, B.; Nguyen, P. The effects of obesity-associated insulin resistance on mRNA expression of peroxisome proliferator-activated receptor-gamma target genes, in dogs. *Br. J. Nutr.* **2007**, *98*, 497–503.
63. Kim, K.Y.; Kim, J.K.; Han, S.H.; Lim, J.S.; Kim, K.I.; Cho, D.H.; Lee, M.S.; Lee, J.H.; Yoon, D.Y.; Yoon, S.R.; *et al.* Adiponectin is a negative regulator of NK cell cytotoxicity. *J. Immunol.* **2006**, *176*, 5958–5964.
64. Holland, W.L.; Miller, R.A.; Wang, Z.V.; Sun, K.; Barth, B.M.; Bui, H.H.; Davis, K.E.; Bikman, B.T.; Halberg, N.; Rutkowski, J.M.; *et al.* Receptor-mediated activation of ceramidase activity initiates the pleiotropic actions of adiponectin. *Nat. Med.* **2011**, *17*, 55–63.
65. Wijesekara, N.; Krishnamurthy, M.; Bhattacharjee, A.; Suhail, A.; Sweeney, G.; Wheeler, M.B. Adiponectin-induced ERK and Akt phosphorylation protects against pancreatic beta cell apoptosis and increases insulin gene expression and secretion. *J. Biol. Chem.* **2010**, *285*, 33623–33631.
66. Weyer, C.; Funahashi, T.; Tanaka, S.; Hotta, K.; Matsuzawa, Y.; Pratley, R.E.; Tataranni, P.A. Hypoadiponectinemia in obesity and type 2 diabetes: Close association with insulin resistance and hyperinsulinemia. *J. Clin. Endocrinol. Metab.* **2001**, *86*, 1930–1935.
67. Ishioka, K.; Omachi, A.; Sagawa, M.; Shibata, H.; Honjoh, T.; Kimura, K.; Saito, M. Canine adiponectin: cDNA structure, mRNA expression in adipose tissues and reduced plasma levels in obesity. *Res. Vet. Sci.* **2006**, *80*, 127–132.
68. Verkest, K.R.; Rand, J.S.; Fleeman, L.M.; Morton, J.M.; Richards, A.A.; Rose, F.J.; Whitehead, J.P. Distinct adiponectin profiles might contribute to differences in susceptibility to type 2 diabetes in dogs and humans. *Domest. Anim. Endocrinol.* **2011**, *41*, 67–73.
69. Tvarijonaviciute, A.; Ceron, J.J.; Holden, S.L.; Cuthbertson, D.J.; Biourge, V.; Morris, P.J.; German, A.J. Obesity-related metabolic dysfunction in dogs: A comparison with human metabolic syndrome. *BMC Vet. Res.* **2012**, *8*, doi:10.1186/1746-6148-8-147.
70. Considine, R.V.; Sinha, M.K.; Heiman, M.L.; Kriauciunas, A.; Stephens, T.W.; Nyce, M.R.; Ohannesian, J.P.; Marco, C.C.; McKee, L.J.; Bauer, T.L.; *et al.* Serum immunoreactive-leptin concentrations in normal-weight and obese humans. *N. Engl. J. Med.* **1996**, *334*, 292–295.
71. Backus, R.C.; Havel, P.J.; Gingerich, R.L.; Rogers, Q.R. Relationship between serum leptin immunoreactivity and body fat mass as estimated by use of a novel gas-phase Fourier transform infrared spectroscopy deuterium dilution method in cats. *Am. J. Vet. Res.* **2000**, *61*, 796–801.
72. Jeusette, I.C.; Lhoest, E.T.; Istasse, L.P.; Diez, M.O. Influence of obesity on plasma lipid and lipoprotein concentrations in dogs. *Am. J. Vet. Res.* **2005**, *66*, 81–86.

73. Tian, Z.; Sun, R.; Wei, H.; Gao, B. Impaired natural killer (NK) cell activity in leptin receptor deficient mice: Leptin as a critical regulator in NK cell development and activation. *Biochem. Biophys. Res. Commun.* **2002**, *298*, 297–302.
74. Sanchez-Margalet, V.; Martin-Romero, C.; Santos-Alvarez, J.; Goberna, R.; Najib, S.; Gonzalez-Yanes, C. Role of leptin as an immunomodulator of blood mononuclear cells: Mechanisms of action. *Clin. Exp. Immunol.* **2003**, *133*, 11–19.
75. Soderberg, S.; Ahren, B.; Jansson, J.H.; Johnson, O.; Hallmans, G.; Asplund, K.; Olsson, T. Leptin is associated with increased risk of myocardial infarction. *J. Intern. Med.* **1999**, *246*, 409–418.
76. Wolk, R.; Berger, P.; Lennon, R.J.; Brilakis, E.S.; Johnson, B.D.; Somers, V.K. Plasma leptin and prognosis in patients with established coronary atherosclerosis. *J. Am. Coll. Cardiol.* **2004**, *44*, 1819–1824.
77. Zhang, F.; Basinski, M.B.; Beals, J.M.; Briggs, S.L.; Churgay, L.M.; Clawson, D.K.; DiMarchi, R.D.; Furman, T.C.; Hale, J.E.; Hsiung, H.M.; *et al.* Crystal structure of the obese protein leptin-E100. *Nature* **1997**, *387*, 206–209.
78. Bodey, A.R.; Michell, A.R. Epidemiological study of blood pressure in domestic dogs. *J. Small Anim. Pract.* **1996**, *37*, 116–125.
79. Mehlman, E.; Bright, J.M.; Jeckel, K.; Porsche, C.; Veeramachaneni, D.N.; Frye, M. Echocardiographic evidence of left ventricular hypertrophy in obese dogs. *J. Vet. Intern. Med.* **2013**, *27*, 62–68.

19

Respiratory Animal Models in the Common Marmoset (*Callithrix jacchus*)

Christoph Curths [1,2], Sascha Knauf [1,2] and Franz-Josef Kaup [1,*]

[1] Pathology Unit, German Primate Center, Leibniz-Institute for Primate Research, Kellnerweg 4, 37077 Göttingen, Germany

[2] Department of Airway Immunology, Fraunhofer Institute for Toxicology and Experimental Medicine, Biomedical Research in Endstage and Obstructive Lung Disease Hannover (BREATH), Member of the German Center for Lung Research, Nikolai-Fuchs-Strasse 1, 30625 Hannover, Germany; E-Mails: ccurths@dpz.eu (C.C.); sknauf@dpz.eu (S.K.)

* Author to whom correspondence should be addressed; E-Mail: fkaup@gwdg.de;

Abstract: Common marmosets (*Callithrix jacchus*) are small non-human primates (NHPs) that are often used for respiratory research. Translational animal models of various pulmonary diseases in marmosets have been developed in favor of models in old world monkeys (OWM, e.g., rhesus or cynomolgus monkeys). The marmoset has the size of a rat (350–450 g), is easier to handle, and the husbandry, care, and management of colonies is much easier compared to OWMs. In contrast to rodents, marmosets provide a high homology to humans, which become especially visible in lung architecture and branching pattern. Features of inflammatory (e.g., COPD) pulmonary diseases can be modeled in marmosets as well the species is used to study bacterial and viral infection. Models for human melioidosis, tuberculosis, anthrax, as well as infections with SARS-associated coronavirus (SARS-CoV), influenza A virus and adenovirus are already established. Toxicological studies often use marmoset monkeys for the advantage of immunological identical twins that are produced by a Callitrichinae-specific placentation type, which ultimately causes blood chimerism. Relatively new approaches in gene therapy use marmosets for respiratory disease research. In this review we will give an overview of existing respiratory marmoset models and their impact on biomedical research.

Keywords: marmoset; non-human primate; animal models; respiratory diseases

1. Introduction

The common marmoset (*Callithrix jacchus*) is a New World primate, native to northeastern Brazil and belongs to the family of the Callitrichidae. The species has several advantages when compared to Old World monkeys (OWM, e.g., rhesus (*Macaca mulatta*) or cynomolgus monkeys (*M. fascicularis*)). Its low body weight (350–450 g), for example, is comparable to the size of a rat (Figure 1) and makes marmosets an easy to handle and economically attractive NHP species for biomedical research [1,2]. Early sexual maturity and high reproductive efficacy allow fast breading capacities and therefore animal supply [3]. Due to hematopoietic chimerism, marmosets but not OWMs, give birth to immunologically identical twins, which facilitates matched control study designs [4]. The absence of herpes virus B (Macacine herpesvirus 1) in new world monkeys (NWMs), a virus that is highly lethal to man and commonly found in Asiatic macaques [2,5], contributes to a relative easy management of marmoset colonies. Table 1 provides an overview about species comparison between marmosets and the classically used Old World monkeys.

Figure 1. Common marmosets (*Callithrix jacchus*) are small non-human primates with a body weight of 350–450 g. Adult marmoset at the facilities of the German Primate Center.

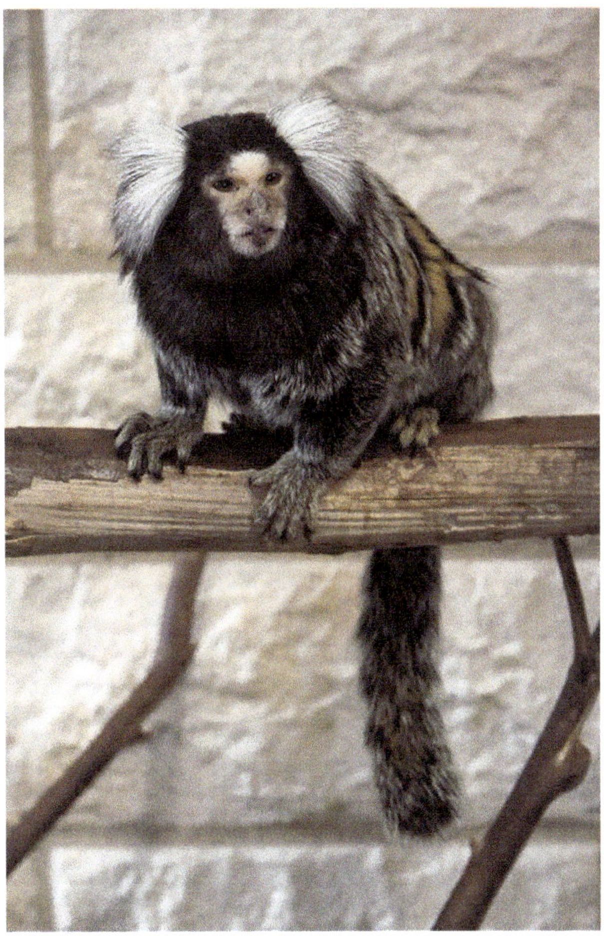

Marmosets are used as a non-rodent species in preclinical toxicology and safety studies. The close homology to humans makes the marmoset a suitable translational model for the human metabolism, enzyme structure and pharmacodynamic effects [3,6]. Furthermore, the high homology of marmoset and human immunological structures provides ground for predictive translational models of human diseases, e.g., to test new human specific biopharmaceuticals that do not find their target(s) in non-primate species [7,8].

The use of marmosets as an animal model for human lung diseases is based on its human-like structure of the lung parenchyma and lung architecture [9]. Similar to humans and in contrast to the monopodial branching pattern in rodents, the marmoset's bronchial tree shows dichotomous branching [10,11]. Marmosets' alveolar size is comparable to other primates and monkey-specific islets of cartilage in the walls of bronchioles as well as highly alveolarized respiratory bronchioles can equally be found in the marmoset [9]. Furthermore, the marmoset's nasal cavity closely resembles the human nasal cavity's morphology, a requirement for translational inhalation studies with a high predictive power for the human situation [12].

A comparable distribution of goblet cells, Clara cells and mixed type secretory cells in the tracheobronchial tree of humans and marmosets is described, whereas there are more Clara cells and less goblet cells in the proximal and distal conducting airway epithelium of marmosets [13]. Another difference from the human situation is the distribution pattern of ciliated cells in the marmoset trachea with ciliated cells almost restricted to cartilage-free regions [14]. Furthermore, ultrastructural alterations of cilia of the respiratory epithelium are a common background finding in marmosets and should be taken into account when analyzing respective data from respiratory studies [15].

Figure 2. Bronchoscopy, a common respiratory technique, is feasible in marmosets. (**A**) The mouth of an adult anesthetized marmoset is opened with a laryngoscope. The bronchoscope is inserted into the trachea and advanced to the main bronchus under video control. Through the bronchoscope the lung can be partially flushed to receive BAL fluid. Bronchoscopic view of (**B**) trachea, (**C**) *bifurcatio tracheae*, (**D**) left and (**E**) right main bronchus. Note the early branching of the tracheal bronchus of the right cranial lobe.

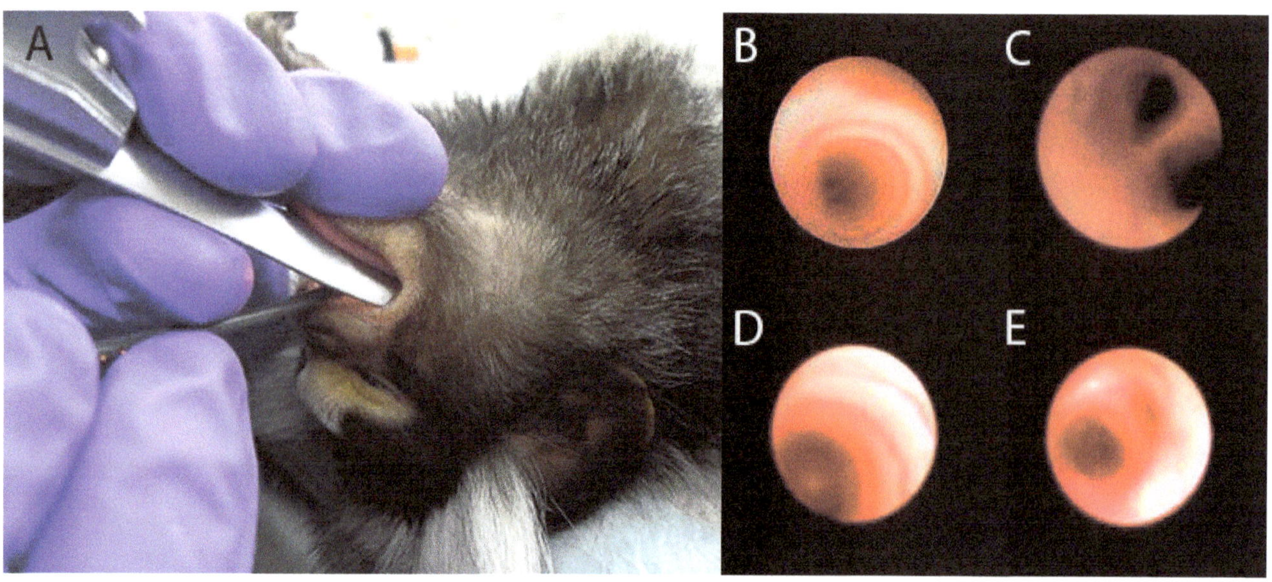

Similarities in human and marmoset neural airway responses, e.g., a comparable reaction towards electrical field stimulation, favor marmosets over rodent models in studies of airway pharmacology [16]. Yet, many aspects are still understudied and contrary results may cause uncertainty in the use of marmoset monkeys. For example, there are conflicting results regarding bronchoconstriction induced by the sensory neuron activator capsaicin in marmosets [16,17]. Despite these pitfalls, human-relevant bronchoconstrictors such as methacholine or histamine, the latter one which is inefficient in rodents, are potent in marmosets [18,19]. At the same time, serotonin, a powerful bronchoconstrictor in rodents, shows no effect in human and marmoset precision-cut lung slices [18], which underlines the importance of species homology for the predictive power of animal models. From the technical point of view, common respiratory techniques such as orotracheal intubation, bronchoscopy and bronchoalveolar lavage (BAL; uni- and bilateral) are well established in marmoset monkeys (Figure 2) [19–21].

2. Models of Lung Inflammation

Due to substantial similarities between the airway wall compartments of NHPs and humans, models of inflammatory lung diseases in nonhuman primates are expected to have advantages over classical rodent models that, to a high degree, lack those morphological similarities [12]. A marmoset model of bleomycin-induced pulmonary fibrosis has been reported to mimic human **adult respiratory distress syndrome (ARDS)** [22]. Transtracheal injection of bleomycin led to pulmonary fibrosis with elevated collagen deposition as well as increased lung lavage desmosine indicating lung elastin destruction [22]. Lung injury was expressed by initial edema, followed by an acute interstitial inflammation [22]. BAL showed a neutrophil dominated cell picture and lung function involved a decrease in lung compliance [22].

To model inflammatory features of human **chronic obstructive pulmonary disease (COPD)** and **acute lung injury (ALI)** a marmoset model of lipopolysaccharide (LPS)-induced acute lung inflammation was established recently [21]. Animals showed, temporarily, a distinct pulmonary inflammation [21]. Inflammation was characterized by an increase of pro-inflammatory cytokines such as tumor necrosis factor alpha (TNF-α) and macrophage inflammatory protein-1 beta (MIP-1β) [21]. High numbers of neutrophils were found in BAL fluid 18 hours post LPS application [21]. In a therapeutic intervention with orally administered anti-inflammatory drugs, dexamethasone and a phosphodiesterase-4 (PDE4) inhibitor (roflumilast), it was shown that lung inflammation could be suppressed significantly [21]. The model therefore provides an interesting approach to test new human specific anti-inflammatory drugs [21]. In addition to this, the same group of researchers characterized the model by comprehensive invasive lung function measurement [19]. Compared to naïve animals, **airway hyperresponsiveness** towards the bronchoconstrictor methacholine occurred post-LPS provocation [19]. Yet, the novel lung function device for marmoset monkeys, that allows inhalation of defined doses of provocative substances and simultaneous (real-time) recording of pulmonary data including key parameters such as lung resistance (R_L) and dynamic compliance (C_{dyn}) [19], makes the marmoset an attractive model for human airway diseases and its treatment.

3. Models of Viral Infection

Marmosets have been utilized several times as a model for viral diseases [2,23]. While these models are not restricted to the respiratory tract, we in the following will focus on respiratory viral infection models. As a consequence of the SARS (Severe Acute Respiratory Syndrome) outbreak in 2002–2003, which killed almost 800 people [24], a marmoset model of the disease was developed that shares features with human SARS. Intratracheal application of **SARS-associated coronavirus (SARS-CoV)** induced an interstitial pneumonia attended by multinucleated syncytia, type 2 pneumocyte hyperplasia, and edema in the lung of infected animals [25]. Similar to human infection, extrapulmonary pathological findings included multifocal hepatitis in all, mild diffuse colitis in most, and mild multifocal lymphocytic myocarditis in some of the infected animals [25]. In addition to the clinical findings, the study showed that marmosets were susceptible to SARS-CoV infection by detection of viral RNA in lung tissue samples and localization of viral antigen in type I pneumocytes, mononuclear alveolar exudate, and multinucleated syncytial cells [25].

Marmosets were likewise susceptible to **influenza A** infection as shown in a study using the human pandemic virus A/California/07/2009 (H1N1pdm) [26]. The virus did not only replicate successfully in infected animals but was also transmitted to a naïve individual in one case [26]. Human-like influenza symptoms such as nasal secretion, sneezing and labored breathing accompanied infection in marmosets [26]. Tissue damage was demonstrated by elevated BAL fluid protein levels [26]. Proof of infection was obtained from recovery of viral RNA from BAL samples and nasal washout samples, using quantitative RT-PCR [26]. Interestingly, sequences of the viral genome isolated from the respiratory tract of infected marmosets revealed that the applied H1N1pdm swarm did only need minimal adaption to cause productive infection, indicating that the species barrier between humans and marmoset influenza infection is low [26]. Anti-H1N1pdm antibodies were detected in serum by hemagglutination inhibition assay [26]. The model seems to provide the exceptional opportunity to study influenza infection in a, for the human situation, highly homologous animal model [26].

Adenovirus infections are known to cause respiratory illness and are responsible for pneumonia outbreaks in humans [27]. Since human and nonhuman primate adenoviruses are closely related there is a risk of interspecies transmission [28,29]. Cross-species infection of marmosets with titi monkey (*Callicebus cupreus*) adenovirus (TMAdV) was shown [30]. Marmosets which were intranasally inoculated with TMAdV, developed clinical signs of acute mild respiratory illness [30]. A sustained infection was proven by positive TMAdV qPCR in nasal swab material and the detection of neutralizing antibody titers against the virus [30]. Animals recovered completely within two weeks [30]. Interestingly, TMAdV infection in titi monkeys produced a fulminant pneumonia with high mortality rates, whereas it caused a mild self-limiting respiratory infection in marmosets which resembled TMAdV infection in humans [30,31]. While the reason for this is, yet, unclear, Titi monkeys and marmosets belong to separate families [32] which could explain differences in clinical manifestations.

4. Models of Bacterial Infection

Several marmoset models of bacterial infection with respiratory implications are described with the objective to mimic the human situation and as alternatives to other nonhuman primates or rodent models. Legionnaires' disease, a severe form of pneumonia, is caused by ***Legionella pneumophila***. The disease is transmitted by inhaling aerosolized contaminated water. Bacteria endure in alveolar macrophages where they cause inflammation [33,34]. Marmosets infected with small particle aerosols of *L. pneumophila* developed pulmonary lesions which resemble those of human Legionnaires' disease [35]. Likewise several days after infection, bronchopneumonia emerging from respiratory and terminal bronchioles and oedemas in the alveoli were observed [35]. Macrophage and polymorphonuclear leukocyte exudation into alveoli occurred and incorporated *L. pneumophila* were demonstrated by electron microscopy [36].

Melioidosis, induced by ***Burkholderia pseudomallei***, is endemic and a considerable cause of mortality in Southeast Asia and northern Australia from where it is disseminating to other areas [37,38]. Treatment is difficult due to lack of vaccines and resistance to many antibiotics [39]. The first NHP animal model for studies of respiratory melioidosis was established in common marmosets by Nelson and colleagues [40]. Marmosets were highly susceptible to airborne infection with *Burkholderia pseudomallei* and developed human-like melioidosis including high mortality [40,41]. The rapidly progressive illness was associated with high fever, decreased activity and dyspnoea [40]. Abnormal liver function enzymes were observed as well as a blood neutrophil increase followed by neutropenia through neutrophil recruitment to the lungs [40]. Ultimately, bacteremia in the animals was observed in conjunction with an extensive bacterial load in the lung [40]. Pathological findings included necrotizing pneumonia, extensive haemorrhage and expanded alveolar oedema in the marmoset lungs [40]. Since melioidosis in the common marmoset resembled human *Burkholderia pseudomallei* infection this animal model is promising to study new therapeutic interventions against the disease [40]. Thus, it is not surprising, that the melioidosis model in marmosets was used to test phosphoantigen treatment towards a T cell subset ($\gamma 9^{+}\delta 2^{+}$) that is exclusively found in primate species [42,43].

For several potentially fatal human infections including anthrax clinical trials in man are not possible which highlights the urgent need for convincing animal models to test antimicrobials and vaccines [44,45]. Especially for testing human anthrax vaccines, NHP models may have benefits over classical rodent models [46]. On the other hand, increased biosafety measures increase costs for housing and managing animals, which is particularly true for experiments with OWMs (e.g., rhesus and cynomolgus monkeys) [44]. Therefore, the marmoset monkey may serve as an attractive alternative to anthrax models in macaques. Aerosol infection with the ***Bacillus anthracis*** Ames strain in marmoset monkeys caused clinical signs of anthrax including dyspnoea, decreased stimuli response and disorientation. Half of the animals had to be put to sleep due to clinical signs of infection 40–140 h post-challenge [44]. Severely infected and therefore euthanized animals showed *B. anthracis* infection in several organs including the spleen and blood [44]. Histopathological results included pulmonary oedema and haemorrhage as it was also observed in NHP and humans as well as acute interstitial pneumonia [44]. Unlike in macaques or humans infection via aerosols caused no signs of meningitis in the common marmoset [44]. Ciprofloxacin, an antibiotic used to treat anthrax in humans [47], was used for therapeutic intervention in infected marmosets and proved to be sufficient to prevent mortality [48].

Limitations of mouse [49] and cynomolgus models of tuberculosis (TB) led to the development of a marmoset model of ***Mycobacterium tuberculosis*** complex infection [50]. Different strains of *M. tuberculosis*, partly emerging and drug resistant, were used to infect marmosets by aerosol exposure [50] which resulted in strain and dose dependent disease progression [50]. The higher virulence of an *M. tuberculosis* Beijing strain compared to the Euro-American lineage in other animal models of TB was reinforced in the marmoset [50]. *In vivo* computed tomography (CT) and positron emission tomography (PET) scans were used to quantify TB lung lesions over the course of infection [50]. Both abnormal lung density, as revealed by CT, and glycolytic activity visualized by 2-deoxy-2-[^{18}F]fluoro-D-glucose (FDG) uptake, increased as *M. tuberculosis* infection progressed [50]. The highest bacterial load was found in the lung, spleen, liver, and lymph nodes of animals infected with *M. tuberculosis* Beijing strain K04 [50]. Infected marmosets exhibited pulmonary lesions and tuberculous pneumonia similar to human TB [50]. Furthermore, the study was interesting because it included chimeric marmoset twins to appraise reproducibility of infection and to assess strain-related differences. Twins infected with the same *M. tuberculosis* strains exhibited almost identical features of disease whereas twin animals exposed to different strains showed disparities specific for the group [50]. Animals infected with an ancient *M. africanum*-like strain for example showed a more extensive extrapulmonary disease and some marmosets infected with the Euro-American lineage developed cavitary disease which is associated with recidivism in humans [50,51]. In fact, marmoset models of TB infection with various *M. tuberculosis* strains include the different characteristics of human TB infection and thus may help to develop new therapeutic strategies to fight the disease.

The severe pulmonary form of leptospirosis (SPFL) associated with pulmonary hemorrhages and respiratory failure causes high mortality rates in humans and represents a particular aggressive form of the emerging zoonosis, which is induced by the spirochete *Leptospira* [52–54]. Marmosets were inoculated intra peritoneal with ***Leptospira interrogans*** serovar Copenhageni which was formerly isolated from a fatal human SPFL case [55]. Infection caused dehydration, weight loss and hepatic injury [55]. Bacteria were recovered from blood samples of infected animals and antibodies against the bacterium indicated seroconversion [55]. Gross pathology revealed hemorrhages on the pleural surface of the lung and histology showed intense intra-alveolar hemorrhages and thickened alveolar septa, caused by inflammatory cellular infiltrates as a response to infection on day 6, 9 and 12 post-inoculation [55]. It was possible to depict leptospiral antigens in the affected areas of lung parenchyma with immunofluorescence techniques [55]. In summary the disease elicited by experimental leptospirosis infection of marmosets with an SPFL-causing serovar resembled human courses of SPFL making the marmoset an attractive model species for human lung disease and pulmonary hemorrhages as a result of leptospirosis in particular [55].

5. Further Models with Respiratory Implications

For the reason that research on toxins needs reliable animal models as a surrogate for human trials [56] toxicological research and work safety is another field where marmoset models are useful. **Sarin**, known as a potent war gas, is an organophosphorus compound which leads to hyperstimulation of muscarinic and nicotinic receptors by inhibiting acetylcholinesterase (AChE) [57]. Beside its unacceptable use as a mass destruction agent, there is a high risk of occupational exposure to low levels of sarin, e.g., for personnel that has to destroy stockpiles or any kind of medical staff which comes into contact with intoxicated victims [58,59]. Long-term low-level exposure to sarin vapor was modeled in marmosets using a novel sensitive apparatus that facilitated vapor generation, exposure in a chamber, and analysis via gas chromatography [58]. Lowest observable effect levels (LOEL) were derived from sarin quantification in the blood [58]. Ascertained LOELs were much lower than previously assumed recommending occupational exposure limits to be re-examined [58].

Another toxin, **Aflatoxin B_1** (AFB_1) is mainly known to promote hepatocellular carcinoma [60]. However, effects of this potent carcinogen are also observed in other parts of the body, such as the respiratory tract [61,62]. To investigate extra-hepatic sites of AFB_1 accumulation and bioactivation in a primate model, marmosets were i.v. injected with radiolabelled ^3H-AFB_1 [63]. Cytochrome P-450-dependent bioactivation of AFB_1 in epithelia of the nasal olfactory mucosa and the upper respiratory tract was observed in marmosets [63] indicating that these tissues were potentially susceptible for AFB_1 related carcinogenicity [63].

Gene therapy is an approach to encounter genetic disorders through replacing deficient by functional genes. In marmoset monkeys, beside hematologic applications [64], gene transfers to the retina facilitated by adeno-associated virus vectors [65], was demonstrated. Furthermore, gene transfer in marmosets was studied to evaluate the potential of this species for gene therapies in **cystic fibrosis** [66]. Results indicated that marmoset lungs were successfully transduced *in vivo* using a VSV-G pseudo-typed HIV-based lentiviral vector [66]. Expression of the LacZ reporter gene was observed 7 days after gene transfer in deep lying conducting airway epithelial cells as well as alveolar epithelial cells [66]. Marmosets may represent a promising model species for gene therapy of human airway diseases such as cystic fibrosis [66]. Also, the high reproductive rate of this NHP species compared to OWMs should not be underestimated and contributes to the use of marmosets in stem cell research and gene therapy.

6. Conclusions

While there are promising translational animal models in marmoset monkeys, the species also has its limitations compared to OWMs. The limited blood sample volume or lower rates of human antibody cross-reactivity are potential drawbacks that need to be considered. However, due to its characteristics, the marmoset monkey is especially attractive when it comes to experiments and models with a high demand of animal numbers or high reproduction rates that are needed to foster a quick generation turnover rate, e.g., in stem cell or gene therapy. Also, the cost-benefit ratio is exceptionally good regarding preclinical studies with the additional advantage of using immunological identical twins for controlled study designs. The marmoset's close homology to humans is especially reflected in its lung architecture and airway branching pattern, which makes it a good model species for human lung diseases. Not only non-infectious, but also infectious disease models have been established in the marmoset with promising results.

Table 1. Species comparison of advantages and disadvantages of macaque (rhesus, cynomolgus) and common marmoset animal models for respiratory diseases.

	Macaques	Common marmosets	Reference
Feature			
Weight	3.0–15.0 kg	0.35–0.45 kg	[1]
Sexual maturity	41–66 months	18–24 months	[1]
Gestation length	24 weeks	21 weeks	[67]
Interbirth interval	12 months	6 months	[67]
Housing requirements (floor area × height)	0.55 m^2 × 1.5 m	2 m^2 × 1.8 m	European Directive 2010/63/EU
Purchase price 2014	~6,000–10,000 €	~3,000–5,000 €	p.c.
Material costs (esp. drug compound) for pharmacology and toxicology studies	high	low	[3]
Hematopoietic chimerism of dizygotic twins	no	yes	[2]
Inter-individual variation of MHC class I and II loci	high	low	[1]
Identical aa residues in average for immunity-related genes compared to human	95 ± 3.4	87 ± 5.4	[7]
Susceptible for viral and bacterial infection with human-relevant pathogens	yes	yes	[23]
Alveolar size	equal		[9]
Highly alveolarized respiratory bronchioles	yes	yes	[9]
Bronchial branching pattern	dichotomous		[10,11]
Presence of Clara cells in the lung	not in trachea and major bronchi	in all airway segments	[13]
Respiratory rate (under anesthesia)	~34 breaths/min	~27 breaths/min	[19]
Latent Herpes Virus B infection	yes	no	[2]
Wasting syndrome in captive colonies	absent	evident	[6]
Methods			
Handling	laborious	easy	[3]
Complete clinical examination	feasible	feasible	[3]
Blood sample volume (*in vivo* every two weeks)	48 mL	2.5 mL	Society for Laboratory Animal Science
Bronchoscopy	yes	yes	[21,68,69]
BAL (uni- and bilateral)	yes	yes	[21,68,69]
BAL flush volume	10–15 mL	2 × 3 mL	[21,68,69]
Lung function assessment	yes	yes	[19,68,69]
Cross-reactivity of human-specific antibodies	frequent	limited	[70]

Conflicts of Interest

The authors declare no conflict of interest.

References and Notes

1. Abbott, D.H.; Barnett, D.K.; Colman, R.J.; Yamamoto, M.E.; Schultz-Darken, N.J. Aspects of common marmoset basic biology and life history important for biomedical research. *Comp. Med.* **2003**, *53*, 339–350.
2. Mansfield, K. Marmoset models commonly used in biomedical research. *Comp. Med.* **2003**, *53*, 383–392.
3. Orsi, A.; Rees, D.; Andreini, I.; Venturella, S.; Cinelli, S.; Oberto, G. Overview of the marmoset as a model in nonclinical development of pharmaceutical products. *Regul. Toxicol. Pharmacol.* **2011**, *59*, 19–27.
4. Sweeney, C.; Ward, J.; Vallender, E.J. Naturally occurring, physiologically normal, primate chimeras. *Chimerism* **2012**, *3*, 43–44.
5. Huff, J.L.; Barry, P.A. B-virus (cercopithecine herpesvirus 1) infection in humans and macaques: Potential for zoonotic disease. *Emerg. Infect. Dis.* **2003**, *9*, 246–250.
6. Smith, D.; Trennery, P.; Farningham, D.; Klapwijk, J. The selection of marmoset monkeys (*callithrix jacchus*) in pharmaceutical toxicology. *Lab. Anim.* **2001**, *35*, 117–130.
7. Kohu, K.; Yamabe, E.; Matsuzawa, A.; Onda, D.; Suemizu, H.; Sasaki, E.; Tanioka, Y.; Yagita, H.; Suzuki, D.; Kametani, Y.; *et al.* Comparison of 30 immunity-related genes from the common marmoset with orthologues from human and mouse. *Tohoku J. Exp. Med.* **2008**, *215*, 167–180.
8. 't Hart, B.A.; Abbott, D.H.; Nakamura, K.; Fuchs, E. The marmoset monkey: A multi-purpose preclinical and translational model of human biology and disease. *Drug Discov. Today* **2012**, *17*, 1160–1165.
9. Barbier, A.; Bachofen, H. The lung of the marmoset (*callithrix jacchus*): Ultrastructure and morphometric data. *Respir. Physiol.* **2000**, *120*, 167–177.
10. Plopper, C.G.; Hyde, D.M. The non-human primate as a model for studying copd and asthma. *Pulm. Pharmacol. Ther.* **2008**, *21*, 755–766.
11. Seidel, V. Morphological investigations on the lung of common marmosets (*Callithrix jacchus*) (in German). Doctoral Thesis, School of Veterinary Medicine, Hannover, Germany, 2012.
12. Wako, K.; Hiratsuka, H.; Katsuta, O.; Tsuchitani, M. Anatomical structure and surface epithelial distribution in the nasal cavity of the common cotton-eared marmoset (*callithrix jacchus*). *Exp. Anim.* **1999**, *48*, 31–36.
13. Seidel, V.; Hoffmann, R.; Braun, A.; Seehase, S.; Knauf, S.; Kaup, F.-J.; Bleyer, M. Distribution and morphology of clara cells in common marmosets (*callithrix jacchus*). *J. Med. Primatol.* **2013**, *42*, 79–88.
14. Hoffmann, R.; Braun, A.; Knauf, S.; Kaup, F.-J.; Bleyer, M. Distribution of ciliated epithelial cells in the trachea of common marmosets (*callithrix jacchus*). *J. Med. Primatol.* **2014**, *43*, 55–58.

15. Hoffmann, R.M.; Kaup, F.-J.; Bleyer, M. Atypical cilia in the respiratory tract of common marmosets (*callithrix jacchus*) with and without concurrent lung disease. *Exp. Lung Res.* **2013**, *39*, 410–414.
16. Schlepütz, M.; Rieg, A.D.; Seehase, S.; Spillner, J.; Perez-Bouza, A.; Braunschweig, T.; Schroeder, T.; Bernau, M.; Lambermont, V.; Schlumbohm, C.; *et al.* Neurally mediated airway constriction in human and other species: A comparative study using precision-cut lung slices (PCLS). *PLoS ONE* **2012**, *7*, e47344.
17. Spina, D.; Matera, G.M.; Riccio, M.M.; Page, C.P. A comparison of sensory nerve function in human, guinea-pig, rabbit and marmoset airways. *Life Sci.* **1998**, *63*, 1629–1642.
18. Seehase, S.; Schlepütz, M.; Switalla, S.; Mätz-Rensing, K.; Kaup, F.-J.; Zöller, M.; Schlumbohm, C.; Fuchs, E.; Lauenstein, H.D.; Winkler, C.; *et al.* Bronchoconstriction in nonhuman primates: A species comparison. *J. Appl. Physiol.* **2011**, *111*, 791–798.
19. Curths, C.; Wichmann, J.; Dunker, S.; Windt, H.; Hoymann, H.G.; Lauenstein, H.D.; Hohlfeld, J.; Becker, T.; Kaup, F.-J.; Braun, A.; *et al.* Airway hyper-responsiveness in lipopolysaccharide-challenged common marmosets (*callithrix jacchus*). *Clin. Sci. (Lond.)* **2014**, *126*, 155–162.
20. Thomas, A.A.; Leach, M.C.; Flecknell, P.A. An alternative method of endotracheal intubation of common marmosets (*callithrix jacchus*). *Lab. Anim.* **2012**, *46*, 71–76.
21. Seehase, S.; Lauenstein, H.D.; Schlumbohm, C.; Switalla, S.; Neuhaus, V.; Forster, C.; Fieguth, H.G.; Pfennig, O.; Fuchs, E.; Kaup, F.-J.; *et al.* Lps-induced lung inflammation in marmoset monkeys—An acute model for anti-inflammatory drug testing. *PLoS ONE* **2012**, *7*, e43709.
22. Idell, S.; Thrall, R.S.; Maunder, R.; Martin, T.R.; McLarty, J.; Scott, M.; Starcher, B.C. Bronchoalveolar lavage desmosine in bleomycin-induced lung injury in marmosets and patients with adult respiratory distress syndrome. *Exp. Lung Res.* **1989**, *15*, 739–753.
23. Carrion, R., Jr.; Patterson, J.L. An animal model that reflects human disease: The common marmoset (*callithrix jacchus*). *Curr. Opin. Virol.* **2012**, *2*, 357–362.
24. Christian, M.D.; Poutanen, S.M.; Loutfy, M.R.; Muller, M.P.; Low, D.E. Severe acute respiratory syndrome. *Clin. Infect. Dis.* **2004**, *38*, 1420–1427.
25. Greenough, T.C.; Carville, A.; Coderre, J.; Somasundaran, M.; Sullivan, J.L.; Luzuriaga, K.; Mansfield, K. Pneumonitis and multi-organ system disease in common marmosets (*callithrix jacchus*) infected with the severe acute respiratory syndrome-associated coronavirus. *Am. J. Pathol.* **2005**, *167*, 455–463.
26. Moncla, L.H.; Ross, T.M.; Dinis, J.M.; Weinfurter, J.T.; Mortimer, T.D.; Schultz-Darken, N.; Brunner, K.; Capuano, S.V., 3rd; Boettcher, C.; Post, J.; *et al.* A novel nonhuman primate model for influenza transmission. *PLoS ONE* **2013**, *8*, e78750.
27. Tsou, T.P.; Tan, B.F.; Chang, H.Y.; Chen, W.C.; Huang, Y.P.; Lai, C.Y.; Chao, Y.N.; Wei, S.H.; Hung, M.N.; Hsu, L.C.; *et al.* Community outbreak of adenovirus, Taiwan, 2011. *Emerg. Infect. Dis.* **2012**, *18*, 1825–1832.

28. Wevers, D.; Metzger, S.; Babweteera, F.; Bieberbach, M.; Boesch, C.; Cameron, K.; Couacy-Hymann, E.; Cranfield, M.; Gray, M.; Harris, L.A.; *et al.* Novel adenoviruses in wild primates: A high level of genetic diversity and evidence of zoonotic transmissions. *J. Virol.* **2011**, *85*, 10774–10784.
29. Ersching, J.; Hernandez, M.I.; Cezarotto, F.S.; Ferreira, J.D.; Martins, A.B.; Switzer, W.M.; Xiang, Z.; Ertl, H.C.; Zanetti, C.R.; Pinto, A.R. Neutralizing antibodies to human and simian adenoviruses in humans and new-world monkeys. *Virology* **2010**, *407*, 1–6.
30. Yu, G.; Yagi, S.; Carrion, R., Jr.; Chen, E.C.; Liu, M.; Brasky, K.M.; Lanford, R.E.; Kelly, K.R.; Bales, K.L.; Schnurr, D.P.; *et al.* Experimental cross-species infection of common marmosets by titi monkey adenovirus. *PLoS One* **2013**, *8*, e68558.
31. Chen, E.C.; Yagi, S.; Kelly, K.R.; Mendoza, S.P.; Tarara, R.P.; Canfield, D.R.; Maninger, N.; Rosenthal, A.; Spinner, A.; Bales, K.L.; *et al.* Cross-species transmission of a novel adenovirus associated with a fulminant pneumonia outbreak in a new world monkey colony. *PLoS Pathog.* **2011**, *7*, e1002155.
32. Perelman, P.; Johnson, W.E.; Roos, C.; Seuanez, H.N.; Horvath, J.E.; Moreira, M.A.; Kessing, B.; Pontius, J.; Roelke, M.; Rumpler, Y.; *et al.* A molecular phylogeny of living primates. *PLoS Genet.* **2011**, *7*, e1001342.
33. Fields, B.S.; Benson, R.F.; Besser, R.E. Legionella and legionnaires' disease: 25 years of investigation. *Clin. Microbiol. Rev.* **2002**, *15*, 506–526.
34. Xu, L.; Luo, Z.Q. Cell biology of infection by legionella pneumophila. *Microbes Infect.* **2013**, *15*, 157–167.
35. Baskerville, A.; Fitzgeorge, R.B.; Broster, M.; Hambleton, P. Histopathology of experimental legionnaires' disease in guinea pigs, rhesus monkeys and marmosets. *J. Pathol.* **1983**, *139*, 349–362.
36. Baskerville, A.; Dowsett, A.B.; Fitzgeorge, R.B.; Hambleton, P.; Broster, M. Ultrastructure of pulmonary alveoli and macrophages in experimental Legionnaires' disease. *J. Pathol.* **1983**, *140*, 77–90.
37. Cheng, A.C.; Currie, B.J. Melioidosis: Epidemiology, pathophysiology, and management. *Clin. Microbiol. Rev.* **2005**, *18*, 383–416.
38. Currie, B.J.; Dance, D.A.; Cheng, A.C. The global distribution of burkholderia pseudomallei and melioidosis: An update. *Trans. R. Soc. Trop. Med. Hyg.* **2008**, *102*(Suppl 1), S1–S4.
39. Choh, L.C.; Ong, G.H.; Vellasamy, K.M.; Kalaiselvam, K.; Kang, W.T.; Al-Maleki, A.R.; Mariappan, V.; Vadivelu, J. Burkholderia vaccines: Are we moving forward? *Front. Cell. Infect. Microbiol.* **2013**, *3*, 5.
40. Nelson, M.; Dean, R.E.; Salguero, F.J.; Taylor, C.; Pearce, P.C.; Simpson, A.J.; Lever, M.S. Development of an acute model of inhalational melioidosis in the common marmoset (*callithrix jacchus*). *Int. J. Exp. Pathol.* **2011**, *92*, 428–435.
41. White, N.J. Melioidosis. *Lancet* **2003**, *361*, 1715–1722.
42. Rowland, C.A.; Laws, T.R.; Oyston, P.C. An assessment of common marmoset (*callithrix jacchus*) gamma9(+) t cells and their response to phosphoantigen *in vitro*. *Cell. Immunol.* **2012**, *280*, 132–137.

43. Laws, T.R.; Nelson, M.; Bonnafous, C.; Sicard, H.; Taylor, C.; Salguero, F.J.; Atkins, T.P.; Oyston, P.C.; Rowland, C.A. *In vivo* manipulation of gamma9(+) t cells in the common marmoset (*callithrix jacchus*) with phosphoantigen and effect on the progression of respiratory melioidosis. *PLoS One* **2013**, *8*, e74789.
44. Lever, M.S.; Stagg, A.J.; Nelson, M.; Pearce, P.; Stevens, D.J.; Scott, E.A.; Simpson, A.J.; Fulop, M.J. Experimental respiratory anthrax infection in the common marmoset (*callithrix jacchus*). *Int. J. Exp. Pathol.* **2008**, *89*, 171–179.
45. Food Drug Administration, H.H.S. New drug and biological drug products; evidence needed to demonstrate effectiveness of new drugs when human efficacy studies are not ethical or feasible. Final rule. *Fed. Regist.* **2002**, *67*, 37988–37998.
46. Fellows, P.F.; Linscott, M.K.; Ivins, B.E.; Pitt, M.L.; Rossi, C.A.; Gibbs, P.H.; Friedlander, A.M. Efficacy of a human anthrax vaccine in guinea pigs, rabbits, and rhesus macaques against challenge by bacillus anthracis isolates of diverse geographical origin. *Vaccine* **2001**, *19*, 3241–3247.
47. Bell, D.M.; Kozarsky, P.E.; Stephens, D.S. Clinical issues in the prophylaxis, diagnosis, and treatment of anthrax. *Emerg. Infect. Dis.* **2002**, *8*, 222–225.
48. Nelson, M.; Stagg, A.J.; Stevens, D.J.; Brown, M.A.; Pearce, P.C.; Simpson, A.J.; Lever, M.S. Post-exposure therapy of inhalational anthrax in the common marmoset. *Int. J. Antimicrob. Agents* **2011**, *38*, 60–64.
49. Mitchison, D.A.; Chang, K.C. Experimental models of tuberculosis: Can we trust the mouse? *Am. J. Respir. Crit. Care Med.* **2009**, *180*, 201–202.
50. Via, L.E.; Weiner, D.M.; Schimel, D.; Lin, P.L.; Dayao, E.; Tankersley, S.L.; Cai, Y.; Coleman, M.T.; Tomko, J.; Paripati, P.; *et al.* Differential virulence and disease progression following mycobacterium tuberculosis complex infection of the common marmoset (*callithrix jacchus*). *Infect. Immun.* **2013**, *81*, 2909–2919.
51. Hamilton, C.D.; Stout, J.E.; Goodman, P.C.; Mosher, A.; Menzies, R.; Schluger, N.W.; Khan, A.; Johnson, J.L.; Vernon, A.N.; Tuberculosis Trials, C. The value of end-of-treatment chest radiograph in predicting pulmonary tuberculosis relapse. *Int. J. Tuberc. Lung Dis.* **2008**, *12*, 1059–1064.
52. Helmerhorst, H.J.; van Tol, E.N.; Tuinman, P.R.; de Vries, P.J.; Hartskeerl, R.A.; Grobusch, M.P.; Hovius, J.W. Severe pulmonary manifestation of leptospirosis. *Neth. J. Med.* **2012**, *70*, 215–221.
53. Silva, J.J.; Dalston, M.O.; Carvalho, J.E.; Setubal, S.; Oliveira, J.M.; Pereira, M.M. Clinicopathological and immunohistochemical features of the severe pulmonary form of leptospirosis. *Rev. Soc. Bras. Med. Trop.* **2002**, *35*, 395–399.
54. Gouveia, E.L.; Metcalfe, J.; de Carvalho, A.L.; Aires, T.S.; Villasboas-Bisneto, J.C.; Queirroz, A.; Santos, A.C.; Salgado, K.; Reis, M.G.; Ko, A.I. Leptospirosis-associated severe pulmonary hemorrhagic syndrome, salvador, brazil. *Emerg. Infect. Dis.* **2008**, *14*, 505–508.
55. Pereira, M.M.; Da Silva, J.J.; Pinto, M.A.; Da Silva, M.F.; Machado, M.P.; Lenzi, H.L.; Marchevsky, R.S. Experimental leptospirosis in marmoset monkeys (*callithrix jacchus*): A new model for studies of severe pulmonary leptospirosis. *Am. J. Trop. Med. Hyg.* **2005**, *72*, 13–20.
56. Levy, A.; Cohen, G.; Gilat, E.; Kapon, J.; Dachir, S.; Abraham, S.; Herskovitz, M.; Teitelbaum, Z.; Raveh, L. Extrapolating from animal studies to the efficacy in humans of a pretreatment combination against organophosphate poisoning. *Arch. Toxicol.* **2007**, *81*, 353–359.

57. Antonijevic, B.; Stojiljkovic, M.P. Unequal efficacy of pyridinium oximes in acute organophosphate poisoning. *Clin. Med. Res.* **2007**, *5*, 71–82.
58. Van Helden, H.P.; Trap, H.C.; Oostdijk, J.P.; Kuijpers, W.C.; Langenberg, J.P.; Benschop, H.P. Long-term, low-level exposure of guinea pigs and marmosets to sarin vapor in air: Lowest observable effect level. *Toxicol. Appl. Pharmacol.* **2003**, *189*, 170–179.
59. Nozaki, H.; Hori, S.; Shinozawa, Y.; Fujishima, S.; Takuma, K.; Sagoh, M.; Kimura, H.; Ohki, T.; Suzuki, M.; Aikawa, N. Secondary exposure of medical staff to sarin vapor in the emergency room. *Intensive Care Med.* **1995**, *21*, 1032–1035.
60. Matsuda, Y.; Wakai, T.; Kubota, M.; Osawa, M.; Sanpei, A.; Fujimaki, S. Mycotoxins are conventional and novel risk biomarkers for hepatocellular carcinoma. *World J. Gastroenterol.* **2013**, *19*, 2587–2590.
61. van Vleet, T.R.; Watterson, T.L.; Klein, P.J.; Coulombe, R.A., Jr. Aflatoxin b1 alters the expression of p53 in cytochrome p450-expressing human lung cells. *Toxicol. Sci.* **2006**, *89*, 399–407.
62. Wilson, D.W.; Ball, R.W.; Coulombe, R.A., Jr. Comparative action of aflatoxin b1 in mammalian airway epithelium. *Cancer Res.* **1990**, *50*, 2493–2498.
63. Larsson, P.; Tjalve, H. Distribution and metabolism of aflatoxin b1 in the marmoset monkey (*callithrix jacchus*). *Carcinogenesis* **1993**, *14*, 1–6.
64. Hibino, H.; Tani, K.; Ikebuchi, K.; Wu, M.S.; Sugiyama, H.; Nakazaki, Y.; Tanabe, T.; Takahashi, S.; Tojo, A.; Suzuki, S.; *et al.* The common marmoset as a target preclinical primate model for cytokine and gene therapy studies. *Blood* **1999**, *93*, 2839–2848.
65. Ivanova, E.; Hwang, G.S.; Pan, Z.H.; Troilo, D. Evaluation of aav-mediated expression of chop2-gfp in the marmoset retina. *Invest. Ophthalmol. Vis. Sci.* **2010**, *51*, 5288–5296.
66. Farrow, N.; Miller, D.; Cmielewski, P.; Donnelley, M.; Bright, R.; Parsons, D.W. Airway gene transfer in a non-human primate: Lentiviral gene expression in marmoset lungs. *Sci. Rep.* **2013**, *3*, 1287.
67. Abee, C.R.; Mansfield, K. *Nonhuman Primates in Biomedical Research*, 2nd ed.; Elsevier: London, UK, 2012; p. 201.
68. Iwashita, K.; Kawasaki, H.; Sawada, M.; In, M.; Mataki, Y.; Kuwabara, T. Shortening of the induction period of allergic asthma in cynomolgus monkeys by ascaris suum and house dust mite. *J. Pharmacol. Sci.* **2008**, *106*, 92–99.
69. Schelegle, E.S.; Gershwin, L.J.; Miller, L.A.; Fanucchi, M.V.; van Winkle, L.S.; Gerriets, J.P.; Walby, W.F.; Omlor, A.M.; Buckpitt, A.R.; Tarkington, B.K.; *et al.* Allergic asthma induced in rhesus monkeys by house dust mite (*dermatophagoides farinae*). *Am. J. Pathol.* **2001**, *158*, 333–341.
70. Jagessar, S.A.; Vierboom, M.; Blezer, E.L.; Bauer, J.; Hart, B.A.; Kap, Y.S. Overview of models, methods, and reagents developed for translational autoimmunity research in the common marmoset (*callithrix jacchus*). *Exp. Anim.* **2013**, *62*, 159–171.

Permissions

All chapters in this book were first published in Veterinary Sciences, by MDPI; hereby published with permission under the Creative Commons Attribution License or equivalent. Every chapter published in this book has been scrutinized by our experts. Their significance has been extensively debated. The topics covered herein carry significant findings which will fuel the growth of the discipline. They may even be implemented as practical applications or may be referred to as a beginning point for another development.

The contributors of this book come from diverse backgrounds, making this book a truly international effort. This book will bring forth new frontiers with its revolutionizing research information and detailed analysis of the nascent developments around the world.

We would like to thank all the contributing authors for lending their expertise to make the book truly unique. They have played a crucial role in the development of this book. Without their invaluable contributions this book wouldn't have been possible. They have made vital efforts to compile up to date information on the varied aspects of this subject to make this book a valuable addition to the collection of many professionals and students.

This book was conceptualized with the vision of imparting up-to-date information and advanced data in this field. To ensure the same, a matchless editorial board was set up. Every individual on the board went through rigorous rounds of assessment to prove their worth. After which they invested a large part of their time researching and compiling the most relevant data for our readers.

The editorial board has been involved in producing this book since its inception. They have spent rigorous hours researching and exploring the diverse topics which have resulted in the successful publishing of this book. They have passed on their knowledge of decades through this book. To expedite this challenging task, the publisher supported the team at every step. A small team of assistant editors was also appointed to further simplify the editing procedure and attain best results for the readers.

Apart from the editorial board, the designing team has also invested a significant amount of their time in understanding the subject and creating the most relevant covers. They scrutinized every image to scout for the most suitable representation of the subject and create an appropriate cover for the book.

The publishing team has been an ardent support to the editorial, designing and production team. Their endless efforts to recruit the best for this project, has resulted in the accomplishment of this book. They are a veteran in the field of academics and their pool of knowledge is as vast as their experience in printing. Their expertise and guidance has proved useful at every step. Their uncompromising quality standards have made this book an exceptional effort. Their encouragement from time to time has been an inspiration for everyone.

The publisher and the editorial board hope that this book will prove to be a valuable piece of knowledge for researchers, students, practitioners and scholars across the globe.

List of Contributors

Pabbati Namrata
Department of Biology and Environmental Science, University of New Haven, West Haven

Jamie M. Miller
Department of Biology and Environmental Science, University of New Haven, West Haven

Madari Shilpa
Department of Biology and Environmental Science, University of New Haven, West Haven

Patlolla Raghavender Reddy
Department of Biology and Environmental Science, University of New Haven, West Haven

Cheryl Bandoski
Department of Biology and Environmental Science, University of New Haven, West Haven

Michael J. Rossi
Department of Biology and Environmental Science, University of New Haven, West Haven

Eva Sapi
Department of Biology and Environmental Science, University of New Haven, West Haven

Alessandra Berry
Section of Behavioural Neurosciences, Department of Cell Biology and Neurosciences, Istituto Superiore di Sanità, Viale Regina Elena 299, Rome 00161, Italy

Veronica Bellisario
Section of Behavioural Neurosciences, Department of Cell Biology and Neurosciences, Istituto Superiore di Sanità, Viale Regina Elena 299, Rome 00161, Italy

Sara Capoccia
Section of Behavioural Neurosciences, Department of Cell Biology and Neurosciences, Istituto Superiore di Sanità, Viale Regina Elena 299, Rome 00161, Italy

Nadia Francia
Section of Behavioural Neurosciences, Department of Cell Biology and Neurosciences, Istituto Superiore di Sanità, Viale Regina Elena 299, Rome 00161, Italy

Enrico Alleva
Section of Behavioural Neurosciences, Department of Cell Biology and Neurosciences, Istituto Superiore di Sanità, Viale Regina Elena 299, Rome 00161, Italy

Francesca Cirulli
Section of Behavioural Neurosciences, Department of Cell Biology and Neurosciences, Istituto Superiore di Sanità, Viale Regina Elena 299, Rome 00161, Italy

Ibrahim Ozmen
Department of Dermatology, Corlu Military Hospital, 59850 Corlu, Tekirdag 59850, Turkey

Rosanna Marsella
Department of Small Animal Clinical Sciences, College of Veterinary Medicine, University of Florida, Gainesville, FL 32610, USA

Anne Schmitt
Pathology Unit, German Primate Center, Leibniz Institute for Primate Research, Kellnerweg 4, 37077 Göttingen, Germany

Kerstin Mätz-Rensing
Pathology Unit, German Primate Center, Leibniz Institute for Primate Research, Kellnerweg 4, 37077 Göttingen, Germany

Franz-Josef Kaup
Pathology Unit, German Primate Center, Leibniz Institute for Primate Research, Kellnerweg 4, 37077 Göttingen, Germany

Alison Diesel
Department of Small Animal Clinical Sciences, College of Veterinary Medicine and Biomedical Sciences, Texas A&M University, College Station, TX 77843, USA

Karen Moriello
Department of Medical Sciences, School of Veterinary Medicine, 2015 Linden Drive West, University of Wisconsin, Madison, WI 53706, USA

Thushara Chakkath
Department of Comparative Biosciences, College of Veterinary Medicine, University of Illinois, Urbana, IL 61802, USA

Sidonie N. Lavergne
Department of Comparative Biosciences, College of Veterinary Medicine, University of Illinois, Urbana, IL 61802, USA

David Bunick
Department of Comparative Biosciences, College of Veterinary Medicine, University of Illinois, Urbana, IL 61802, USA

Levent Dirikolu
Department of Comparative Biosciences, College of Veterinary Medicine, University of Illinois, Urbana, IL 61802, USA

Timothy M. Fan
Department of Veterinary Clinical Medicine, College of Veterinary Medicine, University of Illinois, Urbana, IL 61802, USA

Samuel Frimpong
Department of Agricultural Engineering, Kwame Nkrumah University of Science and Technology, Kumasi, PMB, Ghana

Girma Gebresenbet
Department of Energy and Technology, Swedish University of Agricultural Sciences, Uppsala, 750 07, Sweden

Emmanuel Bobobee
Department of Agricultural Engineering, Kwame Nkrumah University of Science and Technology, Kumasi, PMB, Ghana
Institute for Agricultural Engineering, Agricultural Research Council, Private Bag X519, Silverton, Pretoria, 0127, South Africa

Elias D. Aklaku
Department of Agricultural Engineering, Kwame Nkrumah University of Science and Technology, Kumasi, PMB, Ghana

Ibrahim Hamdu
Department of Agricultural Engineering, Kwame Nkrumah University of Science and Technology, Kumasi, PMB, Ghana

Amanda Loftis
Department of Biomedical Sciences, Ross University School of Veterinary Medicine, P.O. Box 334, Basseterre, St. Kitts, West Indies
Department of Microbiology & Immunology, Midwestern University, Glendale, AZ 85308, USA

Fernanda Castillo-Alcala
Department of Biomedical Sciences, Ross University School of Veterinary Medicine, P.O. Box 334, Basseterre, St. Kitts, West Indies

Lewis Bogdanovic
Department of Biomedical Sciences, Ross University School of Veterinary Medicine, P.O. Box 334, Basseterre, St. Kitts, West Indies
Banfield Pet Hospital, 10520 Trinity Parkway, Stockton, CA 95219, USA

Ashutosh Verma
Department of Biomedical Sciences, Ross University School of Veterinary Medicine, P.O. Box 334, Basseterre, St. Kitts, West Indies

Barbara Natterson-Horowitz
Professor of Medicine, Division of Cardiology, David Geffen School of Medicine at UCLA, Los Angeles, CA 90095, USA

Marc A. C. Silpa
Royal (Dick) School of Veterinary Studies, University of Edinburgh, Easter Bush Campus, Roslin, EH25 9RG, UK

Susan M. Thornton
International Zoo Veterinary Group, Station House, Parkwood Street, Keighley, West Yorkshire, BD21 4NQ, UK

Tamara Cooper
Cornish Seal Sanctuary, Gweek, Nr. Helston, Cornwall, TR12 6UG, UK;

Joanna Hedley
Beaumont Sainsbury Animal Hospital, Royal Veterinary College, Royal College Street, London, NW1 0TU, UK

Karina Klein
Musculoskeletal Research Unit (MSRU), Equine Department, University of Zurich, Winterthurerstrasse 260, CH-8057 Zurich, Switzerland
Graduate School for Cellular and Biomedical Sciences, University of Bern, CH-3012 Bern, Switzerland

Jason Schense
Kuros Biosurgery AG, Technoparkstrasse 1, CH-8005 Zurich, Switzerland

Peter W. Kronen
Musculoskeletal Research Unit (MSRU), Equine Department, University of Zurich, Winterthurerstrasse 260, CH-8057 Zurich, Switzerland
Center for Applied Biotechnology and Molecular Medicine (CABMM), University of Zurich, Winterthurerstrasse 190, CH-8057 Zurich, Switzerland
Veterinary Anaesthesia Services - International (VAS), Zurcherstrasse 39, CH-8400 Winterthur, Switzerland

Nathalie Fouche
Musculoskeletal Research Unit (MSRU), Equine Department, University of Zurich, Winterthurerstrasse 260, CH-8057 Zurich, Switzerland

Mariano Makara
Division of Diagnostic Imaging, Vetsuisse Faculty, University of Zurich, Winterthurerstrasse 258c, CH-8057 Zurich, Switzerland

Katharina Kämpf
Musculoskeletal Research Unit (MSRU), Equine Department, University of Zurich, Winterthurerstrasse 260, CH-8057 Zurich, Switzerland

Thomas Steffen
Orthopaedic Research Laboratory, Department of Surgery, McGill University Hospital Center, 687 Pine Avenue West, Montreal, QC H3A 1A1, Canada

Brigitte von Rechenberg
Musculoskeletal Research Unit (MSRU), Equine Department, University of Zurich, Winterthurerstrasse 260, CH-8057 Zurich, Switzerland
Center for Applied Biotechnology and Molecular Medicine (CABMM), University of Zurich, Winterthurerstrasse 190, CH-8057 Zurich, Switzerland

Caitlin J. Jenvey
School of Animal and Veterinary Sciences, The University of Adelaide, Roseworthy Campus, Roseworthy, SA 5371, Australia

Michael P. Reichel
School of Animal and Veterinary Sciences, The University of Adelaide, Roseworthy Campus, Roseworthy, SA 5371, Australia

Sasha R. Lanyon
School of Animal and Veterinary Sciences, The University of Adelaide, Roseworthy Campus, Roseworthy, SA 5371, Australia

Peter D. Cockcroft
School of Animal and Veterinary Sciences, The University of Adelaide, Roseworthy Campus, Roseworthy, SA 5371, Australia

Heather A. Allen
Center for Food Security and Public Health, College of Veterinary Medicine, Iowa State University, Ames, IA 50011, USA

Hemant Naikare
Texas A&M Veterinary Medical Diagnostic Laboratory, 6610 Amarillo Blvd West, Amarillo, TX 79106, USA

Daniela Bruno
Texas A&M Veterinary Medical Diagnostic Laboratory, 6610 Amarillo Blvd West, Amarillo, TX 79106

Debabrata Mahapatra,
Texas A&M Veterinary Medical Diagnostic Laboratory, 6610 Amarillo Blvd West, Amarillo, TX 79106

Alesia Reinisch,
Texas A&M Veterinary Medical Diagnostic Laboratory, 6610 Amarillo Blvd West, Amarillo, TX 79106

Russell Raleigh
Texas A&M Veterinary Medical Diagnostic Laboratory, 6610 Amarillo Blvd West, Amarillo, TX 79106

Robert Sprowls
Texas A&M Veterinary Medical Diagnostic Laboratory, 6610 Amarillo Blvd West, Amarillo, TX 79106

Thushara Chakkath
Department of Comparative Biosciences, College of Veterinary Medicine, University of Illinois, Urbana, IL 61802, USA

Sidonie Lavergne
Department of Comparative Biosciences, College of Veterinary Medicine, University of Illinois, Urbana, IL 61802, USA

Timothy M. Fan
Department of Veterinary Clinical Medicine, College of Veterinary Medicine, University of Illinois, Urbana, IL 61802, USA

David Bunick
Department of Comparative Biosciences, College of Veterinary Medicine, University of Illinois, Urbana, IL 61802, USA

Levent Dirikolu
Department of Comparative Biosciences, College of Veterinary Medicine, University of Illinois, Urbana, IL 61802, USA

Jessica K. Simmons
Department of Veterinary Biosciences, The Ohio State University, 1925 Coffey Road, Columbus, OH 43210, USA

Said M. Elshafae
Department of Veterinary Biosciences, The Ohio State University, 1925 Coffey Road, Columbus, OH 43210, USA

Evan T. Keller
Department of Pathology and Unit for Laboratory Animal Medicine, School of Medicine, University of Michigan, Ann Arbor, MI 48109, USA

Laurie K. McCauley
Department of Periodontics & Oral Medicine, School of Dentistry, University of Michigan, 1011 N University Avenue, Ann Arbor, MI 48109, USA

Thomas J. Rosol
Department of Veterinary Biosciences, The Ohio State University, 1925 Coffey Road, Columbus, OH 43210, USA

Michelle G. Ritt
Department of Veterinary Clinical Sciences, College of Veterinary Medicine, University of Minnesota, St. Paul, MN 55108, USA

Beth A. Lindborg
Department of Veterinary Population Medicine, College of Veterinary Medicine, University of Minnesota, St. Paul, MN 55108, USA

Timothy D. O'Brien
Department of Veterinary Population Medicine, College of Veterinary Medicine, University of Minnesota, St. Paul, MN 55108, USA
Stem Cell Institute, University of Minnesota, Minneapolis, MN 55455, USA
Masonic Cancer Center, University of Minnesota, Minneapolis, MN 55455, USA

Joseph Bisignano
Department of Veterinary Clinical Sciences, College of Veterinary Medicine, University of Minnesota, St. Paul, MN 55108, USA

Jaime F. Modiano
Department of Veterinary Clinical Sciences, College of Veterinary Medicine, University of Minnesota, St. Paul, MN 55108, USA
Stem Cell Institute, University of Minnesota, Minneapolis, MN 55455, USA
Masonic Cancer Center, University of Minnesota, Minneapolis, MN 55455, USA
Center for Immunology, University of Minnesota, Minneapolis, MN 55455, USA

Margarethe Hoenig
Department of Veterinary Clinical Medicine, College of Veterinary Medicine, University of Illinois at Urbana-Champaign, 1008 W. Hazelwood Drive, Urbana, IL 61802, USA

Christoph Curths
Pathology Unit, German Primate Center, Leibniz-Institute for Primate Research, Kellnerweg 4, 37077 Göttingen, Germany
Department of Airway Immunology, Fraunhofer Institute for Toxicology and Experimental Medicine, Biomedical Research in Endstage and Obstructive Lung Disease Hannover (BREATH), Member of the German Center for Lung Research, Nikolai-Fuchs-Strasse 1, 30625 Hannover, Germany

Sascha Knauf
Pathology Unit, German Primate Center, Leibniz-Institute for Primate Research, Kellnerweg 4, 37077 Göttingen, Germany
Department of Airway Immunology, Fraunhofer Institute for Toxicology and Experimental Medicine, Biomedical Research in Endstage and Obstructive Lung Disease Hannover (BREATH), Member of the German Center for Lung Research, Nikolai-Fuchs-Strasse 1, 30625 Hannover, Germany

Franz-Josef Kaup
Pathology Unit, German Primate Center, Leibniz-Institute for Primate Research, Kellnerweg 4, 37077 Göttingen, Germany